Chemical Carcinogenesis

(in two parts)

Part A

The Biochemistry of Disease

A Molecular Approach to Cell Pathology

A Series of Monographs

Series Editor

Emmanuel Farber

Temple University
Philadelphia, Pennyslvania

Chemical Carcinogenesis

(in two parts)

Part A

Selected Papers Presented at the
World Symposium on Model Studies in Chemical Carcinogenesis, Baltimore, 1972
Held at The Johns Hopkins Medical Institutions, Baltimore, Maryland
October 31—November 3, 1972

Edited by

Paul O. P. Ts'o
The Johns Hopkins University
Baltimore, Maryland

and

Joseph A. DiPaolo
National Cancer Institute
Bethesda, Maryland

MARCEL DEKKER, INC.   New York   1974

MARCEL DEKKER, INC.

305 East 45th Street, New York, New York 10017

LIBRARY OF CONGRESS CATALOG CARD NUMBER: 73-84816

ISBN: 0-8247-6128-6

Current printing (last digit):
10 9 8 7 6 5 4 3 2 1

PRINTED IN THE UNITED STATES OF AMERICA

CONTENTS OF PART A

CONTENTS

CONTENTS

CONTRIBUTORS TO PART A

JOSEPH C. ARCOS, Seamen's Memorial Research Laboratory, U.S. Public Health Service Hospital, New Orleans, Louisiana, and Department of Medicine, Tulane University School of Medicine, New Orleans, Louisiana

WILLIAM M. BAIRD, Chemical Carcinogenesis Division, Chester Beatty Research Institute, Institute of Cancer Research, Royal Cancer Hospital, Fulham Road, London, England

WILLIAM F. BENEDICT, Section of Development Pharmacology, Laboratory of Biomedical Sciences, National Institute of Child Health and Human Development, National Institutes of Health, Bethesda, Maryland[*]

PETER BROOKES, Chemical Carcinogenesis Division, Chester Beatty Research Institute, Institute of Cancer Research, Royal Cancer Hospital, Fulham Road, London, England

W.S. BURNHAM, ICN, Nucleic Acid Research Institute, Irvine, California

NGUYEN BUU-HOI, Institut de Chimie des Substances Naturelles, Centre National de la Recherche Scientifique, Gif-sur-Yvette, France[**]

W.J. CASPARY, Division of Biophysics, Department of Biochemical and Biophysical Sciences, The Johns Hopkins University, Baltimore, Maryland

CYRIL CHAYET, Laboratoire Curie, Fondation Curie — Institut du Radium, Paris, France

---

[*] Present address: Division of Hematology, Children's Hospital of Los Angeles, Los Angeles, California

[**] Deceased

xiii

B. I. COHEN, Department of Radiological Science, The Johns Hopkins University, Baltimore, Maryland[*]

ALLAN H. CONNEY, Director, Department of Biochemistry and Drug Metabolism, Hoffmann-La Roche, Inc. , Nutley, New Jersey

MARTINE CROISY-DELCEY, Institut de Chimie des Substances Naturelles Centre National de la Recherche Scientifique, Gif-sur-Yvette, France

PASCALINE DAUDEL, Laboratoire Curie, Fondation Curie – Institut du Radium, Paris, France

ANTHONY DIPPLE, Chemical Carcinogenesis Division, Chester Beatty Research Institute, Institute of Cancer Research, Royal Cancer Hospital, Fulham Road, London, England

FRANCOISE GACHELIN, Laboratoire Curie, Fondation Curie – Institut du Radium, Paris, France

HARRY V. GELBOIN, Chemistry Branch, National Cancer Institute, National Institutes of Health, Bethesda, Maryland

WOLFGANG GIRKE, Institute of Organic Chemistry, University Frankfurt am Main, West Germany[**]

P. L. GROVER, Chester Beatty Research Institute, Institute of Cancer Research, Royal Cancer Hospital, Fulham Road, London, England

DEZIDER GRUNBERGER, Institute of Cancer Research and Department of Medicine and Biochemistry, Columbia University College of Physicians and Surgeons, New York, New York

JOSEF FRIED, Department of Chemistry and Biochemistry, The Ben May Laboratory for Cancer Research, Chicago, Illinois

ANNE JACQUIER, Laboratoire Curie, Fondation Curie – Institut du Radium, Paris, France

PIERRE JACQUIGNON, Institut de Chimie des Substances Naturelles, Centre National de la Recherche Scientifique, Gif-sur-Yvette, France

[*]Present address: Department of Lipid Research, Public Health Research Institute, New York, New York

[**]Present address: Institute of Organic Chemistry, The Hebrew University, Jerusalem, Israel

DONALD M. JERINA, Laboratory of Chemistry, National Institute of Arthritis, Metabolism and Digestive Diseases, National Institutes of Health, Bethesda, Maryland

N. KINOSHITA, Chemistry Branch, National Cancer Institute, National Institutes of Health, Bethesda, Maryland

MASAHIKA KODAMA, Biophysics Division, National Cancer Center Research Institute, Chuo-ku, Tokyo, Japan

RICHARD E. KOURI, Department of Viral-Chemical Oncology, Micro-biological Associates, Inc., Bethesda, Maryland

GHISLAINE LATAILLADE, Laboratoire Curie Fondation Curie –Institut du Radium, Paris, France

J. C. LEAVITT, Division of Biophysics, Department of Biochemical and Biophysical Sciences, The Johns Hopkins University, Baltimore, Maryland

S. A. LESKO, JR., Division of Biophysics, Department of Biochemical and Biophysical Sciences, The Johns Hopkins University, Baltimore, Maryland

R. J. LORENTZEN, Division of Biophysics, Department of Biochemical and Biophysical Sciences, The Johns Hopkins University, Baltimore, Maryland

ELIZABETH C. MILLER, McArdle Laboratory for Cancer Research, University of Wisconsin Medical Center, Madison, Wisconsin

JAMES A. MILLER, McArdle Laboratory for Cancer Research, University of Wisconsin Medical Center, Madison, Wisconsin

JACQUES MOREAU, Laboratoire Curie, Fondation Curie –Institut du Radium, Paris, France

CIKAYOSHI NAGATA, Biophysics Division, National Cancer Center Research Institute, Chuo-ku, Tokyo, Japan

DANIEL W. NEBERT, Section on Developmental Pharmacology, National Institute of Child Health and Human Development, National Institutes of Health, Bethesda, Maryland

MELVIN S. NEWMAN, Department of Chemistry, The Ohio State University, Columbus, Ohio

ALBERTE PULLMAN, Institut de Biologie Physica-Chimique, Fondation Edmond de Rothschild, Paris, France

JOHN J. ROBERTS, Chester Beatty Research Institute, Institute of Cancer Research, Royal Cancer Hospital, Buckinghamshire, England

L. M. SCHECTMAN, Division of Biophysics, Department of Biochemical and Biophysical Sciences, The Johns Hopkins University, Baltimore, Maryland

DOMINIC SCUDIERO, Department of Microbiology, The University of Chicago, Chicago, Illinois

P. SIMS, Chester Beatty Research Institute, Institute of Cancer Research, Royal Cancer Hospital, Fulham Road, London, England

N. G. STOUT, ICN, Nucleic Acid Research Institute, Irvine, California

BERNARD S. STRAUSS, Department of Microbiology, The University of Chicago, Chicago, Illinois

JEAN E. STURROCK, Chester Beatty Research Institute, Institute of Cancer Research, Royal Cancer Hospital, Buckinghamshire, England[*]

YUSAKU TAGASHIRA, Biophysics Division, National Cancer Center Research Institute, Chuo-ku, Tokyo, Japan

PAUL O. P. TS'O, Division of Biophysics, Department of Biochemical and Biophysical Sciences, The Johns Hopkins University, Baltimore, Maryland

JULIEN L. VAN LANCKER, Department of Pathology, School of Medicine, The Center for the Health Sciences, University of California, Los Angeles, California

KATHERINE N. WARD, Chester Beatty Research Institute, Institute of Cancer Research, Royal Cancer Hospital, Buckinghamshire, England

I. BERNARD WEINSTEIN, Institute of Cancer Research and Departments of Medicine and Biochemistry, Columbia University College of Physicians and Surgeons, New York, New York

JOHN H. WEISBURGER, Experimental Pathology Branch, National Cancer Institute, National Institutes of Health, Bethesda, Maryland[**]

F. J. WIEBEL, Chemistry Branch, National Cancer Institute, National Institutes of Health, Bethesda, Maryland

MANFRED WILK, Section Head, Institute of Organic Chemistry, University of Frankfurt am Main, West Germany

---

[*] Present address: Division of Anesthesia, Clinical Research Centre, Northwick Park Hospital, Harrow, Middlesex, England

[**] Present address: American Health Foundation, New York, New York

CONTENTS OF PART B

IV. CELL TRANSFORMATION AND DIFFERENTIATION

V. MAMMALIAN CELL MUTAGENESIS
AS RELATED TO CARCINOGENESIS

PREFACE

From October 31st to November 3rd, 1972, an International Symposium on "Model Studies in Chemical Carcinogenesis" was held at the Johns Hopkins Medical Institutions, Baltimore, Maryland, with the following four objectives:

(1) Scientists and scholars in chemical carcinogenesis had an opportunity to come together for the exchange of information and ideas with the expectation of finding new directions for future research by examination of past results.

(2) A closer relationship was promoted among the scientists in this field and between the sponsoring agencies of this symposium and the scientific community.

(3) The comprehensive reports and critical reviews presented on the current position and future prospects in the field of chemical carcinogenesis can now be published for use by government agencies, concerned organizations, and individual scientific and medical workers.

(4) The late Professors Antoine Lacassagne and N. P. Buu-Hoi were honored for their contributions to the field of chemical carcinogenesis.

This symposium encompassed a broad range of scientific disciplines, such as chemical physics, organic chemistry, enzymology, biochemistry, cell physiology and genetics, pathology and immunology. The five major areas of discussion were:

(1) Recent advances in chemical carcinogenesis with emphasis on polycyclic hydrocarbons; correlation of the physicochemical, organic, and biochemical studies of the basic mechanism of this abnormal biological process.

(2) Interrelations of chemical, physical, and viral carcinogenesis.

(3) Recent advances in cell transformation and cell mutagenesis.

(4) Prospects in anti-carcinogenesis, such as the nucleic acid repair process and the inhibition of metabolism of carcinogens.

(5) Recent advances in cancer biology, especially in the area of immunology as it relates to the problem of carcinogenesis and possible therapy.

The comprehensive scope of this symposium clearly indicates that advances in the research on chemical carcinogenesis and the solution to the cancer problem depend on a coordinated, multidisciplinary approach.

In 1968, the first international symposium on "Physicochemical Mechanisms of Carcinogenesis" was held in Jerusalem under the auspices of the Israel Academy of Sciences and Humanities. It was especially appropriate that the second international symposium be held in the United States in 1972, the first year of the launching of the "Conquest of Cancer Campaign" in our country. We wish to acknowledge our gratitude to the National Cancer Institute and the Atomic Energy Commission, the two federal agencies most concerned with cancer, which jointly sponsored and financed this symposium (NIH-72-C-1074, AT(49-7)-3107). In particular, we appreciate the support and participation of Dr. Frank J. Rauscher, Jr., Director, and Dr. Umberto Saffiotti, Associate Scientific Director for Carcinogenesis, Division of Cancer Cause and Prevention, of the National Cancer Institute, and of Dr. James L. Liverman, Director, Division of Biomedical and Environmental Research, Atomic Energy Commission.

Assistance of staff members of the National Cancer Institute, Atomic Energy Commission, and the Johns Hopkins Medical Institutions are gratefully acknowledged. To Jean Conley, the symposium secretary, we are indebted for her dedication and most valuable assistance, and to the staff of Marcel Dekker, Inc. for their help and patience in the preparation of this publication.

Paul O. P. Ts'o
The Johns Hopkins University

Joseph A. DiPaolo
National Cancer Institute

Chemical Carcinogenesis

(in two parts)

Part A

I

INTRODUCTION AND MEMORIAL LECTURE

INTRODUCTORY REMARKS ON
DR. JOSEPH C. ARCOS, DR. N. P. BUU-HOI
AND PROF. A. LACASSAGNE

John H. Weisburger[*]

National Cancer Institute
Bethesda, Maryland

I would like to congratulate Professor Ts'o and Dr. DiPaolo for arranging a most useful, timely, and interesting conference on certain facets of chemical carcinogenesis. In these days when there is national interest focused on problems of cancer research and especially so on the important area of the etiology of cancer, it is no doubt rewarding to take stock and examine the current status, so as to be in a position to plan ahead in an efficient and rewarding manner.

I recall with pleasure an earlier such meeting, in which Dr. Ts'o and others here participated. I refer to the 1968 meeting in historic Jerusalem, organized by Dr. Bergman and Dr. Pullman (1). At that time some of us saw a radical change develop in our understanding of certain aspects of chemical carcinogenesis. As a result of the work by several of you here, specifically groups from the Chester Beatty Institute in London and the McArdle Laboratory of the University of Wisconsin, the problem of the activation of the carcinogenic polycyclic aromatic hydrocarbons and of many other chemical carcinogens to key intermediates became clear.

Before exploring further the successes achieved in the last four years as a basis for future programming, it is also timely to look back at some key contributions made by two giants in the field who were lost to medical research forever during the past year.

I was still a student when Professor Antoine Lacassagne discovered the induction of endocrine tumors in mice by estrogen. Lacassagne

[*]Present address: American Health Foundation, New York, New York.

3

has made innumerable further discoveries which will be discussed in detail in just a moment. It was my pleasure to meet Lacassagne many years ago and most recently in his office in Paris two years ago.

Closely associated with Lacassagne for the last 30 years was an even more broadly oriented medical research scientist, our close friend, a wonderful, gentle person, the late Dr. N. P. Buu-Hoi. Our acquaintance was made some 20 years ago when Buu-Hoi and Lacassagne both came to a national meeting in New York City.

Now it gives me great pleasure to introduce the speaker who will discuss "French Research on Chemical Carcinogenesis in the Last Quarter Century, with Special Reference to the Contributions of A. Lacassagne and N. P. Buu-Hoi." Our speaker has been closely associated with our honored French colleagues. After elementary and secondary schooling in Hungary, he earned several degrees in Paris, the first of which was an undergraduate degree in chemical engineering, with honors. The thesis was based on organic synthesis of certain amino acid analogs and their interaction with microorganisms. He went on to the Sorbonne and earned a doctorate in science, magna cum laude, with a dissertation delivered before the College of France, again on a subject of the synthesis and study of the properties of polycyclic hydrocarbon derivatives, and at the same time he wrote a literature thesis with a review on the chemotherapy of leprosy.

Our speaker held a number of positions in France – first in industry, where he developed some novel scientific instruments. He came to the United States in 1953 and spent some years at the important McArdle Laboratory of the University of Wisconsin. He then joined my own professor, the late Francis Earl Ray, in the Cancer Research Laboratory, University of Florida, and since 1960 has been associated with the Research Laboratories of the U.S. Public Health Service Hospital in New Orleans and also with the Department of Medicine of Tulane University where he is now Professor of Medicine. It is my pleasure now to introduce Dr. J. C. Arcos, for his lecture on "French Research on Chemical Carcinogenesis in the Last Quarter Century, with Special Reference to the Contribution of A. Lacassagne and N. P. Buu-Hoi."

REFERENCE

1. Physicochemical Mechanisms of Carcinogenesis (E. D. Bergmann and B. Pullman, eds.), Vol. 1, Israel Academy of Sciences and Humanities, Jerusalem, 1969.

FRENCH RESEARCH ON CHEMICAL CARCINOGENESIS
IN THE LAST QUARTER CENTURY
WITH SPECIAL REFERENCE TO
THE CONTRIBUTIONS OF A. LACASSAGNE AND N. P. BUU-HOI

Joseph C. Arcos[*]

Seamen's Memorial Research Laboratory
U. S. Public Health Service Hospital
New Orleans, Louisiana and
Department of Medicine
Tulane University School of Medicine
New Orleans, Louisiana

INTRODUCTION

Two sad losses marked the years 1971 and 1972 for the world's scientific community. The deaths of Antoine Lacassagne, the grand old man of French cancer research, and of Nguyen Phuc Buu-Hoi conclude a brilliant chapter of French contributions to the study of carcinogenesis and the synthetic chemistry of polynuclear compounds. From the group under their leadership – the most productive and original for the study of the structure-activity relationships of polynuclear carcinogens – came forth an unending stream of publications for over a quarter of a century. However, it would be unjust to their genius not to state immediately that their interest and vision far transcended the field of chemical carcinogenesis, for they were also active and published abundantly in radiobiology, pathology, organic chemistry, pharmacology, therapeutics and epidemiology, and physical- and biochemistry, not directly in relation with the problem of cancer. It is a dizzying thought to consider that the total number of their publications is over 1500.

The broad outline of such a scientific legacy is best seen against the background of the French cancer research establishment and in the light of the personalities and interests of Lacassagne and Buu-Hoi who, from diametrically different national, religious, and family backgrounds, were brought together by fate to carry out this massive work.

---

[*] Recipient of an American Cancer Society Faculty Research Award.

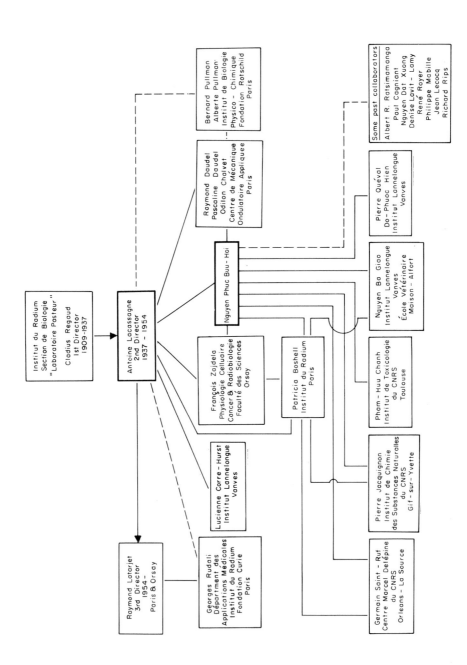

FIG. 1. Interrelationships circa 1970 in the research organization originated by Antoine Lacassagne.

GENERAL TABLEAU OF THE FRENCH RESEARCH ESTABLISHMENT
ON CHEMICAL CARCINOGENESIS

Beginning with Louis XIV in the 16th and 17th century and culminating in the period before World War I, France has become an increasingly centralized country. Economic and cultural strength is concentrated in the capital and essentially all significant political decisions are made in Paris. Science and, in particular, cancer research is no exception.

The two great institutes, where most of cancer research and almost all research on or related to chemical carcinogenesis is carried out, are in Paris: the Radium Institute, its branches and affiliates and the now autonomous research groups which grew out from it, and the "Gustave Roussy" Institute at Villejuif, a suburb of Paris.

The Radium Institute scene was marked between 1937 and 1954 by the towering personality of Lacassagne who laid the foundations of what was destined to become a scientific empire (Fig. 1). His retirement in 1954 was only the beginning of a very active second period of his life. He retained his laboratory at the Radium Institute and, together with Lucienne Corre-Hurst, actively carried out research until shortly before his death; he also took an active interest in the public and organizational aspects of French cancer research as president from 1959 on of the French League Against Cancer. However, branches of his empire continued to grow and expand. In 1954, his erstwhile co-worker, Raymond Latarjet, succeeded him as Director of the Pasteur Laboratories at the Radium Institute and established additional laboratories at the new Science Faculty complex at Orsay. In 1960, Buu-Hoi moved from the Radium Institute to more spacious quarters at the Institute of Chemistry of Natural Substances located in the National Center of Scientific Research laboratory group at Gif-sur-Yvette, about 15 miles from Paris, and in the 1960s, Buu-Hoi established a research group in Orléans-La Source at the Marcel-Delépine Center and another one at the Lannelongue Institute at Vanves, at the southern edge of Paris. The group at Gif-sur-Yvette was supervised by Pierre Jacquignon and the team at Orléans by Germain Saint-Ruf. All organic synthetic work was carried out in these laboratories. Most of the toxologic, pharmacologic, and biochemical studies were carried out by Pham-Huu Chanh at the CNRS toxicological laboratories at Toulouse, and by Nguyen Ba Giao, Pierre Quéval, and Do-Phuoc Hien at the Lannelongue Research Institute at Vanves. In some of the latter studies, Buu-Hoi collaborated with a number of foreign laboratories. François Zajdela, long-time devoted co-worker of Lacassagne, became a Director of Research at the CNRS and established his laboratories at the Science

Faculty complex at Orsay; he carried out much of the pathology involved
in the testing studies, maintained the inbred animal colonies, and
served as consultant to the groups for the designing of biologic experiments. Patricia Boshell, a dedicated associate of Buu-Hoi, acted as
a coordinator of many of these activities as well as scientific editor of
the publications. Georges Rudali, who collaborated extensively with
Lacassagne in the 1940s and early 1950s, became a staff member at the
Department of Medical Applications, the Curie Foundation at the Radium
Institute. The theoretical chemists, brought into the cancer field by
Lacassagne around 1943, the Daudels and the Pullmans, established
their own research groups at the Center of Applied Wave Mechanics
and at the Institute of Physico-Chemical Biology, respectively. Up to
the late 1950s, these two groups collaborated in a number of studies
on chemical carcinogenesis. Subsequently, they followed a course of
action essentially separate from the Radium Institute and independently
acquired international renown in quantum chemistry.

The scene at the second major institute, the "Gustave Roussy"
Institute at Villejuif, was dominated between 1948 and 1960 by the
colorful personality of Charles Oberling. Oberling was first of all a
pathologist, with an absorbing interest in cancer and an almost religious conviction of the viral origin of all tumors. I still recall his
lectures and the subsequent discussions in 1951, in what was my
brief initiation to oncology. He passionately defended the view that
"all that chemical carcinogens do is to activate the viruses present."
Not a very popular proposition those days and somewhat shocking to
those with a chemical bent! His well-known book, The Riddle of Cancer (1), is an inspiring classic, penetrated by his enthusiasm but also
powerfully colored by his scientific convictions. Much of his experimental work on the isolation of various strains of tumors, the viral
transmission of tumors, formation of metastasis, and especially on
filterable fowl leukoses, was carried out in collaboration with Maurice
Guérin. As a pathologist, Oberling was acutely aware of the need for
bolstering the viral studies with morphological evidence, so that in
1948 when he reorganized the institute as the new director succeeding
Gustave Roussy, the founder, he spared no effort to establish a strong
section of electron microscopy, then a new tool. This section was,
from its very inception, under the direction of Wilhelm Bernhard. The
interests and convictions of Oberling – although succeeded by three
consecutive directors since 1960 – left an almost indelible mark on the
scientific strengths and orientations of the different sections. In the
Laboratory of Cellular Biochemistry – initially under the direction of
Éliane Le Breton – Chauveau, Clément, Lacour, the Harrels, Jacob,
Meunier, Moulé, and others investigated lipid alterations, change in
microsomal metabolism and binding to DNA during azo dye carcinogenesis, and enzyme changes in the anaerobic segment of carbohydrate

metabolism. Although only ancillarily related to our topic, I should mention the outstanding textbook — now a classic — The Chemotherapy of Cancers — by George Mathé (2) from the "Gustave Roussy" Institute.

Outside of the Radium Institute and its branches and affiliates, and the "Gustave Roussy" Institute, comparatively little research in the restricted area of our subject — chemical carcinogenesis — was carried out elsewhere in France. Occasional reports were seen, especially in earlier years, from René Truhaut, at the Faculty of Pharmacy of the University of Paris. Some of his work involved investigation of the presence of endogenous carcinogens in human tissues (3), somewhat along the lines of the studies of Shabad and of Hieger. Truhaut, in turn, was much influenced by C. Sannié, at the Department of Chemistry of the Museum of Natural History, whose great interest lay in spectral studies of polycyclic hydrocarbons. A few reports on the complexing of hydrocarbons were seen from the Macromolecular Research Center and the Institute of Physical Biology of the University of Strasbourg, perhaps as a belated flowering of the scientific legacy of the biophysicist, Fred Vlés. I have purposely omitted discussing the International Agency for Research on Cancer in Lyons, which though geographically on French soil, is not a specifically French venture.

CAREER AND WORK OF ANTOINE LACASSAGNE UP TO 1942

Against this background of the French cancer research establishment — which I sketched with very broad strokes — we should now superimpose the two men who so profoundly influenced its advancement. Antoine Lacassagne was born in 1884, in southeastern France, in the country house of his parents in the little village of Villerest, near Roanne, about 50 miles from Lyons. His father was a military physician and a professor of legal medicine at the Faculty of Medicine and Pharmacy of the University of Lyons. Lacassagne grew up in Lyons and his personality and values bore a deep imprint of the social atmosphere of the middle class in that city during the epoch of the Third Republic. He did his secondary schooling at the Lycée Ampère and then entered medical school at the University. As he himself recognized, his choice at that time to enter medicine as a career was much more the result of the influence of his environment than of the true attraction of the profession itself. The year 1908 was a landmark in his life when, at the termination of his formal studies, as an intern of the Lyons Hospitals, he was admitted to the Laboratory of Histology, directed then by Claudius Regaud, to prepare a dissertation. Regaud was deeply involved in exploring a new scientific discipline, radiobiology, and young Lacassagne became fascinated by these investigations. Lacassagne's first scientific work, "Histological and

Physiological Studies of the Effects Produced by X-Rays on the Ovary,"
which he also presented as his dissertation in 1913, contains the seeds
of all his future interests, and served as a gateway to fields that he
persistently explored all his life: radiobiology, pathology, endocrin-
ology, X-ray therapeutics, and experimental oncology.

The years around 1910 were the epoch when the Radium Institute
was established as a cooperative venture between the University of
Paris and the Pasteur Institute. Of the two sections that were set up,
the Section of Physics, administered by the university, was placed
under the direction of Marie Curie. The Section of Biology, administered by the Pasteur Institute, was placed under the direction of
Claudius Regaud, who left Lyons in 1909, barely a year after Antoine
Lacassagne entered his laboratory. However, luckily for science, the
plant had already taken root, and Lacassagne was firmly set in his
determination to pursue his interest in radiobiology. Regaud recognized the exceptional abilities of his student and offered him, at the
termination of his dissertation, a post of assistant supported by a
modest Pasteur Institute fellowship. It is a credit to the idealistic
devotion of Lacassagne to science that he followed this lead, despite
the many unknowns of the venture at that time, rather than remaining
at the University of Lyons with the quasi certainty of a well-delineated
university career. So in 1913, Lacassagne moved to Paris. As a
Pasteur Institute fellow, he took the microbiology curriculum of the
Institute and came under the influence of a rare constellation of exceptional teachers: Émile Roux, discoverer of the serum therapy of diph-
theria; Elie Metchnikoff, discoverer of immunity and phagocytosis;
Charles Nicolle, famous for his investigations on typhoid and Maltese
fever; Amédé Borrel, the proponent of the virus theory of cancer as
early as 1903; and others. At the same time Lacassagne helped Regaud
in the building and organization of the Pasteur Pavillion, the main
building housing the Biology Section.

The outbreak of World War I meant a four-year interruption in
Antoine Lacassagne's career, which he spent as an auxiliary physician
with the armies of the Western powers. On his discharge in 1919, he
immediately returned to Paris. He was then appointed Chief of Laboratories and became the principal associate of Regaud. From then on
his advancement was assured. He became Deputy Director of the
Pasteur Laboratory in 1923 and succeeded Regaud on his retirement in
1937. His scientific accomplishments, which were considerable,
received many honors, prizes, and recognitions in France and abroad
(see, e.g., Refs. 4-6).

Antoine Lacassagne is among the most original and productive
radiobiologists of our time. In radiotherapy, he continued the major

work of Regaud, and in systematic and painstaking work between 1920 and 1939, established the exact anatomo-pathologic effects of ionizing radiations on normal and malignant tissues. This rapidly led to new and improved schemas and procedures of treatment of cancer in man by X rays, radium, and radioisotopes, which became universally employed.

In fundamental radiobiology, his classic work, carried out around 1928 in collaboration with the physicist Fernand Holweck, is the mathematical interpretation of the dose-response curves of radiation effect on homogeneous populations of monocellular organisms, mainly yeast. About 10 years later, he extended these studies to bacteriophages in collaboration with Eugene Wollman. This work gave birth to the "quantal theory," known later as the "target theory" of radiation effect. In the course of these quantitative studies, he was the first to observe the lag period of radiation death on Polytoma uvella and to describe the decrease of radiosensitivity in anaerobiosis. From his collaboration with Jeanne Lattès around 1924 was born the definite methodology of what became known as autoradiography, which gave a powerful impetus to the development of many branches of biology and has been compared in importance to electrophoresis, chromatography, and density gradient centrifugation (5, 6).

In experimental oncology, Lacassagne contributed extensively to the methodology of the experimental production of tumors by irradiation and to the understanding of their histogenesis. For example, it became known, owing to his studies on tumorigenesis by radon, that a necrotic zone is established in the immediate vicinity of the tube inserted in the animal, and the tumors arise in the next zone of tissue surrounding the tube, where the radiation particles have lost enough of their energy to allow the cells to survive but can still bring about critical cellular lesions. In 1930, in collaboration with R. Vinzent, Lacassagne reported the first instance of cocarcinogenesis in a study of the tumor response of infected foci following irradiation; very low doses of radiation were without effect on normal tissues but did induce tumors in the regions of inflammation. In 1942-1943, with Raymond Latarjet, he studied the combined action of X rays and ultraviolet radiations with polycyclic hydrocarbons on mouse skin and established the critical role of the pilosebaceous follicles in the genesis of epitheliomas. In these investigations they could also demonstrate the sensitizing effect of tissue oxygen toward X rays. Although from 1954 on he became increasingly engaged in problems of chemical carcinogenesis, he continued to maintain a deep interest in radiation carcinogenesis through recent years (e.g., Refs. 7 and 8).

Lacassagne's epoch-making discovery was the demonstration between 1932 and 1936 of the carcinogenic action of estrogenic hormones

(see Ref. 9 for review). It was known at that time, for a number of
years since the classical investigations of Lathrop and Loeb, that
removal of the ovaries in female mice at an early age prevents the
onset of mammary tumors in susceptible inbred strains. This could
also be confirmed with the Radium Institute inbred strain, which had
a high incidence of spontaneous mammary carcinomas. In males of
the same strain, castration followed by implantation of ovary tissue
brought about the appearance of mammary tumors, just as in the females.
Hence, mammary tumorigenesis depended on some substance produced
by the ovary. Estrone and other ovarian hormones became available at
that time owing to the synthetic work of Girard. Lacassagne knew that
estrone brought about active cell proliferation in the female primary
and secondary sex organs and that the hormone appeared at sufficiently
large concentration to produce this effect only at regular, periodic
intervals. He then reasoned that maintenance of continuous stimulation of the tissues for a long period of time by repeated injection of
estrone could induce tumor growth. Indeed, he found that injection of
estrone brought about close to 100% mammary tumor incidence in male
mice belonging to a strain in which only the females normally showed
a high incidence of this tumor. In males of a strain in which the

Estrone   Equiline   Equilenine

females have only a low spontaneous incidence, repeated injections of
estrone produced only a low incidence of mammary tumors. This was
the first instance of a naturally occurring pure chemical compound as
the cause of induced cancer. In later studies, Lacassagne found that
equiline, equilenine, estradiol, and stilbestrol possess qualitatively
the same tumorigenic effect. It appeared puzzling to him that the
tumorigenicity of estrone, equiline, and equilenine decrease in this
order despite the increasingly aromatic character that makes these
structures more akin to the aromatic hydrocarbons. We now know that,
despite increasing aromatization, the overall molecular thickness
increases in this order because of the conformation of the remainder of
the steroid nucleus. Subsequently, Lacassagne demonstrated that
estrone is tumorigenic also toward tissue targets other than the ovary
and that testosterone inhibits estrone-induced mammary tumorigenesis.
We should remember that these discoveries were epochmaking not only
for fundamental cancer research. Together with "Haddow's paradox,"
that is of the association of tumorigenic and tumor-inhibitory properties
in carcinogenic compounds, firmly established a few years later, they

paved the way for the hormone-therapy of human malignancies worked out by Charles Huggins.

THE ELECTRONIC THEORY OF OTTO SCHMIDT AND
ITS INFLUENCE ON FRENCH CANCER RESEARCH

The year is 1939. Dark clouds are gathering, fearful and bloody years are to follow for France and for the most of humanity! The entrails of History are pregnant with unspent malignant energies preparing one of those periodic upheavals. The History of Science is also pregnant with new developments as Antoine Lacassagne's prepared mind faces unusual circumstances. For prepared he was! The electronic theory of molecular structure was still in its infancy, and at any rate little of it distilled down to the organic chemists and essentially none to the biologists. But Lacassagne's whole scientific past in radiobiology made him acutely aware of the importance of subatomic particles, and his own studies on hormonal carcinogenesis as well as the then unfolding panorama of the polycyclic hydrocarbon carcinogens made him conscious of the peculiar structural pattern of polynuclear compounds. So his mind was ready to see the promise of Otto Schmidt's magisterial synthesis, which he was destined to guide to flowering. Let Lacassagne himself tell us in his First Kennaway Memorial Lecture (10): "Now, during the Second World War, when France was occupied and only German publications reached us, my attention was attracted by an article by a chemist named Otto Schmidt expounding a theory which appeared to furnish a mathematical explanation of carcinogenesis by polycyclic hydrocarbons, applicable equally to radiation carcinogenesis and even to viruses! The fact that I could not follow Schmidt's reasoning made me the more curious. I questioned the chemists among my friends; each referred me to another more versed in these matters; until finally I met a young theoretical chemist, Raymond Daudel, who was kind enough to take an interest in this work. The author explained the differences in the activity of polycyclic hydrocarbons by calculations of wave mechanics. We were thus concerned with a quantum theory, and since, twenty years earlier, my friend the great physicist, Holweck, and I had been among the first to explain the biological action of radiations by quantum theory, I was tempted to try to confirm, by experiment, Otto Schmidt's purely speculative idea."

Otto Schmidt was an industrial research chemist at the I. G. Farbenindustrie central laboratories in Ludwigshafen, who published substantially on theoretical and experimental problems of catalysis. He devoted the last three years of his life to a theoretical study of the polycyclic hydrocarbons (11-15; reviews 16, 17); as far as I could ascertain, he died in 1941.

Schmidt proposed that ionizing radiations, chemical carcinogens, and carcinogenic viruses bring about an alteration of the chemical structure of one or more of the critical macromolecules in the cell; this alteration would be the result of a well-defined chemical reaction akin to a mutation. Since the energy of photons in the lowest energy carcinogenic radiation is of the order of 3.4 eV, the chemical reaction brought about by the radiation must require an energy of activation of the same order of magnitude or greater. The structural alteration leading to carcinogenesis would be the result of one or several activations, each requiring an energy of at least 3.4 eV. Schmidt considered an enolization reaction involving the structural backbone, the polypeptide chain, in proteins:

$$
\begin{array}{ccc}
\text{N-H} & \text{N-H} & \text{N} \\
| & | & \| \\
\text{C=O} \xrightarrow{h\nu} & \text{C-O-H} \longrightarrow & \text{C-O-H} \\
| & \| & | \\
\text{H-C-NH-} & \text{C-NH-} & \text{H-C-NH-} \\
| & | & | \\
\text{R} & \text{R} & \text{R}
\end{array}
$$

Following Schmidt's hypothesis, radiations could produce such keto-enol rearrangements by directly providing the energy for the reaction. Chemical carcinogens would further the same reaction by lowering catalytically the energy required. Almost all the carcinogens known in Schmidt's time were aromatic compounds, and among them the carcinogenic polycyclic hydrocarbons were numerically overwhelming. Hence, the suggestion was at hand that the catalytic property of these compounds might be due to their specific electron distribution, in particular to the presence of certain molecular regions rich in π electrons. (To understand the penchant of Schmidt for using protein structure rather than nucleic acid structure as the foundation of his hypothesis, one must remember that it was not before the late 1940s that the role of nucleic acids as the carriers of transmissible genetic information was established beyond doubt.)

Using a highly simplified theoretical treatment, Schmidt hypothesized that benzene, containing six π electrons, and naphthalene, containing 10 π electrons, represent self-contained entities within the whole electron distribution of larger polycyclic hydrocarbons. The electron distributions of these benzenic and naphthalenic entities occupy toric volumes and, thus, every hydrocarbon may be divided into regions (Fig. 2). This "parcelling off" results in the appearance of large and small zones. The π electron density is higher in the compressed narrow B zones than in the A zones. Schmidt attributed

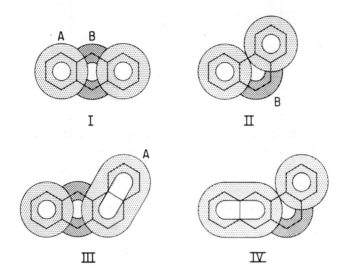

FIG. 2.   Toroid regions of polycyclic hydrocarbons following the "box model" of Otto Schmidt.

carcinogenic activity precisely to the presence of such high-electron-density regions. With a highly simplified variant of the LCAO method, Schmidt calculated the electron densities of meso regions in several hydrocarbons and came to the conclusion that the electron density in these zones must be at or above 0.44 electrons/$\mathring{A}^2$ for the enolizing catalytic activity to become operative.   In this conceptual framework, meso methyl substitution transforms the very weakly active 1, 2-benz-anthracene to the highly potent 9, 10-dimethyl-1, 2-benzanthracene because it further compresses the meso-anthracenic toroid zones and thereby raises the electron density well beyond the threshold.   On the other hand, introduction of a nitrogen heteroatom generally brings about a lowering of carcinogenic activity because, owing to the attraction of the electrons toward the more electronegative heteroatom, there is "decompression" of electron density in these high-energy zones.

Later, Daudel (16) gave an explicit form to the postulated enolizing catalytic activity of hydrocarbons due to high π-electron density regions (Fig. 3).   Consider — following Daudel — that an electron doublet representing one of the two bonds of the C=O double bond is localized in region 1 and a hydrocarbon molecule arrives in the vicinity so that its zone of high electron density overlaps with region 2.   Because the electrons are indistinguishable from each other, the high

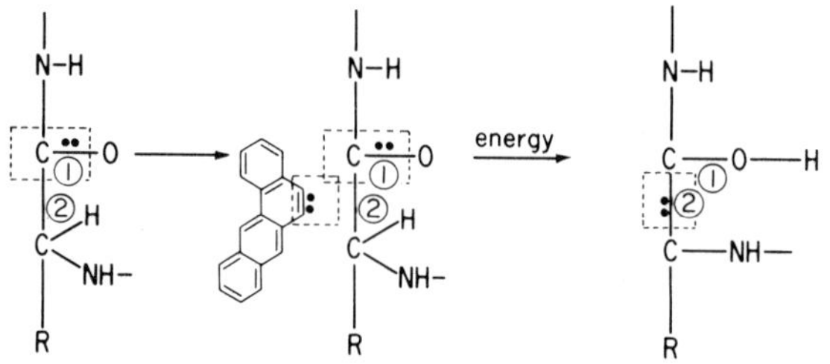

FIG. 3. Enolizing catalytic activity of polycyclic hydrocarbons toward proteins, postulated by Otto Schmidt, as interpreted by R. Daudel.

electron-density region represents an "energy tunnel" which facilitates the shift of the electron doublet from region 1 to region 2 so that a minute excitation energy, such as can be provided by a small thermic shock or a chemical perturbation in the metabolic environment, suffices to bring about isomerization.

Despite the great originality of the basic idea, Schmidt's technique was rudimentary. Its most flagrant contradiction was that, depending on how the "parcelling off" by toric volumes was carried out, when hydrocarbons more complex than anthracene or phenanthrene were used, the "electron-rich" region may be either in the meso-anthracenic or in the meso-phenanthrenic position. This is illustrated in Fig. 2 on 1, 2-benzanthracene (formulas III and IV). Moreover, his method of calculation could not account for the large changes of electron density due to substituents distant from a particular molecular region.

A different approach to this question was taken in 1941 by Svartholm (18) at the Wenner-Gren Institute, who attempted to correlate carcinogenic activity not so much with π-electron density per se but rather with the ability of the molecule to undergo addition reactions. From calculations carried out by the valence-bond method, Svartholm concluded that the meso-phenanthrenic region is particularly apt to undergo addition reaction in 1, 2-benzanthracene, 1, 2, 5, 6-dibenzanthracene, and 3, 4-benzopyrene. The ideas of Schmidt and Svartholm were destined to exert considerable influence on the research orientation of Lacassagne and his associates and through them upon concepts and experimental approaches throughout the world.

ESTABLISHMENT OF THE RADIUM INSTITUTE TEAM.
CONTRIBUTION OF THE QUANTUM CHEMISTS

It was evident to Lacassagne that the magnitude of the task of putting to test and exploring the corollaries of Schmidt's theory would require an interdisciplinary group composed of biologists, pathologists, and theoretical and organic chemists. So Raymond Daudel's joining the Radium Institute was followed by others . Raymond and Pascaline Daudel, and Bernard Pullman and Alberte Bucher (later Mrs. Pullman) were to become the leading figures of the theoretical chemistry branch. They soon made considerable contributions to the quantum chemical explanation of hydrocarbon carcinogenesis (see reviews, e. g., Refs. 19 and 20); their contributions became an important stimulus for new experimental approaches. Besides their theoretical work on the mechanism of carcinogenesis by aromatic hydrocarbons, the Daudels and the Pullmans published profusely in fundamental and applied quantum chemistry (e. g., Refs. 21-23). Although the association of the theoretical chemists with the rest of the Radium Institute group became tenuous in the later years, they continued to make important contributions to the problem of carcinogenesis. In 1943, Georges Rudali and around 1947 François Zajdela joined to carry out the biologic and pathologic studies. A most crucial step was the acquisition, in 1944, of a brilliant organic chemist, Nguyen Phuc Buu-Hoi, who with the years became the principal associate of Lacassagne and co-leader of the group.

Very early, the Daudels came to the realization that the most fertile avenue for formal mathematical exploration is represented by a synthesis of the basic assumptions of Schmidt and Svartholm. Thus, they proposed that a meso-phenanthrenic region rich in π electrons but also especially prone to undergo addition reactions with growth-controlling cell constituents would be the critical structural feature of carcinogenic hydrocarbons (16, 17, 24). This is illustrated with 1, 2, 5, 6-dibenzanthracene (Fig. 4).

Using improved quantum mechanical methods, the Daudels and the Pullmans, as well as Odilon Chalvet, observed correlations between the rank of carcinogenic activities of certain polycyclic hydrocarbons and various theoretical indexes that have been developed to characterize the electronic properties of the meso-phenanthrenic region. Up

TABLE 1

Evolution of the Quantum Mechanical Parameters Defining the
Electronic Characteristics of Polynuclear Hydrocarbons

Static indexes (based on an isolated molecule in the absence of charge perturbation)

	earliest ideas (1943-1945)	A. Pullman, 1947	Buu-Hoi, Daudel, Daudel, Lacassagne, Lecocq, Martin, and Rudali, 1947
"Total charge"	$q_1 + q_2$	$2p_{12} + F_1 + F_2 + q_1 + q_2$	$2p_{12} + F_1 + F_2 + q_1 + q_2 + p_1 + p_2$

$$p_2 \underset{q_2}{\overset{q_1}{\bullet}} p_1$$
$$F_2 \quad p_{12} \quad F_1$$

Dynamic indexes (based on the molecule in a reacting state, ready to be engaged in bond formation)

1. Combined electron localization indexes
   (A. Pullman, 1954)

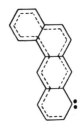

Carbon localization

Bond localization
$BLE + CLE_{min} < 3.31\,\beta$

Para localization
$PLE + CLE_{min} > 5.66\,\beta$

requirements for carcinogenicity

2. Electrophilic potential barrier (for benzacridines)
(Chalvet and Sung, 1960)

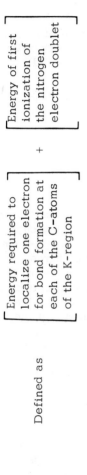

Defined as
$$\left[\begin{array}{l}\text{Energy required to}\\ \text{localize one electron}\\ \text{for bond formation at}\\ \text{each of the C-atoms}\\ \text{of the K-region}\end{array}\right] + \left[\begin{array}{l}\text{Energy of first}\\ \text{ionization of}\\ \text{the nitrogen}\\ \text{electron doublet}\end{array}\right]$$

3. Indexes based on reaction kinetics
(O. Chalvet, R. Daudel, and Moser, 1958)

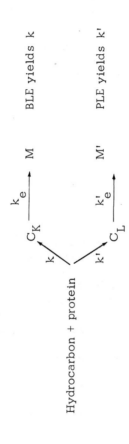

$$\text{Hydrocarbon + protein}$$

$$C_K \xrightarrow{k_e} M \quad \text{BLE yields } k$$

$$C_L \xrightarrow{k'_e} M' \quad \text{PLE yields } k'$$

Thus, $C_K \text{max} = [K]$ and $C_L \text{max} = [L]$, and the maximum amount of hydrocarbon bound via the K- and L-regions, respectively, may be calculated.

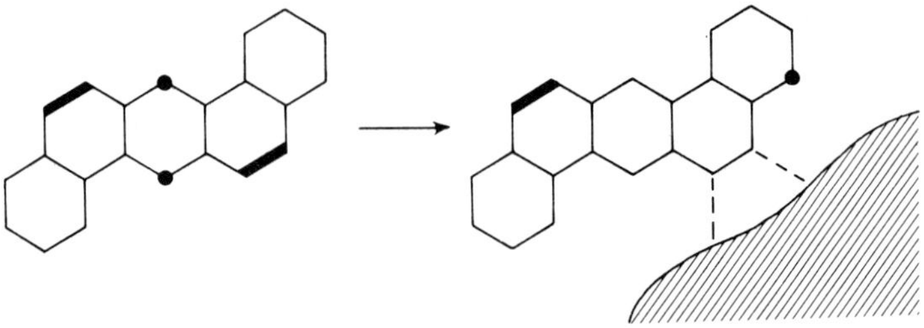

FIG. 4.   Schematic representation of the linking of a 1, 2, 5, 6-
dibenzanthracene molecule to a cell constituent by way of the meso-
phenanthrenic region (following P. Daudel and R. Daudel).

until about 1954, the mobile bond index, free valence index, and
electric charge index were used singly or in various combinations.
The success of the theory and the underlying mathematical apparatus
is best indicated by the fact that in some instances it allowed the
prediction of carcinogenic activity (e. g., 25). The progress of the gradual
refinement of these theoretical indexes is shown in Table 1.   In one
of the earliest reports, carcinogenic activity was related to the net
electric charge of the K-region.   However, this was soon replaced by
a more complex definition of the "total charge" (also called "charge
density").   The use of electric charge alone is not applicable to
unsubstituted hydrocarbons comprising only aromatic six-membered
rings in which every carbon atom has unit electric charge.   In 1947, A.
Pullman (26) proposed a definition of the charge containing as components the mobile bond index of the meso-phenanthrenic region (p_{12}),
and the free valence indexes and net electric charges of the two carbon
atoms (F_1, F_2 and q_1, q_2).   Buu-Hoi et al. (27) noted that the correlations
are improved if the mobile bond indexes of the bonds adjacent to the
meso-phenanthrenic bond (p_1 and p_2) are included in the expression of
the "total charge."   In 1954, A. Pullman (28, review 29) proposed relating
the carcinogenic activity of polycyclic hydrocarbons to the reactivity
of the meso-phenanthrenic region and to the reactivity of the meso-
anthracenic region by combined electron localization indexes.   These
indexes, unlike the expression of the "total charge," describe the
molecule in a dynamic reacting state ready to be engaged in bond formation.   Thus, these were termed dynamic indexes in contradistinction
to the expressions describing the "total charge" which characterize
the molecule in a quasi-isolated state, in the absence of charge perturbation by neighboring molecules.   Thus, the expressions of the
"total charge" are static indexes.   In 1960, Chalvet and Sung (30)
attempted to correlate the electrophilic potential barrier of some benzacridines with their carcinogenic activity, predicated on the idea that
the heteroatom is also involved in the cellular interaction leading to

carcinogenesis. In 1958, Chalvet et al. (31-33) introduced a set of indexes based on the kinetics of binding of a hydrocarbon molecule by way of the meso-phenanthrenic region, leading to carcinogenesis, or by way of the meso-anthracenic region, in which case carcinogenesis would not be initiated. These evidently can only serve as a most sketchy illustration of the considerable productivity of the two groups of quantum chemists in relation to the problem of carcinogenesis. Publications on this subject have continued uninterrupted through recent years (34-37). The work of the Pullmans and Daudels made popular the terms K-region for the meso-phenanthrenic region and L-region for the meso-anthracenic region. It is also customary to distinguish a region of metabolic perhydroxylation par excellence, named M-region.

BACKGROUND OF NGUYEN PHUC BUU-HOI
AND HIS CAREER UNTIL 1945

Nguyen Phuc Buu-Hoi was born in 1915 in Hué, the ancient capital of Vietnam. He was a member of the Vietnamese royal family, a descendant of the emperors Gia Long and Minh Mang, who founded and consolidated the Nguyen dynasty in the early 19th century. His father, Ung Uy, headed the Private Council of the imperial family until 1945. On his mother's side he descends from the Ho Dac's, another illustrious family of Vietnam.

Like all upper-class Vietnamese, Buu-Hoi grew up steeped in two cultures. The traditional Vietnamese way of life which, as in all cultures in the Chinese sphere, is deeply imbued with Confucian, Buddhist, and Taoist elements, and, on the other hand, the Western culture imported by the French. Buu-Hoi's own mother heavily leaned toward Buddhist beliefs and philosophy.

He did his secondary schooling at the Lycée "Albert Sarraut" in Hanoi, which under the French colonial administration was the capital and the largest city. Subsequently, he studied for a degree in Pharmacy at the University of Hanoi and audited courses simultaneously at the Faculty of Medicine. From his early youth he gravitated toward science;

as he puts it in a later autobiographical summary, "because of the desire of his mother and partly because of his own belief in the human value of science . . . " (38). Buu-Hoi was 20 when, with his degree freshly acquired, he left for Paris never to return to Vietnam as a resident. He would, from then on, see his native country only on short visits.

Barely a few days after his arrival in Paris, an event took place which further motivated him to pursue a scientific career. A journalist friend of his family took him to a tea party given by Jean Perrin, the physicist of Nobel fame, where he met an unusual concentration of scientific notoriety: Prince de Broglie, another past Nobelist, as well as Dr. and Madame Joliot-Curie, who had just been awarded their prize, and other contemporary great figures of French science. But he relates that, "What impressed me then the most was that all that concentration of science was paralleled by an equal concentration of kindness and universal open mindedness" (39).

At the university, he followed the regular curriculum toward the doctorate. He studied for a "Licence ès Science" degree while working as an Intern of Pharmacy at the Paris hospitals. Then, after a short period spent in the Institute of Chemical Physics with Jean Perrin, he was admitted to the laboratory of Pauline Ramart-Lucas for his doctoral work on the spectrophotometry of organic compounds.

At the outbreak of World War II, he volunteered in the French army and served until the defeat. The armistice found him in Toulouse in 1940 where he was greatly helped by the physicist, Paul Langevin, whom he met at Jean Perrin's memorable tea party. With his aid, he entered the occupied northern zone of France and returned to Paris. He became a member of the research staff of the National Center of Scientific Research (CNRS) in 1941, and at the liberation of France was appointed "Maître de Conférence" (equivalent to Assistant Professor) at the famous École Polytechnique by the Provisional Government. At about the same period, in 1944, he met Antoine Lacassagne who was then establishing his interdisciplinary team. Jacquignon (40) writes in his obituary of Buu-Hoi: "No one will ever know what happened at the first meeting of these two men, respectively 29 and 60 years old, and coming from backgrounds and cultures so different yet complementary; no one will ever know since neither of them was — by natural reserve or modesty — prolix of confidences. What is certain is that from that time was born in them a mutual esteem and admiration, growing with time, and leading to innumerable communications and reports at congresses, colloquia, and symposia throughout the world. "

Although they had already begun publishing together in 1944-1945, Buu-Hoi did not formally join the Radium Institute until 1947 when he became head of the newly established Department of Organic and Medicinal Chemistry and Maître de Recherches at the CNRS. In 1962, he reached the top of the CNRS-supported research hierarchy with his promotion to Director of Research.

The scientific accomplishments of Buu-Hoi are immense. Although an organic chemist by training and of world-wide renown, he had the intuitive intelligence coupled with a vast memory which enabled him to grasp the essentials of a biological problem sometimes only remotely related to organic chemistry. It is in his laboratory at the École Polytechnique that he truly began his research career with investigations on chaulmoogric and hydnocarpic acids, which were then the only products used for the treatment of leprosy. In a few years, he established himself as an international authority on the chemotherapy of leprosy. Together with Paul Cagniant, Albert Ratsimamanga (now the ambassador of Madagascar to France), and others, he delineated the role of the cyclopentene ring, of the double bond thereof, and of the chain length, in the toxicity and leprostatic activity of these compounds. My awareness of Buu-Hoi and my admiration for his work dates from 1947 when, browsing in a scientific bookstore in Munich, I came across some past issues of the Angewandte Chemie, containing a series of reviews by Lennartz (41), from the Frankfurt-am-Main Georg Speyer Haus, "On the Syntheses of Higher Aliphatic Compounds. " My imagination was fired by the elegance, or should I say romance, of some of the syntheses carried out by Buu-Hoi and his colleagues.

Although from the time of his meeting with Lacassagne, Buu-Hoi's main preoccupation was chemical carcinogenesis, throughout his career he continued to devote substantial efforts to the chemotherapy of leprosy — his "first love" — and associated it with the chemotherapy of tuberculosis (e.g., 42-51). An important finding that should be singled out in the latter field was his observation that the multiplication of Mycobacterium tuberculosis is strongly inhibited by hydrazides. This was subsequently of crucial importance for Domagk in his discovery of the tuberculostatic drug, isoniazide. In addition to the above fields, Buu-Hoi and his associates carried out investigations on a wide range of problems of therapeutic and biologic interest, for example, the synthesis and testing of anti-inflammatory nonsteroid compounds, substituted sex hormones, antidiabetic agents, anticoagulant substances and their potentiation, treatment of hypertension by methyl-DOPA, antioxidants and the chemoprophylaxy of aging, odor and chemical constitution, the toxicity of dioxine. Many honors and prizes recognized his accomplishments (40, 52-55).

It is probably safe to say that Prince Buu-Hoi was the most prestigious intellectual that Vietnam has produced since the French
conquest of the country in the second half of the 19th century — a
somewhat legendary personage to many of his countrymen. On this
account and as a scion of the most illustrious family of his country,
both Vietnams vied for him. North Vietnam's president, Ho Chi Minh,
named him in 1947 Rector of the University of Hanoi, an appointment
he did not take up. He acted as a science advisor to South Vietnam's
late President Ngo Dinh Diem, who in 1960 appointed him Director of
the Atomic Energy Establishment of Vietnam. He was instrumental in
the establishment of an Atomic Energy Research Center — geared toward
the medical and agricultural uses of atomic energy — including a nuclear
reactor in Dalat in 1963. He represented the Republic of South Vietnam
as an ambassador-at-large to several African countries and to the
United Nations in 1963, until the death of President Diem. He was
involved in several missions attempting to establish peace in Vietnam.
Some aspects of his public life related to Vietnam are discussed in
two excellent monographs (56, 57) by his devoted friend, Ellen J. Hammer,
an American-born political scientist and expert on Vietnamese affairs.

WORK OF LACASSAGNE, BUU-HOI, ZAJDELA, AND THEIR ASSOCIATES: A PERSPECTIVE

Aside from the reports published in collaboration with the theoretical chemists on aspects of hydrocarbon carcinogenesis related to
quantum mechanics, the principal study areas were (a) the structure-
activity relationships of polynuclear carcinogens and (b) the influence
of various agents (carcinogens and inactive compounds) on carcinogenic activity; the latter category also includes work by Lacassagne
and Corre-Hurst on hormonal influences upon carcinogenesis. Before
opening the curtain on their accomplishments, I should mention, in
passing, that Buu-Hoi (58) was the first to propose that noncovalent
forces play a role in the carcinogenicity of chemical agents.

Table 2 presents some types of polycyclic systems that have been
synthesized and tested for carcinogenic activity. The effect of methyl
substitutions on 1, 2-benzanthracene has been explored mainly in
relation to the finding of the early workers, listed in Hartwell's first
compendium and unexpected in view of the quantum mechanical results,
that methyl derivatives that bear the substituent in the benz ring have
only trace activity or are inactive (59).

A very intriguing recent finding of Buu-Hoi and Giao (60) was that
total deuteration of 9, 10-dimethyl-1, 2-benzanthracene close to
doubled the potency of the already highly carcinogenic compound.

Since extensive deuteration increases the life span of triplet states of aromatic hydrocarbons, Buu-Hoi and Sung (61) regarded this as evidence for nonradiative photochemical energy transfer, in which the hydrocarbon acts as an energy transfer catalyst to, and denaturation of, cellular macromolecules.

The Radium Institute group has synthesized and tested some "steranthrenes, " which result from the joining of five- and/or six-membered alicyclic rings to 1, 2-benzanthracene. These were of interest because of the postulated transformation of cholesterol to the fundamental "steranthrene" nucleus. All "steranthrenes" tested (62, 63) were found to be potent carcinogens. In connection with the possibility that naturally occurring sterols may be carcinogenic, they have also tested apocholic acid. In line with the earlier reports of other investigators that deoxycholic acid is a weak carcinogen, apocholic acid was found to possess moderate activity (64). The group has also synthesized (in collaboration with Daub) and tested a number of mono-, di-, and trimethyl derivatives of 3, 4-benzopyrene (65).

The group has confirmed the assumption that the 6- and 12-positions

TABLE 2
Some Types of Alternant Polynuclear Homocyclic Systems Investigated

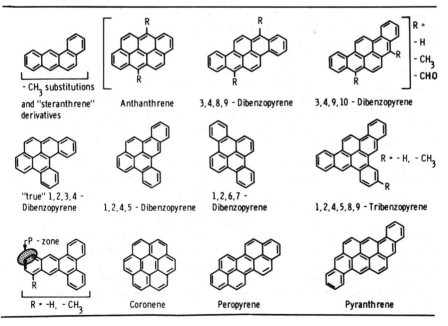

in anthanthrene are analogous to meso-anthracenic positions. Indeed, substitution at these site(s) by one and two methyl group(s) create increasingly carcinogenic compounds. Formyl groups are more effective than the methyls in potentiating carcinogenic activity (66-68). However, a theoretical interpretation of these substituent effects becomes most problematic in the light of the finding in 1971 of Bahna et al. (69) that anthanthrene also becomes a potent carcinogen by aza replacement of the —CH= groups in the 6- and 12-positions.

Testing the five isomeric dibenzopyrenes under standardized conditions showed that, with the exception of 1, 2, 6, 7-dibenzopyrene which is inactive, all are potent agents able to induce subcutaneous sarcomas in mice (66, 68, 70-73). The group has made the interesting discovery that methyl or formyl substitution of 3, 4, 8, 9-dibenzopyrene in the 5- and 5, 10-positions increasingly reduces carcinogenic activity; similar observations were made when these substituents were introduced into 3, 4, 9, 10-dibenzopyrene (67, 68, 70) or into 1, 2, 3, 4-dibenzopyrene (74). Since the sites of substitution are comparable to meso-anthracenic positions, it is remarkable that in the dibenzo-pyrenes, methyl substitution brings about a diametrically opposite effect than in the 1, 2-benzanthracene series.

1, 2, 3, 4-Dibenzanthracene has always been regarded as a crucial instance with respect to the requirement of a K-region for carcino-genicity in aromatic hydrocarbons. This compound has no K-region and, indeed, in most (but not all) testing studies it has been found inactive. Also the Radium Institute group found 1, 2, 3, 4-dibenzanthra-cene inactive in their standard test system in XVII nc/Z-strain mice; however, it is a most interesting development that introduction of a methyl group in the 5-position transforms this inactive hydrocarbon to a moderately potent carcinogen (75). The interpretation given to this finding was (76) that, as a result of the substitution, a reactive region (called P-region) arises (corresponding to the 7- and 8-positions) which performs the same role in cellular interactions as the typical K-region in other hydrocarbons.

A great variety of large-size and "hypercondensed" hydrocarbons were explored; for example, naphtho [2', 3':3, 4] pyrene and phenanthro [2', 3':3, 4] pyrene (77), coronene, 1, 2-benzocoronene, pyranthrene (78, 79), 1, 12-benzoperylene (80), peropyrene and periflanthene (79), 1, 2, 4, 5, 8, 9-tribenzopyrene and its 2'-methyl derivative (74, 78), some of which are shown in Table 2. The latter methyl derivative and the above phenanthro-pyrene are the largest molecular-size hydrocarbons known to display carcinogenic activity. These very large-size carcinogenic molecules are of a troublesome significance for different hypotheses attempting to link carcinogenicity with intercalation into DNA.

A different approach to the exploration of the molecular geometry required for carcinogenicity consisted in the "opening" of several rings in the polynuclears and the testing of highly elongated electron-rich structures. Again another approach is the testing of partially hydrogenated compounds. Partial hydrogenation, although it does bring about a less drastic change in overall geometry, does in most instances abolish the coplanarity of planar aromatics. For example, a variety of diarylacetylenes and diarylpolyacetylenes, even though they are high conjugated and rich in π electrons, were found non-carcinogenic by Buu-Hoi et al. (81). The effect of partial hydrogenation on carcinogenic activity appears to depend entirely on the extent of alteration of coplanarity. Thus, Lacassagne and his associates found that meso-hydrogenated 3, 4, 8, 9- and 3, 4, 9, 10-dibenzopyrene — which remain essentially coplanar — retain their potency virtually unchanged; on the other hand, hydrogenation of a lateral ring, such as in 3, 4-benzopyrene or in some benzacridines, leads to buckled structures and brings about considerable loss of activity (82).

At about the time when the synthesis of the dibenzopyrenes was carried out, Buu-Hoi and his associates discovered that polynuclear hydrocarbons undergo drastic molecular rearrangements under the catalytic effect of AlCl$_3$ (Table 3). Reinvestigation of the compound, regarded until then as 1, 2, 3, 4-dibenzopyrene, indicated that it was actually 2, 3, 5, 6-dibenzofluoranthene (83, 84). The "true" 1, 2, 3, 4-dibenzopyrene, prepared by an unequivocal synthetic route not involving AlCl$_3$, is a quite potent carcinogen (72) while 2, 3, 5, 6-dibenzofluoranthene is only a weak to moderately active carcinogenic hydrocarbon.

The migration of the phenyl group under the action of AlCl$_3$ from the sterically more hindered 9-position to the sterically less hindered 10-position in 1, 2-benzanthracene is, however, only a particular instance of these rearrangements. The organic synthesis group at Gif-sur-Yvette was fascinated by the fact that the AlCl$_3$-catalyzed rearrangements can involve not only migration of substituents but also drastic rearrangements of the fundamental aromatic skeleton itself, as shown in Table 4. For example, 1, 2-benzanthracene can rearrange to chrysene, and 1, 2, 7, 8-dibenzanthracene to picene by passing through an intermediate stage as 1, 2, 5, 6-dibenzanthracene. At the same time the picene formed condenses with benzene used as solvent to yield 1, 2, 4, 5, 8, 9-tribenzopyrene (85-88).

Table 5 shows the nonalternant hydrocarbons hitherto tested. With the exception of fluoranthene itself and the compounds marked by an asterisk, these results are to be credited to the Radium Institute group (68, 89). The numbers under the formulas are the Iball Indexes for a ready comparison of the carcinogenicities. Nonalternant hydro-

TABLE 3
Establishment of Structure of the "True" 1, 2, 3, 4-Dibenzopyrene

carbons — those, for example, that possess in their skeleton a pentagonal ring — have electronic properties different from alternant hydrocarbons. In nonalternants the net electric charges are not unitary, and this results in the appearance of an appreciable dipole moment even in the absence of substituents. The fluoranthene skeleton is a powerful "carcinophilic" structure since a number of highly active compounds are found in this series. Nevertheless, though a pronounced angular arrangement of the rings always provides for higher activity, the presence of a true K-region is not a condition sine qua non for carcinogenicity, as is clearly indicated by the activity of 11, 12-benzofluoranthene (center formula). Molecular size and shape appear to be a limiting factor. A most interesting development was the finding that azuleno[5, 6, 7-cd]phenalene, a deep-green, highly oxidizable, nonbenzenoid hydrocarbon, as well as its methyl derivative, are carcinogens of potency approaching that of 3, 4-benzopyrene (90).

In the course of their work, the Radium Institute group was led to compare aromatic hydrocarbons with various heteroaromatic analogs. They found that heterocycles containing nitrogen, sulfur, oxygen, or even arsenic, may replace homocyclic aromatic rings in carcinogenic polycyclic hydrocarbons with no loss or only partial loss of activity

TABLE 4
Some AlCl₃-Catalyzed Rearrangements of Polynuclear Hydrocarbons

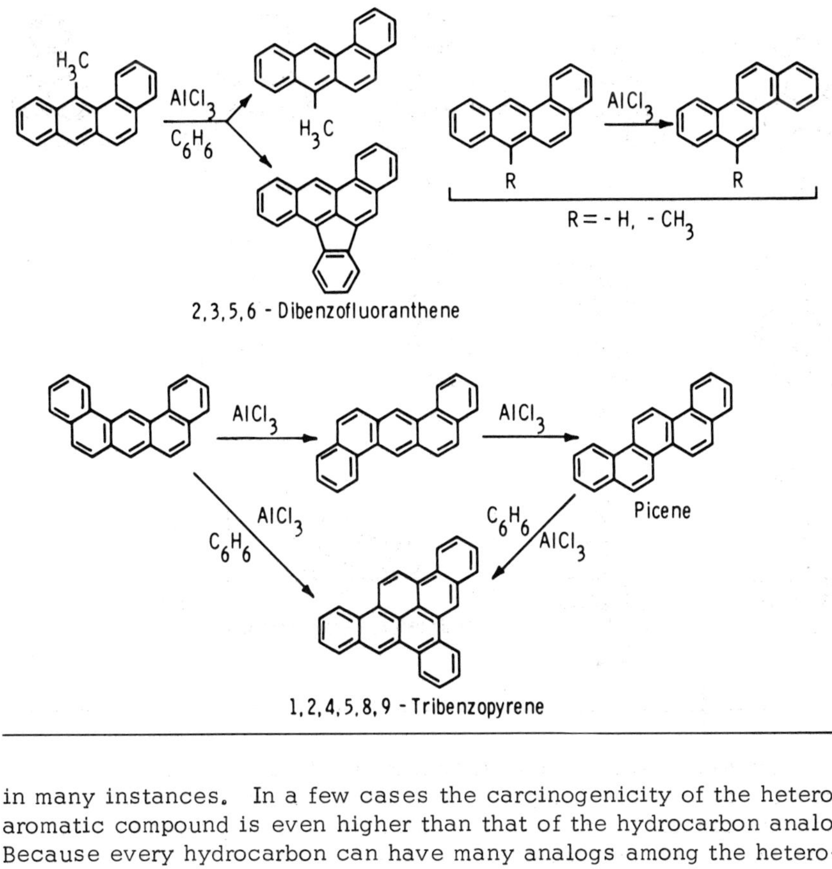

2,3,5,6 - Dibenzofluoranthene

R = - H, - CH₃

1,2,4,5,8,9 - Tribenzopyrene

in many instances. In a few cases the carcinogenicity of the heteroaromatic compound is even higher than that of the hydrocarbon analog.
Because every hydrocarbon can have many analogs among the heteroaromatic compounds, a great variety of carcinogenic compounds are
found in the latter group. For example, considering the lateral benzo
ring only in 3, 4-benzopyrene, four aza analogs are possible; aza
substitution in 3, 4-benzofluoranthene can yield 12 isosters.

Table 6 exemplifies the variety of heteroaromatics with nitrogen
replacement studied by the Paris group. The compounds in the first
row are structural analogs of 1, 2-benzanthracene, 3, 4-benzopyrene,
1, 2, 3, 4-dibenzophenanthrene, and 3, 4- and 11, 12-benzofluoranthene,
respectively. In general, these aza polynuclears are more likely to
possess carcinogenic activity if they are isosteric with hydrocarbons
of high potency; this is most striking with the two aza benzofluoranthenes.

TABLE 5

Nonalternant Hydrocarbons: Benzofluoranthenes and Azulenophenalenes[a]

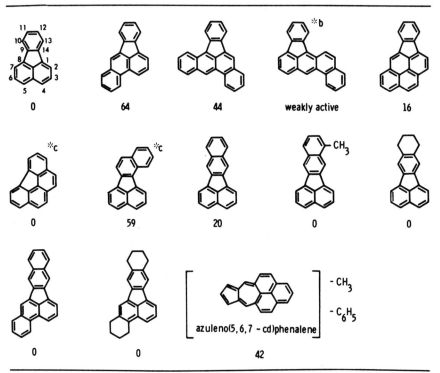

[a]Complete listing of benzofluoranthenes tested for carcinogenic activity up to 1972. Except when otherwise stated, the numbers under the formulas represent the Iball Indexes based on the average incidence of subcutaneous sarcomas in male and female mice (XVII nc/Z strain, Paris Radium Institute).

[b]Naphtho[1', 2':3, 2]fluoranthene (also known as 15, 16-benzo-dehydrocholanthrene); tested by early workers, see in J. L. Hartwell, Survey of Compounds Which Have Been Tested for Carcinogenic Activity. USPHS Publication No. 149. Washington, D.C., 1951, p. 329.

[c]Iball Index is based on the epithelioma + papilloma incidence obtained by skin painting on random-bred female Swiss mice [E. L. Wynder, Brit. Med. J., 317 (1959-1), and E. L. Wynder and D. Hoffmann, Cancer, 12, 1194 (1959)].

TABLE 6

Examples of Nitrogen Heteroaromatics Studied: Aza Analogs of Hydrocarbons, Benzacridines, Benzo- and Naphtho-pyridocarbazoles and β-Carbolines

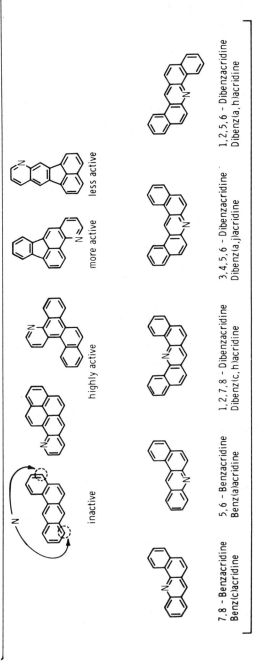

The second row in Table 6 shows the two angular benzacridine isomers and the three angular dibenzacridine isomers. The carcinogenicity of these and of their derivatives has been investigated by the Radium Institute group in considerable detail. This is probably the one structural category where their contribution to synthetic organic chemistry and to the structure–activity relationship in carcinogenesis is the most massively overwhelming; it is best compared to the exhaustive coverage of the 4-nitroquinoline-N-oxide area by Japanese investigations. In 1956 the Paris group summarized their investigations in a review on "The Relation between Carcinogenic Activity and the Physical and Chemical Properties of Angular Benzacridines" (91).

Many substances of high carcinogenic activity are found in the 7, 8-benzacridine series in contrast with the weak activity of analogous compounds in the 5, 6-benzacridine series; similarly, the derivatives so far explored in the 3, 4, 5, 6-dibenzacridine series are only weak to moderately carcinogenic. In the latter two molecular skeletons, which are precisely the ones not favorable to high levels of carcinogenicity, the heteroatom is in a sterically exposed position — on the outer periphery of the molecule; this could favor increased interaction with water and high rate of excretion. However, the relation they found experimentally between the pK and carcinogenic activity (92), and between the theoretically calculated electrophilic potential barrier and carcinogenic activity (30), suggests that the heteroatom may itself be involved in interactions leading to carcinogenesis.

Among the many compounds in this series, the Paris group has synthesized and tested two compounds of special stereochemical interest that should be pointed out. In 10-isopropyl-3, 4, 5, 6-dibenzacridine the isopropyl group does not overlap with the lateral benz rings, but is rigidly "nested" in the unoccupied space between them, so that the two methyl groups point toward the same face of the molecular plane. Rotation of the isopropyl group is totally blocked and there is only slight strain, which is distributed over the molecular frame. Thus, despite what may be concluded from a summary observation of the formula, there is little departure from coplanarity; consistent with this the compound manifest appreciable activity toward the mouse skin. The weak but definite carcinogenic activity of 10-n-butyl-1, 2, 5, 6-dibenzacridine — one of the bulkiest carcinogenic molecules known — points to a distinct difference from the analogous benzanthracene series in which, for alkyl groups in the meso-anthracenic position, there is complete cutoff of carcinogenic activity beyond ethyl.

From the late 1950's, the Radium Institute group focused its attention to other heteroaromatics (see below) and only occasional reports (e. g. , Refs. 93 and 94; in review 68) on benzacridine derivatives appeared. [I should also mention at this point their substantial studies on the carcinogenicity of derivatives of carbazole (95).] Increasingly their interest shifted to polynuclears containing two nitrogen atoms, the benzo- and naphtho-derivatives of pyridocarbazole and of β-carboline (96-98, review 68). These compounds are exemplified in the last row of Table 6. Introduction of the second nitrogen atom can powerfully potentiate the carcinogenicity of the parent dibenzocarbazole. Several compounds in the pyridocarbazole series have been found to be potent carcinogens; however, activity appears to be highly sensitive to increase in size. The β-carboline skeleton is, as a rule, much less favorable to carcinogenicity; in these, the second nitrogen is para with respect to the biphenylic linkage, very drastically modifying the resonance as compared with the parent dibenzocarbazole.

The heteroaromatics prepared and tested that contain sulfur, selenium, or arsenic, alone or in association with nitrogen, are exemplified in Table 7. In the first row of compounds sulfur replaces a meso-phenanthrenic region. Their weak activity or inactivity would appear to be consistent with the requirement for a formal K-region. However, the inactivity of these particular molecules may be entirely fortuitous and could well be due to the specific positional relationship of the two heteroatoms and the excessive polarity — unfavorable in these polynuclear types — contributed by them. Indeed, we know from an earlier work of Waravdekar and Ranadive (99) that analogs of

9,10-dimethyl-1,2,5,6-dibenzanthracene and 9,10-dimethyl-1,2,7,8-dibenzanthracene, in which both K-regions are replaced by a sulfur bridge, are sarcomatogenic agents of potency entirely comparable with that of the most active hydrocarbons. Clearly then, not enough is known of the electronic characteristics of these complex molecules and of the type of interactions they may undergo with cell constituents.

In the second row of Table 7 the nitrogen- and sulfur-containing pseudoazulenes tested (100) by the Paris group are exemplified. The pseudoazulenes are compounds π- isoelectronic with azulene. The first compound in the row is highly active, despite the presence of the two heteroatoms, in both the conjugated dienic form as shown (Iball Index 30) and in the dihydrogenated form (Iball Index 63). One should note in this molecule a positional relationship of N and S different from that seen in the inactive and weakly active compounds in the first row. Removal of the lateral benzo ring (as indicated) brings about loss of activity.

With the intention of establishing a connecting link between the polynuclear aromatics and the aflatoxins, which are polynuclear lactones, the Paris group has synthesized and tested a series of derivatives of 5-oxo-isochromeno-indole and 6-oxo-chromenoquinoline (101,102). The first compound shown in Table 8, a benzo derivative of oxo-isochromeno-indole, produces pulmonary tumors in all mice

TABLE 7
Heteroaromatics with Sulfur, Selenium, and Arsenic Replacements

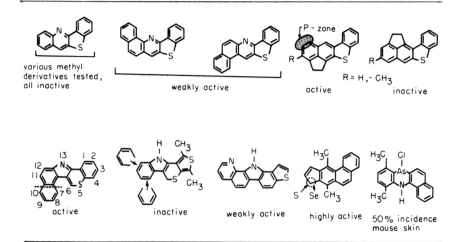

by oral administration, besides being one of the most potent sarcomatogenic agents known by subcutaneous administration. The lateral
benzo ring, delineated in the formula, is required for its activity.

Converging lines of evidence suggest that carcinogenic activity in
this series depends on the reactivity of the lactone ring, which
appears to be enhanced by electron withdrawal from the ester bond
toward the pyrrole nitrogen, owing to its electronegativity. This is
indicated, for example, by the abolishment of activity by methyl
substitution in the 12-position, as well as by the weak activity or
inactivity of the other compounds shown in Table 8.

The great variety of heteroaromatics displaying carcinogenic
activity and the number of exceptions to the classical interpretation
of the electronic theory led Buu-Hoi to propose a "newer picture" of
a carcinogenic hydrocarbon (68). Daudel and Daudel (20) have pointed
out subsequently that the term K-region has been used — historically
speaking — in a too restricted way and that any bond with a low enough
ortho-localization energy should be regarded as a K-region, irrespec-
tive of whether it coincides with meso-phenanthrenic positions.
Already in 1950 Buu-Hoi envisioned that van der Waals forces may
play a role in some instances (58). While covalent binding is no

TABLE 8
Intraring Replacements by Oxygen and Nitrogen: Polynuclear Lactones

highly sarcomatogenic   weakly active   isochromenone

inactive   inactive   chromenone

doubt of paramount importance in carcinogenicity by many chemical
agents — and these were the first to be detected because of the
inherent stability of the bond — it is possible that for an equally
great number of carcinogens various noncovalent interactions will be
found ultimately to play a critical role.

From the mass of sometimes contradictory experimental evidence
and the maze of interpretations, there emerges a fascinating yet
simple picture of a carcinogenic hydrocarbon so aptly described by
Buu-Hoi (68):

"The conjugated frame offers certain sites and areas of
high π-electron densities, hence a greater covalent and
noncovalent reactivity, through which the interaction with
cell components is facilitated; in many instances, there is
a meso-phenanthrenic K-zone, whose involvement in the
metabolic degradation of the carcinogen has been experimentally established but whose existence is essential neither
for protein-binding nor for carcinogenicity. Where meso-
anthracenic L-zones are present, their reactivity does not
necessarily preclude carcinogenicity. Replacement of =CH—
groups by tervalent nitrogen heteroatoms may have a positive
or a negative effect on the carcinogenicity, depending on the
number and the position of the nitrogen atoms and on the nature
of the molecule; when several nitrogen heteroatoms are present,
the prime importance of their position in relation to one another
suggests that they act as centers for binding with cell components, in place of, or in conjunction with, other zones of
biochemical interaction.

"Where there are substituents, these may be either
electron-donating or electron-accepting groups (except acid
functions), and their contribution to the carcinogenicity may
be positive or negative, depending on the type of molecule.
In the case of alkyl substituents, lengthening of the chain
has an adverse effect on activity, owing to increase in the
encumbrance area of the carcinogen, the degree of loss of
activity depending on the site of substitution. The introduction of substituents with acid hydroxyl groups (carboxyl,
sulfonic acid, and phenolic functions) invariably results in a
sharp decrease or total loss of carcinogenicity — an effect
which must be due to a departure from the "normal" molecular
orientation of the carcinogen within cellular lipid structures,
produced by the strong hydrophilic radical.

"These, then, are the basic physico-chemical characteristics which are to be borne in mind when formulating or
assessing general theories on the mode of interaction of polycyclic aromatic hydrocarbons and their heterocyclic analogs

with cell components. The electronic theory of carcinogens which has proved of such great value in the past, as a guide in the search for active compounds through the maze of organic chemistry, can probably continue to play that role if through adequate refinements and/or modifications it can integrate the new experimental data. "

This summary review of the accomplishments of the Paris group on structure-activity relationships would not be balanced without mentioning their reports on the carcinogenicity of 4-nitroquinoline-N-oxide derivatives (103), on the production of plant tumors by a nitrosamine (104), on the metabolism and protein binding of poly-nuclears (105-108) and effect of the latter on DNA replication and transcription (109), on the effect of various carcinogens on the hatching of shrimp eggs (110), etc. Beginning in the mid 1960's, Buu-Hoi focused his interest increasingly on the structural facets of polynuclears that govern their ability to induce microsomal enzyme synthesis, using zoxazolamine and dicoumarol hydroxylation as standard test systems (111-118). Particularly interesting results obtained in collaboration with our laboratory were the findings (119, 120) that there is an optimum molecular size of polycyclic hydro-carbons for both the induction of aminoazo dye N-demethylase synthesis and the repression of dimethylnitrosamine-demethylase synthesis, as shown in Fig. 5. These distribution curves are in a mirror-image relationship (Fig. 6), which led to the proposal that the hydrocarbons act on repressor proteins of gene action and that the group of operons coding for inducible enzymes and the group of operons coding for repressible enzymes are in a cascade relationship (120, 121).

Finally, a massive amount of work has been carried out in the last 15 years, especially by Lacassagne and Corre-Hurst, on anti- and cocarcinogenesis and on antagonism and synergism between carcino-gens, as well as on the effect of steroid hormones and other endocrine factors on carcinogenesis. This is presented in tabular form in Table 9. Historically, this was originated by the discovery, in the early 1940's, by Lacassagne, the Daudels, and Buu-Hoi, of the competitive antagonism between strong and weak polycyclic hydrocarbon carcino-gens in tumor induction on the mouse skin.

CLOSING NOTE

Let us, in parting, contemplate the contrast of the two men whose personalities left such a characteristics stamp on the endeavors of the Radium Institute group.

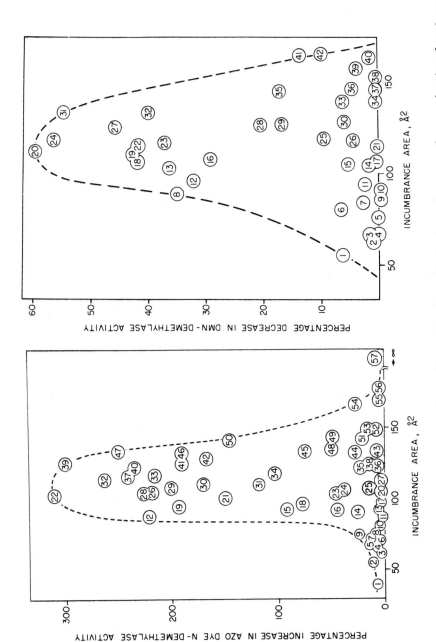

Fig. 5. Molecular size-dependent effect of polycyclic hydrocarbons on the synthesis of aminoazo dye N-demethylase and DMN-demethylase in the rat liver (identification numbers correspond to the hydrocarbons given in the references cited).

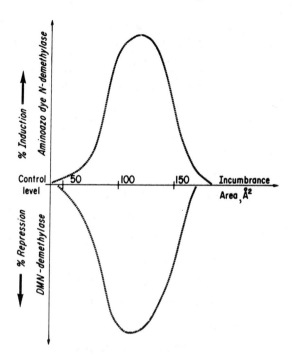

FIG. 6. Mirror-image relationship of the molecular size-dependent effect of polycyclic hydrocarbons in inducing aminoazo dye N-demethylase and repressing DMN-demethylase.

Antoine Lacassagne (Fig. 7) bore the mark of the social atmosphere of tolerance, probity, and uprightness of the earlier part of the Third French Republic. In describing the era of Ernest Kennaway's and his own upbringing, he writes: "We came to maturity during the thirty years preceding the outbreak of the First World War, in a period when the cultivated middle classes, both in Britain and in France, enjoyed complete independence of mind and liberty of action . . . It was a period when one could go round the world without a passport, stay at any hotel without filling up a form for the police, profess oneself an agnostic in the political as well as the religious sense without risk of being thought a revolutionary and suspected of a plot to endanger the safety of the State and of society . . . We both grew up in an atmosphere where a respect for individual liberty and a veneration for scientific progress were looked on as articles of faith . . . " (10).

With a colorful and very fitting term, his successor describes (5) Lacassagne's bearing as that "d'un gentilhomme de cape et d'épée, " that untranslatable expression best approximated by the old-fashioned but very highest British meaning of "gentleman. " One of the most

TABLE 9
Combined Effect of Carcinogens with Inactive or
Other Active Compounds

(a) Anti- and cocarcinogenesis[a, b]			
Carcinogen	Second agent	Effect	Reference
4-Dimethylamino azobenzene	Cholic acid	0	122
	Litocholic acid	0	122
	α-Naphthylisothiocyanate	-	123
	β-Naphthylisothiocyanate	--	123
	p-Hydroxyacetophenone	--	124
	m-Hydroxyacetophenone	-	125
	3-Allyl-4-hydroxyacetophenone	-	125
	p-Hydroxypropiophenone	-	124
	p-Hydroxybutyrophenone	-	124
	2, 4, 5-Trihydroxybutyrophenone	0	125
	Metopirone[c]	0	126
	o-p'-DDD[d]	--	127, 128
	N-Methyl-3, 5-dimethyl-benzheparide-amide	-	128
	Iproniazide[e]	-	129
	Reserpine	+	129-131
	Yohimbine	0	132
	Chloropromazine	0	130
	Chloramphenicol	--	133
	Various steroid hormones[f]		134-139: rev. 140
2-Acetylamino-fluorene	Tolbutamide[g]	+	141, 142
	Diazoxide[h]	-	142
	Tolbutamide + diazoxide	0	142

TABLE 9 (continued)

(a) Anti- and cocarcinogenesis (continued)

Carcinogen	Second agent	Effect	Reference
Diethyl- nitrosamine	p-Hydroxyacetophenone	0	143
	p-Hydroxypropiophenone	0	143
	p-Hydroxybutyrophenone	0	143
	o-p'-DDD[d]	0	143
	Reserpine	-	144, 145
	Yohimbine	0	132

(b) Antagonism and Synergism

Carcinogen 1	Carcinogen 2	Effect	Reference
20-Methylcholanthrene	1, 2, 5, 6-Dibenzo-fluorene	Antagonism[i]	146, 147
20-Methylcholanthrene	Chrysene	Weak antago-nism[i]	147
1, 2, 5, 6-Dibenzanthra-cene	1, 2, 5, 6-Dibenzacridine	Antagonism[i]	147, 148
9, 10-Dimethyl-1, 2-benzanthracene	1, 2-Benzanthracene	Antagonism[i]	149
9, 10-Dimethyl-1, 2-benzanthracene	3, 4, 5, 6-Dibenzo-phenothiazine[j]	Strong promotion	149
20-Methylcholanthrene	2-Aminochrysene (also known as 6-amino-)	Antagonism[k]	150

TABLE 9 (continued)

(b) Antagonism and Synergism (continued)

Carcinogen 1	Carcinogen 2	Effect	Reference
9, 10-Dimethyl-1, 2-benzanthracene	4-Dimethylamino-azobenzene	No mutual influence on respective effects[b]	151
4-Dimethylaminoazo-benzene	4'-Methyl-4-dimethylaminoazo-benzene	Synergism[b]	152
4-Dimethylaminoazo-benzene	Ethionine	Antagonism[b]	153
4-Dimethylaminoazo-benzene	Griseofulvin	No effect[b] (some increase in no. of cancer foci)	154

Footnotes to Table 9

[a]Complete suppression or considerable retardation of the carcinogenic effect, (--); moderate inhibition, (-); promotion, (+); no effect, (0).

[b]By oral administration.

[c]2-Methyl-1, 2-bis(3-pyridyl)-1-propanone.

[d]o-p'-Dichlorodiphenyldichloroethane.

[e]1-Isonicotinyl-2-isopropyl hydrazine.

[f]By oral or parenteral administration.

[g]N-(Sulfonyl-p-methylbenzene)-N'-n-butyl-urea.

[h]3-Methyl-7-chloro-1, 2, 4-benzothiadiazine-1-dioxide.

[i]By skin painting.

[j]Not known to be carcinogenic.

[k]20-Methylcholanthrene by skin painting and 2-aminochrysene by oral administration.

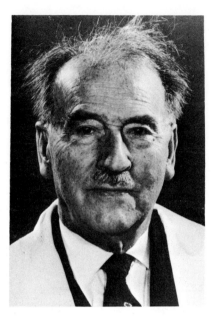

FIG. 7. Antoine Lacassagne in the late 1960's.

salient character traits of Lacassagne was his exceptional self-discipline. Early, he established for himself a strict but very balanced way of life. He was an early riser and kept long working hours; he did not believe in weekly rest or holidays, except for two yearly periods of vacation — in spring and early fall — liberally filled with physical exercise, at his small farm in Villerest, adjacent to his family's country house where he was born. An even pace and a recollected, serene attitude marked his way and rhythm of working. He had a prodigious memory for the scientific literature, observations, events, and people, even in his later years.

In other respects he was very much rooted in the French cultural traditions. At his Paris home and the Villerest country house, he surrounded himself with pieces of art and memorabilia of the Lacassagne clan. Despite his absorption in his work, he kept very much abreast of political and cultural events. He was much attached to family traditions, and was a sophisticated connoisseur of the culinary art which he regarded as an element of cultural expression inseparable from the whole (6). Perhaps for these same reasons he was close to nature, and during the years — without ever getting discouraged — continued to reforest the arid hills on his Villerest property (6).

His attitude toward his fellow men was marked by true simplicity, tolerance, and friendliness. He easily accorded his trust to individuals and chose to overlook as much as he could their weaknesses.

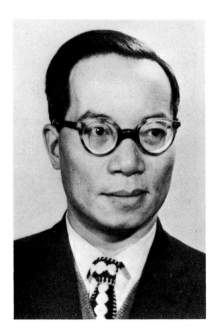

FIG. 8. Nguyen Phuc Buu-Hoi in 1971.

Though it must be said that he hated false sophistication tending to
cover up cracks in the essence.

He was much less optimistic, if not sometimes frankly pessimistic,
regarding nations and mankind in general. As a radiobiologist he was
acutely aware of the dangers of radioactive pollution and actively
participated in various movements for its control. He had the deep
conviction that one should always act in the direction of progress
even if this brings trouble on one's own head (6).

From his childhood in Lyons — as a late echo of the best standards
of the medieval guilds — he retained his appreciation for conscientious
work, well done for its own sake. He defined himself as a kind of lay
monk whose religion was a rationalistic, very cartesian scientific
world-view. He never married. He shunned small talk and mundane
happenings. He carefully, almost jealously, maintained to the very
end the image of that personality that he willed himself to be.

In contrast to the methodical personality of Lacassagne imbued
with cartesian reasonableness, Buu-Hoi (Fig. 8) was sensitive, artistic,
highly intuitive, enlivened by a touch of flamboyance and dry wit.
He was born a royal prince and member of a family most prestigious

in his society. This has contributed, in his young years, to establishing that very secure inner core of self-identity that helped him in his career to overcome difficult times and frustrations —often with a smile — and led him to be unstintingly generous and kind toward his students and friends. No doubt Confucian elements in his upbringing must have further deepened his high sense of obligation toward his family, nation, and those who depended on him. Still quite a young man, but already a scientist of repute, he became the elected spokesman of the 25,000 Vietnamese living in France at the end of World War II and as a member of the royal family served in the Vietnamese delegation at the Fontainebleau peace conference with France. As a man primarily absorbed in his scientific pursuits, he did not relish but he did not shun what he felt were his political obligations; he regarded these, with truly Confucian equanimity, as a duty — that he was born into — toward his family and his divided country, and which he must carry out to the best of his ability.

On the other side of the ledger, Buu-Hoi knew very well the debt he owed to France and to Western culture, which was the nurturing soil of his intellectual life. He was, using the term coined by Robert Guillain, bi-civilized. He practiced two civilizations at the same time. In many respects, he became very much a Frenchman; he had a great appreciation for the beautiful and good things life has to offer, as well as for the more earthy pleasures of the culinary art. He was an exemplary father to his children, living in France, who are the issues of the two cultures. He went to great lengths to motivate them and to implant in them an appreciation for the humanitarian and cultural value of science.

Although a multilingual speaker and writer, and an excellent and widely sought lecturer, in social intercourse he was soft-spoken, courteous, and modest; he had a warm boyish smile that lit up on his serious, slightly sad face as sunshine breaking through the clouds. Behind that boyish smile lay a giant intellect, coupled with an encyclopedic memory. As the conversation turned toward his favorite subjects, the structure-activity relationships of carcinogens and other pharmacologically active agents, or synthetic organic chemistry, I have often seen him suddenly enliven and intellectual sparks of ideas, new plans, and interpretations begin to fly. He literally endowed organic compounds with life. While a quantum chemist may see organic compounds through the formal crystalline beauty of matrices, these structures acquired a lifelike dynamism and fluidity in Buu-Hoi's mind as he "felt" the geometry of the molecules and the interaction forces reaching out from them. He was an intuitive pharmacologist in the best Ehrlichian sense. I always felt that that intuition was somehow connected in him with the sense of wonder of the eternal child and his fantasies.

In many of us, this internal child withers away with the years. He managed somehow to keep his child very much alive, who, peeping out the window to the Unknown, kept on perceiving and discovering new things . . .

While, as a result of his scientific renown and political prestige, influence accrued to him, he decried those who sought science for power's sake. He was, behind the prestige, fundamentally an idealist and to some extent a romantic. He sought understanding truly for satisfying his innate curiosity and his thirst for the peculiar brand of beauty shrouded in the symbols of science.

Lacassagne and especially Buu-Hoi lived in times and in an atmosphere of perpetual scientific and political change. Yet both, from their respective cultural vantage points, were very much aware of the unchanging elements of human nature and of the limitations of human societies, perhaps because they shared that character trait of the great, pride tempered by inner humility. The acquaintance with and friendship of these men, and of a number of their co-workers, gave me the privilege of a ring-side seat in a stirring and colorful contemporary chapter in the History of Science. Lacassagne and Buu-Hoi fought valiantly to conquer territories from the Unknown. But perhaps more importantly, they have set examples for many, to be inspired by and to follow. They have left us a parcel of that spiritual heritage which is ". . . beyond love and hate, beyond profit and loss, beyond honor and dishonor. Thus it is the most valuable treasure in all the world. "

REFERENCES

1. C. Oberling, The Riddle of Cancer, Yale Univ. Press, New Haven, Conn. , 1952.
2. G. Mathé, La Chimiothérapie des Cancers (leucémies, hémato-sarcomes, tumeurs solides), 2nd ed. , L'Expansion Sci. Française, Paris, 1966.
3. R. Truhaut, Les Facteurs Chimiques de Cancérisation, Soc. Ed. Enseignement Supérieur, Paris, 1950.
4. A. Haddow, Professor Antoine Lacassagne — An obituary, Nature, 235, 291 (1972); Cancer Res., 32, 1093 (1972); UICC Bull. Cancer, 10, [1], 5 (1972).
5. R. Latarjet, Antoine Lacassagne 1884-1971, Ann. Inst. Pasteur, 122, 69 (1972).

6. F. Zajdela, In Memoriam — Antoine Lacassagne 1884-1971, Bull. Cancer, 59, 1 (1972).

7. A. Lacassagne, La leucémogénèse par radiations, J. Radiol. Electrol., 43, 803 (1962).

8. A. Lacassagne, Contributions de la radiobiologie aux progrès de la cancérologie, Minerva Radiol. Fisioterap. e Radiobiol., 10, 191 (1965).

9. A. Lacassagne, Les Cancers Produits par des Substances Chimiques Endogènes, Hermann, Paris, 1950.

10. A. Lacassagne, Kennaway and the carcinogens, Nature, 191, 743 (1961).

11. O. Schmidt, Die Beziehungen zwischen Dichterverteilung bestimmter Valenzelektronen (B-Elektronen) und Reaktivität bei aromatischen Kohlenwasserstoffen, Z. Phys. Chem., B39, 59 (1938).

12. O. Schmidt, Die Charakterisierung der einfachen und Krebs erzeugenden aromatischen Kohlenwasserstoffe durch die Dichteverteilung bestimmter Valenzelektronen (B-Elektronen), Z. Phys. Chem., B42, 83 (1939).

13. O. Schmidt and H. Schmidt, Weitere Untersuchungen zum Kastenmodell — Zylinderring, Kompression der B-Elektronen. (Dritte Mitteilung über Dichteverteilung und Energiespektrum der B-Elektronen), Z. Phys. Chem., B44, 185 (1939).

14. O. Schmidt, Beiträge zum Mechanismus der Anregungsvorgänge in der krebskranken und gesunden Zelle. (Vierte Mitteilung über Dichteverteilung und Energiespektrum der B-Elektronen), Z. Phys. Chem., B44, 194 (1939).

15. O. Schmidt, Charakterisierung und Mechanismus der Krebs erzeugenden Kohlenwasserstoffe, Naturwissenschaften, 24, 146 (1941).

16. R. Daudel, Les théories physicochimiques du cancer, Rev. Sci., 84, 37 (1946).

17. P. Daudel and R. Daudel, Application de la mécanique ondulatoire à l'étude du mécanisme de l'action des substances cancérigènes sur les tissus, Biol. Méd., 39, 201 (1950).

18. N. Svartholm, Electronic distribution and chemical reactivity in condensed unsaturated hydrocarbons, Arkiv Kemi, Mineral. Geol., 15A, No. 13 (1941-1942).

19. A. Pullman and B. Pullman, Cancérisation par les Substances Chimiques et Structure Moléculaire, Masson, Paris, 1955.

20. P. Daudel and R. Daudel., Chemical Carcinogenesis and Molecular Biology, Interscience (Wiley), New York, 1966.

21. B. Pullman and A. Pullman, Les Théories Electroniques de la Chimie Organique, Masson, Paris, 1952.

22. A. Pullman and B. Pullman, Quantum Biochemistry, Wiley, New York, 1963.

23. R. Daudel, The Fundamentals of Theoretical Chemistry, Pergamon, New York, 1968.
24. P. Daudel and R. Daudel, Sur l'éventualité de la formation d'un complexe entre les corps cancérigenes et les tissus soumis à leur action, Bull. Soc. Biol., 31, 353 (1949).
25. P. Daudel, R. Daudel, and N.P. Buu-Hoi, Le problème de la prévision du pouvoir carcinogène des substances chimiques, Acta Union Intern. Contra Cancrum, 7, 91 (1950).
26. A. Pullman, Contribution a l'étude de la structure électronique des molécules organiques. Étude particulière des hydrocarbures cancérigènes, Ann. Chim., 2, 5 (1947).
27. N.P. Buu-Hoi, P. Daudel, R. Daudel, A. Lacassagne, J. Lecocq, M. Martin, and G. Rudali, Sur une tentative de prévision du pouvoir cancérigène des substances chimiques, Compt. Rend., 225, 238 (1947).
28. A. Pullman, Structure électronique et activité cancérogène des hydrocarbures aromatiques, Bull. Soc. Chim. France, 21, 595 (1954).
29. A. Pullman and B. Pullman, Electronic structure and carcinogenic activity of aromatic molecules, Advan. Cancer Res., 3, 117 (1955)
30. O. Chalvet and S.S. Sung, Sur la théorie quantique du mécanisme de la cancérisation par les substances chimiques. Le cas des benzacridines et de leurs dérivés méthylés. Compt. Rend., 251, 2092 (1960).
31. O. Chalvet, R. Daudel, and C. Moser, Sur le théorie quantique du mécanisme de la cancérisation par les substances chimiques, Compt. Rend., 246, 3457 (1958).
32. O. Chalvet, R. Daudel, and C. Moser, A note on the interaction of carcinogenic molecules with cellular protein, Cancer Res., 18, 1033 (1958).
33. O. Chalvet, P. Daudel, R. Daudel, C. Moser, and G. Prodi, "Some Applications of Wave Mechanics and the Radioindicator Method to the Study of Carcinogenesis" in Wave Mechanics and Molecular Biology, (L. DeBroglie, ed.), Addison-Wesley, Reading, Mass., 1966, p. 106.
34. A. Pullman, "The Theory of Chemical Carcinogenesis and the Problem of Hydrocarbon-Protein Interaction" in Biopolymers, Suppl. "Quantum Aspects of Polypeptides and Polynucleotides," Symp. No. 1 (M. Weissbluth, ed.), Interscience (Wiley), New York, 1964, p. 47.
35. B. Pullman, "Aspects of the Electronic Structure of the Nucleic Acids in Relation to the Theories of Mutagenesis and Carcinogenesis" in Biopolymers, Suppl. "Quantum Aspects of Polypeptides and Polynucleotides," Symp. No. 1 (M. Weissbluth, ed.), Interscience (Wiley), New York, 1964, p. 141.

36. A. Pullman and B. Pullman, "A Quantum Chemist's Approach to the Mechanism of Chemical Carcinogenesis" in Physico-Chemical Mechanisms of Carcinogenesis (E. D. Bergmann and B. Pullman, eds.), Israel Academy of Science and Humanities, Jerusalem, 1969, p. 9.

37. R. S. Umans and B. Pullman, The mechanism of binding polycyclic aromatic hydrocarbons to nucleic acids: A theoretical investigation, Intern. J. Quantum Chem., 5, 575 (1971).

38. N. P. Buu-Hoi, Recent developments in the chemistry of organic carcinogens, Record Chem. Progr., 13, 23 (1952).

39. N. P. Buu-Hoi, "Causerie sur 'France-Vietnam' faite au Club du Faubourg à Paris, le 17 Mars 1964. "

40. P. Jacquignon, Nécrologie — N. P. Buu-Hoi 1915-1972, Bull. Périodique Ligue Nat. Franc. contre Cancer, 49 (194), 30 (1972).

41. T. A. Lennartz, Synthesen höherer aliphatischer Verbindungen, Angew. Chem., 59, 10, 49, 77 (1947).

42. A. R. Ratsimamanga, N. P. Buu-Hoi, G. Dechamps, H. LeBihan, F. Binon, and M. Nigeon-Dureuil, Activité antituberculeuse in vivo de quelques dérivés de la thiosemicarbazide, Compt. Rend. Soc. Biol., 146, 354 (1952).

43. N. P. Buu-Hoi, The selection of drugs for chemotherapy research in leprosy, Intern. J. Leprosy, 22, 16 (1954).

44. N. P. Buu-Hoi, Ng. Ba-Khuyen, and N. D. Xuong, Six mois de chimiothérapie antilèpreuse au Sud Vietnam avec le 4, 4'-diaminodiphénylsulfoxide et le 4, 4'-diethoxythiocarbanilide, Bull. Acad. Nat. Méd., 139, 275 (1955).

45. N. P. Buu-Hoi, New developments in the chemotherapy of leprosy, Bull. Calcutta School Trop. Med., 3, 133 (1955).

46. M. Welsch, N. P. Buu-Hoi, P. Danthinne, and N. D. Xuong, Structure moléculaire et activité tuberculostatique dans le groupe des dérives de la thiourée, Experientia, 12, 102 (1956).

47. N. P. Buu-Hoi, Ng. Ba-Khuyen, and N. D. Xuong, Chimiothérapie antilèpreuse au Sud-Vietnam avec les thiocarbanilides seuls ou associés au 4, 4', -diaminodiphénylsulfoxide, et avec une thiosemicarbazone, Bull. Acad. Nat. Méd., 141, 204 (1957).

48. N. P. Buu-Hoi, T. V. Bang, T. T. Kim Mong-Don, and N. D. Xuong, Résultats à court terme d'un traitement de la lèpre par le 4, 4'-diisoamyloxythiocarbanilide, Chemotherapia, 2, 122 (1961).

49. N. P. Buu-Hoi, Tran-Van-Bang, and N. D. Xuong, Activité anti-lèpreuse importante de la 4, 4'-dihydroxydiphénylsulfone, Bull. Acad. Nat. Méd., 146, 78 (1962).

50. N. P. Buu-Hoi, Activité antilèpreuse considérable du 2-mercaptobenzimidazole: Observations préliminaires, Chemotherapia, 7, 27 (1963).

51. N. P. Buu-Hoi, Le-Khac-Quyen, and N. D. Xuong, Five years experience in upper South Vietnam with dialide, and comparison with DDSO, Leprosy Rev., 36, 105 (1965).

52. P. Jacquignon, Un grand savant disparaît: N. P. Buu-Hoi, Chim. Thérap. (Europ. J. Medicinal Chem.), 7, 178 (1972).

53. J. Weisburger, Obituary — Professor N. P. Buu-Hoi, Nature, 237, 470 (1972).

54. G. Lambelin, In Memoriam Professor N. P. Buu-Hoi, Arzneimittel-Forsch., 22, 950 (1972).

55. J. C. Arcos, In Memory of Nguyen Phuc Buu-Hoi 1915-1972, Cancer Res., 32, 2856A (1972).

56. E. J. Hammer, The Struggle for Indochina, Stanford Univ. Press, Stanford, Calif., 1954.

57. E. J. Hammer, Vietnam Yesterday and Today, Holt, Rinehart & Winston, New York, 1966.

58. N. P. Buu-Hoi, L'intervention des forces de van der Waals dans les phénomènes de cancérisation chimique, Acta Union Intern. Contra Cancrum, 7, 68 (1950).

59. A. Lacassagne, F. Zajdela, N. P. Buu-Hoi, and O. Chalvet, Contribution a l'étude de pouvoir cancérogène de quelques homologues méthylés du 1, 2-benzanthracène, Bull. Cancer, 49, 312 (1962).

60. N. P. Buu-Hoi, and N. B. Giao, Enhancement of the carcinogenicity of 7, 12-dimethylbenz[a]anthracene through replacement of hydrogen by deuterium: A new biological isotope effect, Naturwissenschaften, 58, 371 (1971).

61. N. P. Buu-Hoi, and S. S. Sung, A non-radiative photochemical model for polycyclic aromatic hydrocarbon-induced carcinogenesis, Naturwissenschaften, 57, 135 (1970).

62. A. Lacassagne, E. Buchta, D. Kiessling, F. Zajdela, and N. P. Buu-Hoi, Particular carcinogenic activity of F-nor-steranthrene, Nature, 200, 183 (1963).

63. A. Lacassagne, F. Zajdela, N. P. Buu-Hoi, E. Buchta, and D. Kiessling, Specificity of carcinogenic action of F-nor-steranthrene hydrocarbons, Naturwissenschaften, 53, 583 (1966).

64. A. Lacassagne, N. P. Buu-Hoi, and F. Zajdela, Carcinogenic activity of apocholic acid, Nature, 190, 1007 (1961).

65. A. Lacassagne, F. Zajdela, N. P. Buu-Hoi, O. Chalvet, and G. H. Daub, Activité cancérogène élevée des mono-, di-, et trimèthylbenzo[a]pyrène, Intern. J. Cancer., 3, 238 (1968).

66. A. Lacassagne, N. P. Buu-Hoi, and F. Zajdela, Relation entre structure moléculaire et activité cancérogène dans trois séries d'hydrocarbures aromatiques hexacycliques, Compt. Rend., 246, 1477 (1958).

67. A. Lacassagne, N. P. Buu-Hoi, F. Zajdela, and D. Lavit-Lamy,

Sur le pouvoir cancérogène des aldéhydes dérivés de l'anth-
anthrène, et des 3, 4:8, 9 et 3,4:9, 10-dibenzopyrènes, Compt.
Rend., 252, 1711 (1961).

68. N. P. Buu-Hoi, New developments in chemical carcinogenesis by
polycyclic hydrocarbons and related heterocycles: A review,
Cancer Res., 24, 1511 (1964).

69. L. Bahna, V. Podaný, and A. Godàl, 6, 12-Diazaanthanthrene
(acridino[2, 1, 9, 8-klmna]acridine) — a new polycyclic
carcinogen, Neoplasma, 18, 591 (1971).

70. A. Lacassagne, F. Zajdela, N.P. Buu-Hoi, and H. Chalvet, Sur
l'activité cancérogène du 3, 4:9, 10-dibenzopyrène et de
quelques-uns de ses dérivés, Compt. Rend., 244, 273 (1957).

71. A. Lacassagne, N.P. Buu-Hoi, F. Zajdela, and D. Lavit-Lamy,
Activité cancérogène élevée du 1, 2:3, 4-dibenzopyrène et
1, 2:4, 5-dibenzopyrène, Compt. Rend., 256, 2728 (1963).

72. A. Lacassagne, N.P. Buu-Hoi, and F.A. Vingiello, The true
dibenzo[a, 1]pyrene, a new, potent carcinogen, Naturwissenschaften, 55, 43 (1968).

73. A. Lacassagne, F. Zajdela, and N.P. Buu-Hoi, Sur la différence
de susceptibilité entre les sexes, dans la production de
sarcomes par les hydrocarbures polycycliques, chez les souris
XVII, Compt. Rend. Soc. Biol., 152, 1312 (1958).

74. A. Lacassagne, N.P. Buu-Hoi, F. Zajdela, and D. Lavit-Lamy,
Activité cancérogène de dérivés substitués du 1, 2:3, 4-
dibenzopyrène, du 1, 2:4, 5-dibenzopyrène, et du 1, 2:4, 5:8, 9-
tribenzopyrène, Compt. Rend., 259, 3899 (1964).

75. A. Lacassagne, N.P. Buu-Hoi, and F. Zajdela, Absence de
propriété sarcomogène chez le dibenzo [a, c]anthracène; nette
activité de son dérivé 10-méthylé, Europ. J. Cancer, 4, 123
(1968).

76. N. P. Buu-Hoi, Biochemical properties of compounds derived from
polycyclic aromatic systems by replacement of benzene rings by
equivalent sulfur heterocycles, Quart. Rept. Sulfur Chem., 5,
9 (1970).

77. A. Lacassagne, N.P. Buu-Hoi, and F. Zajdela, Activité cancérogène d'hydrocarbures polycycliques dérivés du naphthacène,
Compt. Rend., 250, 3547 (1960).

78. A. Lacassagne, N.P. Buu-Hoi, F. Zajdela, and D. Lavit-Lamy,
Sur le pouvoir cancérogène de quelques hydrocarbures condensés
renfermant plus de six cycles benzèniques, Compt. Rend., 252
826 (1961).

79. A. Lacassagne, N.P. Buu-Hoi, F. Zajdela, and G. Saint-Ruf,
Sur le pouvoir cancérogène de deux hydrocarbures aromatiques
à sept cycles, Compt. Rend., 266D, 301 (1968).

80. A. Lacassagne, N.P. Buu-Hoi, and F. Zajdela, Sur l'activité

cancérogène de dérivés méthylés du pérylène et du 1,12-
benzopérylène, Compt. Rend., 245, 991 (1957).

81. N.P. Buu-Hoi, F. Zajdela, K.-E. Schulte, and P. Mabille,
    Absence d'activité cancérogène chez des hydrocarbures
    aromatiques acétyléniques fortement conjugués, Bull. Cancer,
    50, 105 (1963).

82. A. Lacassagne, N.P. Buu-Hoi, F. Zajdela, and P. Jacquignon,
    Faible réduction du pouvoir cancérogène par hydrogénation de la
    molécule d'hydrocarbures; forte réduction dans le cas des
    benzacridines, Compt. Rend., 251, 1322 (1960).

83. D. Lavit-Lamy and N.P. Buu-Hoi, The true nature of "dibenzo-
    [a,1]pyrene" and its known derivatives, Chem. Commun.
    (1966), 92.

84. N.P. Buu-Hoi, O. Périn-Roussel, and P. Jacquignon, An unequiv-
    ocal synthesis of dibenzo[a,1]pyrene, Chem. Commun. (1968),
    718.

85. N.P. Buu-Hoi and D. Lavit-Lamy, Un nouveau type de réarrange-
    ment moléculaire: l'isomérisation du méthyl-10 benzo-1,2
    anthracène en méthyl-6 chrysène, Bull. Soc. Chim. France,
    (1961), 1657.

86. D. Lavit-Lamy and N.P. Buu-Hoi, Isomérisation des hydro-
    carbures aromatiques polycycliques sous l'action du chlorure
    d'aluminium. — IV. Réarrangements moléculaires dans la
    cyclodéshydrogénation du phényl-12 benzo[a]anthracène, Bull.
    Soc. Chim. France (1966), 2613.

87. D. Lavit-Lamy and N.P. Buu-Hoi, Isomérisation des hydro-
    carbures aromatiques polycycliques sous l'action du chlorure
    d'aluminium — V. Réarrangements moléculaire du méthyl-12
    benzo[a]anthracène en méthyl-7 benzo[a]anthracène, Bull. Soc.
    Chim. France (1966), 2619.

88. N.P. Buu-Hoi, O. Périn-Roussel, and P. Jacquignon, Réarrange-
    ments moléculaires du dibenzo[a,j]anthracène sous l'action du
    chlorure d'aluminium, Bull. Soc. Chim. France (1970), 1194.

89. A. Lacassagne, N.P. Buu-Hoi, F. Zajdela, D. Lavit-Lamy, and
    O. Chalvet, Activité cancérogène d'hydrocarbures aromatiques
    polycycliques à noyau fluoranthène, Acta Unio. Intern. Contra
    Cancrum, 19, 490 (1963).

90. N.P. Buu-Hoi, N.B. Giao, and C. Jutz. Carcinogenicity of a
    nonbenzenoid hydrocarbon, azuleno[5,6,7-cd]phenalene, and
    derivatives, Naturwissenschaften, 57, 499 (1970).

91. A. Lacassagne, N.P. Buu-Hoi, R. Daudel, and F. Zajdela, The
    relation between carcinogenic activity and the physical and
    chemical properties of angular benzacridines, Advan. Cancer
    Res., 4, 315 (1956).

92. M. Pagès-Flon, N.P. Buu-Hoi, and R. Daudel, Étude d'une

relation entre pK et pouvoir cancérogène pour deux séries de benzacridines, Compt. Rend., 236, 2182 (1953).

93. N.P. Buu-Hoi, F. Zajdela, O. Roussel, and L. Petit, Activité cancérogène de quatre dérivés de la benzacridine linéaire, Bull. Cancer, 52, 49 (1965).

94. A. Lacassagne, N.P. Buu-Hoi, F. Zajdela, N.B. Giao, P. Jacquignon, and M. Dufour, Nouvelle étude de l'influence exercée par la nature et le nombre des substituants, sur l'activité cancérogène des benzacridines angulaires, Compt. Rend., 267D, 981 (1968).

95. A. Lacassagne, N.P. Buu-Hoi, F. Zajdela, and N.D. Xuong, Relations entre la structure moléculaire et l'activité cancérogène dans la série du carbazole, Bull. Cancer, 42, 3 (1955).

96. A. Lacassagne, N.P. Buu-Hoi, F. Zajdela, F. Périn, and P. Jacquignon, A new family of potent carcinogens: Benzo-pyridocarbazoles, Nature, 191, 1005 (1961).

97. A. Lacassagne, N.P. Buu-Hoi, F. Zajdela, P. Jacquignon, and F. Périn, Relations entre structure moléculaire et activité cancérogène chez les benzopyridocarbazoles et les composés polycycliques analogues, Compt. Rend., 257, 818 (1963).

98. A. Lacassagne, N.P. Buu-Hoi, F. Zajdela, O. Périn-Roussel, P. Jacquignon, F. Périn, and J.-P. Hoeffinger, Activité sarcomogène chez deux nouveaux types d'hétérocycles: les benzocarbolines et les thiénopyridocarbazoles, Compt. Rend., 271D, 1474 (1970).

99. S.S. Waravdekar and K.J. Ranadive, Biological testing of sulfur isosters of carcinogenic hydrocarbons, J. Natl. Cancer Inst., 18, 555 (1957).

100. F. Zajdela, N.P. Buu-Hoi, P. Jacquignon, A. Croisy, and F. Périn, Carcinogenic activity of polycyclic pseudoazulenes containing both nitrogen and sulfur heterocycles, J. Natl. Cancer Inst., 46, 1257 (1971).

101. A. Lacassagne, N.P. Buu-Hoi, F. Zajdela, P. Jacquignon, and M. Mangane, 5-Oxo-5H-benzo[e]isochromeno[4,3-b]indole, a new type of highly sarcomagenic lactone, Science, 158, 387 (1967).

102. A. Lacassagne, N.P. Buu-Hoi, F. Zajdela, C. Stora, M. Mangane, and P. Jacquignon, Sur les propriétés cancérogènes du 5-oxo-5H-benzo[e]isochromeno[4,3-b]indole et de ses dérivés et analogues: Relations entre structure et activité, Compt. Rend., 272D, 3102 (1971).

103. A. Lacassagne, N.P. Buu-Hoi, F. Zajdela, J.-P. Hoeffinger, and P. Jacquignon, Structure and carcinogenicity in some derivatives of 4-nitroquinoline N-oxide, Life Sci., 5, 1945 (1966).

104. R. Garrigues, N. P. Buu-Hoi, and A. Ramé, Production de
     tumeurs végétales par action de la N-méthyl-N-nitrosoaniline,
     composé cancérogène chez l'animal, Compt. Rend., 273, 1123
     (1971).
105. M. Chenon, P. Daudel, A. Lacassagne, J. Willeput, and F.
     Zajdela, Etude de l'élimination de dérivés cancérogènes de
     benzacridines angulaires, marqués par du radiocarbone,
     Compt. Rend., 247, 2070 (1958).
106. P. Daudel, G. Prodi, and B. Chenon, Sur un phénomène d'inhibi-
     tion au cours de la fixation de certains hydrocarbures aromatiques
     sur les protéines cellulaires, Compt. Rend., 248, 3238 (1959).
107. P. Daudel, G. Vallée, and R. Vasquez, Fixation sur les protéines
     cellulaires de dérivés cancérogènes de benzacridines angulaires
     marquées par du radiocarbone, Compt. Rend., 248, 1880 (1959).
108. P. Daudel, B. Chenon, N. P. Buu-Hoi, P. Jacquignon, A.
     Lacassagne, G. Prodi, G. Vallée, R. Vasquez, and F. Zajdela,
     Relation entre le pouvoir cancérogène des molécules conjuguées
     et leur fixation sur les protéines cellulaires, Bull. Soc. Chim.
     Biol., 42, 135 (1960).
109. P. Daudel, F. Lutcher, M. Croisy-Delcey, J. Moreau, P.
     Jacquignon, and N. P. Buu-Hoi, Effet de substances cancéro-
     gènes sur la réplication et la transcription in vitro des acides
     désoxyribonucléiques. Effet d'hydrocarbures aromatiques
     bromométhylés, Compt. Rend., 270D, 2394 (1970).
110. N. P. Buu-Hoi and P. -H. Chanh, Effect of various types of car-
     cinogens on the hatching of Artemia salina eggs, J. Natl.
     Cancer Inst., 44, 795 (1970).
111. N. P. Buu-Hoi and D. P. Hien, Induction of zoxazolamine
     hydroxylase synthesis in rats by means of 6-aminochrysene,
     Naturwissenschaften, 53, 435 (1966).
112. N. P. Buu-Hoi, D. P. Hien, and C. Jutz, Similarity in a biological
     effect of benzo[a]pyrene and of an azulene analogue thereof,
     Naturwissenschaften, 54, 470 (1967).
113. N. P. Buu-Hoi, D. P. Hien, and G. Saint-Ruf, Induction par les
     indophénazines de la synthèse de la zoxazolamine hydroxylase
     chez le rat. Relations entre structure chimique et activité,
     Compt. Rend., 264D, 2414 (1967).
114. N. P. Buu-Hoi, and D. P. Hien, Action des dibenzacridines et de
     leurs analogues sur la synthèse de la zoxazolamine-hydroxylase
     et de la dicoumarol-hydroxylase chez le rat; non-identité de
     ces deux systèmes enzymatiques adaptatifs, Compt. Rend.,
     264D, 153 (1967).
115. N. P. Buu-Hoi, D. P. Hien, A. Ricci, and P. Jacquignon,
     Activité inductrice importante de pseudo-azulènes polycycliques
     sur la synthèse de la zoxazolamine-hydroxylase chez le rat:

Relations entre structure moléculaire et activité, Compt. Rend., 265D, 714 (1967).

116. N. P. Buu-Hoi and D. P. Hien, The effect of benzocarbazoles and benzacridines on the paralysing action of zoxazolamine; Structure/activity relationships, Biochem. Pharmacol., 17, 1227 (1968).

117. N. P. Buu-Hoi and D. P. Hien, Zoxazolamine-hydroxylase inducing effect of polycyclic aromatic hydrocarbons. Relationships between structure and activity, and degree of correlation with carcinogenicity, Biochem. Pharmacol., 18, 741 (1969).

118. N. P. Buu-Hoi and D. P. Hien, Un effet biologique nouveau de certain hydrocarbures polycycliques aromatiques et de leurs analogues hétérocycliques: l'Inhibition de l'hydroxylation de la zoxazolamine chez le rat, Compt. Rend., 268D, 423 (1969).

119. J. C. Arcos, A. H. Conney, and N. P. Buu-Hoi, Induction of microsomal enzyme synthesis by polycyclic aromatic hydrocarbons of different molecular sizes, J. Biol. Chem., 236, 1291 (1961).

120. M. F. Argus, R. T. Valle, N. Venkatesan, N. P. Buu-Hoi, and J. C. Arcos, Molecular size-dependent effects of polynuclear hydrocarbons on mixed-function oxidases: Possible action on cascade-coupled operons, Proc. Europ. Biophys. Congr. (Vienna), 1st, 1 (EI/38), 187 (1971).

121. N. Venkatesan, J. C. Arcos, and M. F. Argus, Induction and repression of microsomal drug-metabolizing enzymes by polycyclic hydrocarbons and phenobarbital: Theoretical models, J. Theoret. Biol., 33, 517 (1971).

122. A. Lacassagne, N. P. Buu-Hoi, and L. Hurst, Étude comparative du foie de rats recevant l'acide cholique ou l'acide litho-cholique seuls, ou associés avec du jaune de beurre, Tumori, 53, 43 (1967).

123. A. Lacassagne, L. Hurst, and N. D. Xuong, Inhibition, par deux naphthylisothiocyanates, de l'hépatocancérogènèse produite, chez le rat, par le p-diméthylamino-azobenzène (DAB), Compt. Rend. Soc. Biol., 164, 230 (1970).

124. A. Lacassagne, N. P. Buu-Hoi, L. Hurst, and N. B. Giao, Inhibition complète, par la p-hydroxyacétophénone, de l'activité cancérogène du jaune de beurre sur le foie du rat, Compt. Rend., 258, 5763 (1964).

125. A. Lacassagne, N. P. Buu-Hoi, R. Ferrando, and N. B. Giao, Influence de trois cétones phénoliques sur l'activité cancérogène du p-diméthylaminoazobenzène sur le foie du rat, Compt. Rend., 260, 287 (1965).

126. A. Lacassagne and L. Hurst, La métopirone n'inhibe pas la cancérisation du foie du rat par le p-diméthylaminoazobenzène, Compt. Rend., 261, 2263 (1965).

127. A. Lacassagne and L. Hurst, Inhibition par l'o-p'-dichloro-
     diphényldichloroéthane de l'action cancérogène du jaune de
     beurre chez le rat, Compt. Rend., 256, 5474 (1963).
128. A. Lacassagne and L. Hurst, Action du N-monométhylbenzhéparide-
     amide et de l'o-p'-dichlorodiphényldichloroéthane, seuls ou
     associés, sur la cancérisation du foie du rat par le p-
     diméthylaminoazobenzène, Compt. Rend., 260, 4285 (1965).
129. A. Lacassagne and L. Hurst, Effets opposés de l'iproniazide et
     de la résérpine sur la cancérisation du foie par le p-diméthyl-
     aminoazobenzène, Compt. Rend., 263, 701 (1966).
130. A. Lacassagne, L. Hurst, and A. J. Rosenberg, Influence de la
     chlorpromazine et de la résérpine sur la cancérisation du foie
     chez le rat, Compt. Rend., 249, 903 (1959).
131. L. Hurst, A. Lacassagne, and A. J. Rosenberg, Action de la
     résérpine sur la cancérisation du foie chez le rat, Compt.
     Rend. Soc. Biol., 152, 441 (1958).
132. A. Lacassagne, N. P. Buu-Hoi, and N. B. Giao, Contrairement à
     la résérpine, la yohimbine ne modifie pas la cancérisation
     chimique du foie chez le rat, Compt. Rend., 270D, 746 (1970).
133. A. Lacassagne and L. Hurst, Action retardatrice du chloramphénicol
     sur le processus de cancérisation du foie du rat par le p-
     diméthylaminoazobenzène (DAB), Bull. Cancer, 54, 405 (1967).
134. A. Lacassagne and L. Hurst, Influence de la désoxycorticostérone
     et de l'hydrocortisone sur la cancérisation du foie du rat par
     le p-diméthylaminoazobenzène (DAB), Compt. Rend., 257,
     1576 (1963).
135. A. Lacassagne and L. Hurst, Influence de l'administration
     simultanée de résérpine et d'un corticoide, sur la cancérisa-
     tion du foie du rat par le p-diméthylaminoazobenzène (DAB),
     Compt. Rend., 257, 1658 (1963).
136. A. Lacassagne, M. F. Jayle, L. Hurst, and J. R. Pasqualini,
     Influence de différents corticostéroides sur la cancérisation
     du foie du rat par le p-diméthylaminoazobenzène (DAB), Compt.
     Rend., 262D, 2117 (1966).
137. A. Lacassagne, M. F. Jayle, and L. Hurst, Influence exercée
     par différents oestrogènes sur la cancérisation du foie du rat
     par le para-diméthyl-amino-azobenzène (DAB), Compt. Rend.,
     267D, 137 (1968).
138. A. Lacassagne, M. F. Jayle, and L. Hurst, Action des stéroides
     en C21 sur la cancérisation du foie du rat par le para-
     diméthyl-aminoazo-benzène (DAB), Compt. Rend., 268D, 740
     (1969).
139. A. Lacassagne, M. F. Jayle, and L. Hurst, Actions inhibitrice
     de la prégnénolone sur la cancérisation du foie, et favorable
     au développement de tumeurs de la glande interstitielle du

testicule, chez des rats intoxiqués par le para-diméthyl-
aminoazobenzene (DAB), Compt. Rend., 272D, 174 (1971).

140. A. Lacassagne, "Examples of the Action of Steroid Hormones on
the Development of Certain Experimental Tumors, " Proc.
Intern. Congr. Hormonal Steroids, 1st, Vol. 2, Academic Press,
New York, 1965, p. 379.

141. A. Lacassagne and L. Hurst, Quelques éléments de comparaison
de l'action hépatocancérogène du 2-acétylaminofluorène chez
le rat, avec celle du p-diméthylaminoazobenzène et de la
diéthylnitrosamine, Bull. Cancer, 54, 171 (1967).

142. A. Lacassagne and L. Hurst, Influence de sulfamides hypo- ou
hyperglycémiants sur la cancérisation du foie du rat par le
2-acétylaminofluorène, Bull. Cancer, 56, 397 (1969).

143. A. Lacassagne, N. P. Buu-Hoi, N. B. Giao, and R. Ferrando,
Absence d'effets inhibiteurs des cétones phénoliques du type
de la p-hydroxypropiophénone, ainsi que de l'o-p'-
dichlorodiphényldichloroéthane, sur la cancérisation du foie
du rat par la diéthylnitrosamine, Compt. Rend., 262, 1498
(1966).

144. A. Lacassagne, N. P. Buu-Hoi, N. B. Giao, L. Hurst, and R.
Ferrando, Comparaison des actions hépatocancérogènes de la
diéthylnitrosamine et du p-diméthylaminoazobenzène, Intern.
J. Cancer, 2, 425 (1967).

145. A. Lacassagne, N. P. Buu-Hoi, N. B. Giao, and R. Ferrando,
Action retardatrice de la résérpine sur la cancérisation du
foie du rat par la diéthylnitrosamine, Bull. Cancer, 55, 87
(1968).

146. A. Lacassagne, N. P. Buu-Hoi, and P. Cagniant, Association
d'hydrocarbures polycycliques et mécanisme de la cancérisation, Compt. Rend. Soc. Biol., 138, 16 (1944).

147. A. Lacassagne, N. P. Buu-Hoi, and G. Rudali, Inhibition of the
carcinogenic action produced by a weakly carcinogenic hydrocarbon on a highly active carcinogenic hydrocarbon, Brit. J.
Exp. Pathol., 26, 5 (1945).

148. A. Lacassagne, N. P. Buu-Hoi, R. Daudel, and G. Rudali,
Réduction de l'activité d'un hydrocarbure cancérigène par un
autre hydrocarbure associé, Compt. Rend. Soc. Biol., 138,
282 (1944).

149. G. Rudali, N. P. Buu-Hoi, A. Lacassagne, and J. Lecocq,
Variations du pouvoir cancérigène du 9:10-diméthylbenzanthra-
cène en fonction de quelques facteurs physiques et chimiques,
Compt. Rend. Soc. Biol., 140, 234 (1946).

150. G. Rudali, N. P. Buu-Hoi, and A. Lacassagne, Sur quelques
effets biologiques du 2-amino-chrysène, Compt. Rend., 236,
2020 (1953).

151. A. Lacassagne and L. Hurst, Influence réciproque du 7, 12-
       diméthylbenz(a)anthracène (DMBA) et du para-diméthylamino-
       azobenzène (DAB) administrés simultanément à des rats, Bull.
       Cancer, 56, 169 (1969).
152. L. Corre-Hurst, N. P. Buu-Hoi, R. Royer, and B. Bizzini,
       Compétitions et synergies dans la production de cancers du
       foie chez le rat par des azoïques de constitution chimique
       voisine de celle du jaune de beurre, Bull. Cancer, 40, 397
       (1953).
153. A. Lacassagne and L. Hurst, Effets, sur le foie et le testicule,
       de l'éthionine associée au jaune de beurre, Bull. Cancer, 57,
       365 (1970).
154. A. Lacassagne and L. Hurst, Effets de la griséofulvine sur la
       cancérisation du foie par le p-diméthylaminoazobenzène,
       Compt. Rend., 263, 93 (1966).

PART II

CHEMICAL AND ENZYMATIC ASPECTS
OF CHEMICAL CARCINOGEN
ACTIVATION AND METABOLISM

Chapter 1

SOME CURRENT THRESHOLDS OF RESEARCH IN
CHEMICAL CARCINOGENESIS

James A. Miller
and
Elizabeth C. Miller

McArdle Laboratory for Cancer Research
University of Wisconsin Medical Center
Madison, Wisconsin

Chemical carcinogenesis was first noted in man two centuries ago
in the observations of Hill on snuff users and of Pott on London chimney sweeps (1, 2). The experimental confirmation of the latter observation and the first induction of cancer by pure chemicals occurred in
the first third of this century. The past forty years have encompassed
the discoveries of a wide variety and large number of chemicals,
viruses, and radiations that can induce cancer in mammalian species.
Now, as we enter the last third of this century, it would be fitting if
chemical carcinogenesis could emerge as a unified body of knowledge
and as a principal contributor to the control of cancer in man.

Every field of scientific inquiry undergoes transitions in which
collections of facts and hypotheses rapidly begin to be sorted out and
basic concepts and principles emerge. This happened a long time ago
in organic chemistry and in descriptive biology, and everyone here
has seen it occur in biochemistry and molecular biology. These are
the principal fields that underlie chemical and, indeed, all forms of
carcinogenesis. It appears that the time is ripe for the facts and
hypotheses in carcinogenesis to crystallize into concepts and principles that will provide an understanding of the malignant transformations of cells at the molecular level and that hopefully will lead to
means of controlling these processes. The thresholds of research in
chemical carcinogenesis discussed below are among those that seem
due for great increases in understanding in the near future.

61

CHEMICAL CARCINOGENESIS IN MAN

Epidemiologic studies led to the discovery of the chemical carcinogens for the human, which are shown in Table 1. The carcinogenicities of these agents were detected in studies of small population
groups which had received high exposures for many years. All these
agents are also carcinogenic in experimental animals. A probable
addition to this list is diethylstilbestrol. Recent studies (3) strongly
suggest that the use of this drug 15 to 20 years ago in cases of
threatened abortion has resulted in the development of vaginal carcinomas in some of the female offspring. This appears to be the
first instance of transplacental chemical carcinogenesis in man; many
such instances are known in experimental animals. In this chemical
age it appears likely that carcinogenesis in man following gross industrial or medical exposures to certain chemicals will continue to be
found. However, while such cases and the data in Table 1 are important in showing that man is susceptible to the carcinogenic activity
of a variety of chemicals and chemical classes, there are more
general environmental aspects of chemical carcinogenesis in man that
promise to be far more important.

Let us consider several features of the occurrence of cancer in
man. Despite the great preponderance of mesenchymal tissue over
epithelial tissue in the human body, 90% of the so-called "spontaneous" cancer in adult man is derived from epithelial tissues, and only
10% occurs in the mesenchymal tissues. Furthermore, one-half or
more of this excess of epithelial cancer occurs in the epithelium that

TABLE 1
Chemicals Recognized as Carcinogens in
the Human (and experimental animals)

Soots, tars, oils	Skin, lungs
Cigarette smoke	Lungs, other sites
Betel nut	Buccal mucosa
2-Naphthylamine, benzidine	Urinary bladder
4-Aminobiphenyl, 4-nitrobiphenyl	Urinary bladder
N, N-Bis(2-chloroethyl)-2-naphthylamine	Urinary bladder
Bis(2-chloroethyl)sulfide	Lungs
Nickel compounds	Lungs, nasal sinuses
Chromium compounds	Lungs
Asbestos	Lungs, pleura

is in contact with man's environment, viz., the skin epithelium, the epithelial lining of the gastrointestinal tract, and the bronchial epithelium in the lungs. Exposure to ultraviolet light is the principal etiologic agent for practically all cases of skin cancer, but environmental chemicals, both natural and manmade, appear to be important causative agents at other sites. The roles of cigarette smoke inhalation and, to a lesser extent, of general air pollution in the induction of cancer of the lung appear to be established. The role of chemical factors in the etiology of most human cancers is still obscure, but the findings of the cancer epidemiologists in the past two decades point to the importance of chemicals in the etiology of certain tumors of the gastrointestinal tract and of tumors at some other sites (4, 5). Consider first the encouraging statistics on the continual fall in the incidence of primary stomach cancer in the United States since 1930, so that the incidence now is about one-third of that in 1930 and the trend is still downward. These data indicate that for this tissue site favorable changes in environmental factors — possibly dietary — occurred in the 1920's or earlier. On the other hand, the incidence of primary colon cancer in the United States is among the highest in the world. In Japan the opposite situation exists, viz., the incidence of stomach cancer is the highest in the world and the incidence of colon cancer is low. That environmental factors are operative in the etiology of these cancers is shown by the experience of Japanese migrants to the United States (6). Such migrants, especially in the second generation, exhibit large reductions in the incidence of stomach cancer, but they also show large increases in the incidence of colon cancer. These and other findings with migrant populations and the large differences in the incidence of other important human cancers from country to country (7) and within countries (5, 8) have led to the conclusion that a high percentage, perhaps as much as 90%, of human cancer has a strong environmental element in its etiology (4). Genetic factors have been largely discounted in these considerations because of the short time in which the changes in incidence have occurred. Likewise, variations in carcinogenic radiations, other than ultraviolet light (9, 10), are not considered to be large enough to explain the differences seen. So chemical carcinogens and, possibly, viruses appear to be the culprits. Consequently, chemicals in the environment — in food, water, air, drugs, etc. — have come under great suspicion as contributors to the processes that result in the formation of cancers during the long lifespan of modern man. These chemicals probably include not only manmade but also naturally occurring compounds. Research in the past two decades has uncovered an increasing list of carcinogens that occur naturally in fungi and green plants (11, 12). These considerations on the occurrence of cancer in man serve to emphasize the importance of this topic. Model systems, especially

with epithelial cells in vitro, are required for further elucidation of
the molecular reactions involved in the induction and maintenance of
the malignant state. Systems are needed in which the malignant
transformation of human cells can be observed and studied. From
these studies and from studies on the metabolism of chemical carcinogens, sensitive systems for the detection and monitoring of chemical
carcinogens in all parts of man's environment should emerge. Con-
current efforts must be made to reduce the exposure of man to environmental carcinogens and to reduce in vivo the carcinogenic impact of
those chemicals that cannot be avoided (5).

THE ELECTROPHILIC NATURE OF THE ULTIMATE REACTIVE AND CARCINOGENIC FORMS OF CHEMICAL CARCINOGENS

The chemical carcinogens now comprise a large and structurally
diverse group of synthetic and naturally occurring organic and inorganic compounds with various species and tissue selectivities (13,
14). The majority of these agents are low molecular weight (< 500)
organic molecules. The more important organic carcinogens include
the polycyclic aromatic hydrocarbons, aromatic amines and aminoazo
dyes, 4-nitroquinoline-1-oxide, dialkyl nitrosamines, alkyl nitrosamides, polychlorinated aliphatic and alicyclic hydrocarbons, aflatoxins,
pyrrolizidine alkaloids, ethionine, urethane, cycasin, and a wide
array of alkylating agents. The known inorganic chemical carcinogens
consist of a small group of compounds of certain metals (beryllium,
cadmium, chromium, cobalt, lead, and nickel) and certain complex
silicates (asbestos). Many classes of organic compounds and many
metals and their compounds remain to be tested for their carcinogenic
potentials.

The wide structural variety of chemical carcinogens has raised the
suspicion that any chemical given chronically at high dosage levels
would induce cancer in some animals. This concept is not supported
by the negative results obtained in long-term tests with many compounds (15-17). Specific examples are presented in a recent study
of 120 pesticides of varied structure in two sensitive strains of mice
(18). Only 10% of these compounds, which were selected for their
toxicity as pesticides, showed carcinogenic activity in lifetime tests
at high levels of administration.

In the induction of tumors it appears axiomatic that chemical carcinogens must react, directly or indirectly, with critical molecules in
cells. Early in the study of the carcinogenic aminoazo dyes and the
polycyclic aromatic hydrocarbons, in vivo covalent binding of these
carcinogens to macromolecules was noted in tissues susceptible to
their carcinogenic action. Since then, many covalent bindings of chemical

carcinogens, or of significant parts of their structures, with nucleic acids and proteins of tumor-susceptible tissues in vivo and in vitro have been observed (12), and in several cases good correlation exists between the amount of macromolecular binding and carcinogenicity. There are also exceptions to these correlations in that some weak or apparently noncarcinogenic compounds show extensive binding. However, no exceptions are known in which a well-studied carcinogen has failed to bind in vivo to macromolecules of the target tissue. In this respect it is of interest that Svoboda et al. (19) showed that actinomycin D, which is well known to bind very tightly but non-covalently to DNA in vitro, produced mesotheliomas upon i.p. injection into rats. While it is possible that a covalent binding takes place in vivo (for instance, through the aromatic amine chromophore), the possible importance of the noncovalent binding is suggested by the observation that actinocylgramicidin S, which has the same chromophore but a different peptide cycle than actinomycin D, binds only weakly to DNA and was not carcinogenic in the same tests. While much more work needs to be done, this interesting case points to the possibility that tight noncovalent bindings of carcinogens may be as important as covalent reactions in the induction of neoplasia.

The nature of the interactions in vivo of chemical carcinogens with tissue components such as proteins and nucleic acids has become much clearer in the past decade. While no common structural feature is evident among chemical carcinogens, it is now clear that the ultimate reactive forms of most, if not all, of these structures are electrophilic (electron-deficient) reactants (14, 20). The carcinogenic alkylating agents are electrophiles per se (Fig. 1), but the majority of chemical carcinogens are not reactive as such and must be metabolized to electrophilic forms. Thus the majority of chemical carcinogens are potential alkylating, arylating, arylaminating, or arylamidating agents. In addition, a few acylating agents, which are also electrophilic reactants, have been found to be carcinogenic (21, 22). The ultimate reactive electrophilic forms of the chemical carcinogens combine with nucleophilic (electron-rich) groups in proteins and nucleic acids and thus give rise to covalently bound derivatives (Fig. 2). These reactive, strongly electrophilic forms of chemical carcinogens are presumably also the ultimate carcinogenic forms of these agents. This has been demonstrated for one aromatic amide (2-acetylaminofluorene) and for the alkylating agents. Thus, some of the latter compounds are of such simple structure, i.e., dimethyl sulfate, that they appear incapable of yielding any reactive forms except alkylating species.

No reactive nucleophilic form of a carcinogen has been noted so far. These findings appear to be a consequence of the fact that cellular components such as nucleic acids, proteins, and other

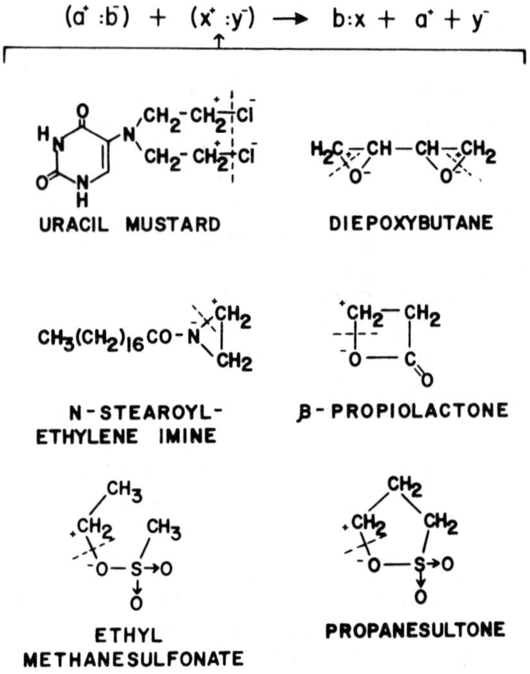

$$(\overset{+}{a}:\overset{-}{b}) + (\overset{+}{x}:\overset{-}{y}) \longrightarrow b{:}x + \overset{+}{a} + y^-$$

URACIL MUSTARD

DIEPOXYBUTANE

N-STEAROYL-
ETHYLENE IMINE

β-PROPIOLACTONE

ETHYL
METHANESULFONATE

PROPANESULTONE

FIG. 1. Some carcinogenic alkylating agents. Most of these agents react with tissue nucleophiles (ab) by the S_N2 reaction shown at the top.

structures contain many more strongly nucleophilic centers than electrophilic centers. While multitudinous covalent bond-breaking and covalent bond-making events occur in cell metabolism, the electrophiles and nucleophiles formed and joined in these operations are under tight and highly ordered control at enzyme surfaces. These metabolic species do not wander about the cell. In contrast, the strongly reactive electrophilic forms of chemical carcinogens are capable of attacking nucleophiles in the cell with less discrimination and without the aid of enzymes. Some of these attacks evidently initiate the malignant transformation. Other attacks and a variety of enzymatic reactions lead to the destruction or inactivation of a portion of the doses of chemical carcinogens.

These aspects of chemical carcinogenesis are illustrated by the metabolic activation and deactivation of the versatile carcinogen 2-acetylaminofluorene (AAF) (Fig. 3). This compound is first N-hydroxylated to a proximate carcinogen (14). In rat liver this proximate carcinogen is esterified to the very reactive and highly mutagenic sulfuric acid ester (14, 23, 24), and close correlations

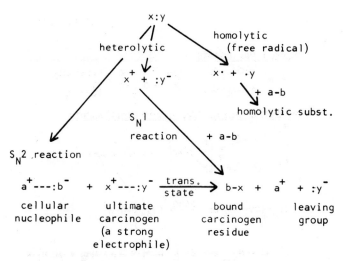

FIG. 2. Bond-breaking mechanisms in chemical carcinogens (xy) that yield electrophiles that could form covalently bound carcinogen residues through substitution reactions. The S_N2 reaction probably predominates in vivo.

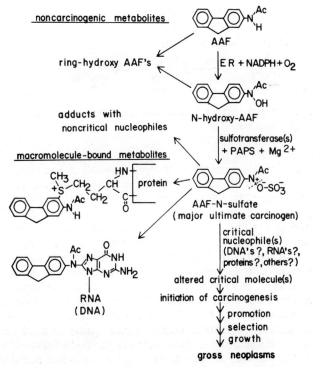

FIG. 3. Major routes of the activation and deactivation of 2-acetylaminofluorene in the male rat liver.

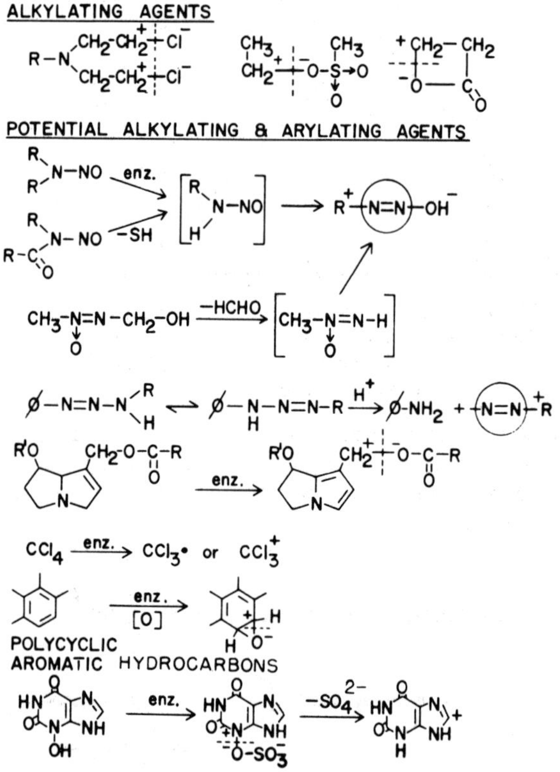

FIG. 4. Probable ultimate reactive and carcinogenic metabolites of certain carcinogens.

between the activity of this enzymatic esterification system and the carcinogenicity and reactivity of N-hydroxy-AAF in rat liver indicate that the sulfuric acid ester is its major ultimate reactive and carcinogenic form in liver (23). This conclusion is greatly strengthened by the findings that both the amounts of hepatic macromolecule-bound fluorene derivatives and the hepatic tumor incidence due to N-hydroxy-AAF are decreased by administration of acetanilide or p-hydroxy-acetanilide (apparently by competition for available sulfate) and that these inhibitions can be prevented by the simultaneous administration of sulfate (25, 26). However, further studies in our laboratory and in other laboratories have shown that a variety of other metabolic activation pathways are open to N-hydroxy-AAF in rodent tissues. The carcinogenic activity of this compound, especially in nonhepatic tissues where the sulfotransferase activity for N-hydroxy-AAF has not been demonstrated, may be due to some of these other possible active forms, e. g. , other esters of N-hydroxy-AAF, esters of N-hydroxy-2-aminofluorene (27), free nitroxide radicals (28), and the glucuronides of N-hydroxy-AAF and of N-hydroxy-2-aminofluorene (29-31). Similar activation mechanisms are presumably involved in the reactivity and carcinogenicity of other aromatic amines and amides, aromatic nitro compounds (which can be reduced to the hydroxylamines), and 3-hydroxyxanthine (32, 33) (Fig. 4).

Figure 4 presents examples of the metabolic activation of some other carcinogens to probable ultimate reactive and carcinogenic forms. The simplest cases of activation of chemical carcinogens include the potential alkylating agents such as the alkylnitrosamides, which require only reaction with a nucleophilic compound (e. g. , —SH, —NH$_2$, water) to yield an unstable monoalkylnitrosamine that then rearranges spontaneously to an alkyldiazonium hydroxide (34). Similarly, the dialkylnitrosamines (35) and aryldialkyltriazenes (36) require only enzymatic dealkylation by the mixed function oxygenases to yield unstable intermediates which decompose to the alkyldiazonium hydroxides. The hepatocarcinogenic pyrrolizidine alkaloids appear to be activated through oxidative dehydrogenation to pyrrole derivatives which are very reactive allylic esters (37-39).

Recent studies have shown the metabolic formation of epoxides of the carcinogenic polycyclic hydrocarbons (40, 41). While the epoxides are intermediates in the deactivation of the carcinogen via reaction with water, glutathione, or other noncritical nucleophiles, they also react readily with proteins and nucleic acids and appear, at least in cell culture systems, to be responsible for a major fraction of the macromolecule-bound derivatives of the hydrocarbons (42, 43). The epoxides which have been tested have shown very limited carcinogenic activity in intact animals (44-46), very possibly because they are dissipated by extracellular reactions. The K-region epoxides which have been studied in cell cultures are, in most cases, much more active in the induction of malignant transformation and are also stronger mutagens for certain mammalian cells than the parent hydrocarbons or the corresponding phenols or dihydrodiols (47-52). Thus, it appears very likely that epoxides of the hydrocarbons are important ultimate carcinogenic metabolites of the polycyclic hydrocarbons. The multiplicity of phenolic and dihydrodiol derivates which are excreted in the urine of animals administered certain of the polycyclic hydrocarbons and which are formed in in vitro incubations indicate that each hydrocarbon may be epoxidized at a number of sites. With one exception (benz(a)anthracene-8, 9-epoxide), all of the epoxides which have been studied for transforming ability and mutagenicity have been K-region epoxides; this non-K-region epoxide did not transform hamster or mouse cells under conditions where the isomeric K-region epoxide was active (48, 49).

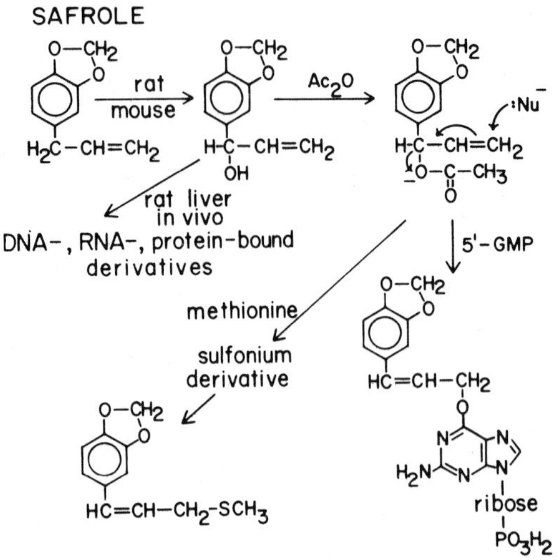

FIG. 5. Metabolic activation of the naturally occurring carcinogen safrole to 1'-hydroxysafrole and the reactivity of 1'-acetoxysafrole with methionine and 5'-guanylic acid.

In each of the cases for which information is available, the ulti-mate carcinogenic forms of the chemical carcinogens appear to be electrophilic reactants, and we have generalized the situation to suggest that the ultimate carcinogenic forms of most, if not all, chemical carcinogens are probably electrophilic reactants (14, 20). We have used this generalization to aid in the prediction of the natures of the metabolic activations for carcinogenesis of a number of classes of chemicals.

Thus, in considering the structure of safrole, a component of a number of essential oils from plant materials and a hepatocarcinogen for rats and mice, we were impressed by the possibility that safrole might be converted into a proximate carcinogen by 1'-hydroxylation and that this allylic and benzylic alcohol would become strongly electrophilic upon esterification. Recent studies by Borchert and Wislocki in our laboratory (53, 54) have shown that 1'-hydroxysafrole (Fig. 5) is indeed a metabolite of safrole in rats and mice and is excreted in the urine as a conjugate which can be cleaved by β-glucuronidase. Furthermore, 1'-hydroxysafrole is a stronger hepato-carcinogen for both rats and mice than is safrole. 1'-Hydroxysafrole also induces some papillomas of the forestomach when fed to mice; these tumors were rare in control animals or in safrole-treated rats or mice. Esterification of 1'-hydroxysafrole with acetic anhydride converts 1'-hydroxysafrole into an electrophilic reactant that yields adducts with nucleic acids, various nucleosides, and methionine (Fig. 5). This synthetic ester is also more active than 1'-hydroxy-safrole in the induction of tumors of the forestomach on feeding and in the induction of sarcomas at the site of repeated injections in rats.

The generalization that metabolism to electrophilic metabolites may be a prime factor in the carcinogenicity of chemicals thus facilitated the elucidation of the nature of at least one proximate carcinogenic form of safrole and should have similar utility in the examination of the proximate and ultimate carcinogenic forms of other carcinogenic chemicals of interest to man.

NATURE OF THE CRITICAL TARGETS OF ULTIMATE CARCINOGENS

Since the growth of tumors into clones of large numbers of similar cells appears to require at least a quasipermanent alteration in phenotype of the tumor as compared with the cell of origin, most investigators are biased toward the idea that the critical target(s) of chemical carcinogens must be one or more of the informational macromolecules. The further bias that chemical carcinogenesis is a mutagenic event has led some investigators to the more restrictive hypothesis that carcinogenesis must result from alterations in DNA. While each of these points of view has merit, the true nature of the critical target is not known in any instance of chemical carcinogenesis; we cannot even cite strong evidence that it must always be a macromolecule.

The electrophilic structure of most ultimate carcinogens places emphasis on nucleophilic centers in cellular constituents as targets of the chemical carcinogens. Such nucleophilic centers are available in both the nucleic acids and proteins (Fig. 6), and, as noted above, both nucleic acid- and protein-bound derivatives of chemical carcinogens are formed in target tissues on administration of chemical carcinogens. As one approach to determining the class of molecules to which the critical target(s) belong, attempts have been made to correlate the levels of specific protein-, DNA-, and RNA-bound carcinogen derivatives with the likelihood of tumor development with that carcinogen. The first of these studies was that of Miller and Miller (55) who correlated the total amounts of hepatic protein-bound aminoazo dyes with susceptibility to aminoazo dye hepatocarcinogenesis in the rat. This approach was extended by Sorof and his colleagues (56, 57) who showed that the major share of the soluble protein-bound dye was associated with specific slightly basic ("h") proteins. Litwak et al. (58) have more recently reported that one of these "h" proteins is also a steroid-, 3-methylcholanthrene-, and bilirubin-binding protein. Sugimoto and Terayama (59) introduced new complexity into these studies by their report that the properties

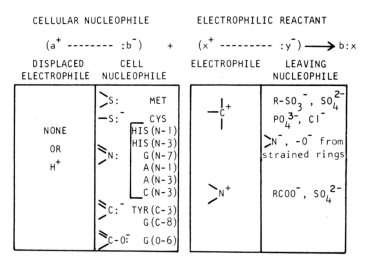

FIG. 6. Cellular nucleophiles known to be attacked in vivo by electrophilic metabolites of chemical carcinogens.

of the dye-binding proteins (or the proteins to which the dyes are bound) change on continued administration of hepatocarcinogenic aminoazo dyes.

Brookes and Lawley (60) correlated the levels of binding of certain polycyclic hydrocarbons to mouse skin DNA with the carcinogenic potencies of the hydrocarbons, while Heidelberger and his associates (43, 61, 62) have noted discrepancies between the extent of hydrocarbon binding in vivo or in vitro to DNA and carcinogenicity. Heidelberger et al. (61, 63) have also emphasized correlation between the extent of the binding of polycyclic hydrocarbons to the "h" proteins of mouse skin and their carcinogenicities. On administration of β-propiolactone to mouse skin, the extent of binding to DNA, but not to protein or RNA, has been correlated with the ability of this alkylating agent to initiate skin papillomas in studies by Boutwell and his associates (64).

The rather extensive studies on the fluorenyl-bound derivatives in the liver after administration of AAF or N-hydroxy-AAF have shown that the macromolecule-bound derivatives tend to be present at higher levels in livers susceptible to carcinogenesis than in those which are less susceptible (65, 66). However, later studies, especially those of Kriek (67), have emphasized the importance of considering the structures of the bound residues. Thus, in Kriek's studies with N-hydroxy-2-AAF the binding of 2-acetylaminofluorene residues to hepatic RNA (ribosomal) correlated much better with susceptibility to hepatic carcinogenesis than did the binding of 2-acetylaminofluorene residues to DNA or the binding of 2-aminofluorene residues to DNA or RNA. These conclusions were supported by analogous finding with N-hydroxy-4-acetylaminobiphenyl (68).

Studies on the levels of alkylated bases in DNA and RNA from the tissues of animals treated with various methylating or ethylating agents have not led to any firm conclusions on the importance of these substitutions to the carcinogenic events (69, 70). Comparisons of different tissues, species, or methylating or ethylating agents with susceptibility to carcinogenesis have not always correlated well with the level of total alkylation of DNA or RNA by the carcinogen. However, it is well known, especially from the studies of Lawley (71), that although N-7-alkylation of guanine is the major reaction, alkylating agents attack a number of sites on the purine and pyrimidine bases of nucleic acids. Recent studies by Loveless (72) and Lawley and Thatcher (73) indicate that the relative amounts of alkylation at various sites differ with the alkylating agent; thus, analyses for the total amounts of alkylation or analyses only for N-7 alkylation of guanine are too crude. In fact, the latter authors have evidence which suggests that the level of O-6 alkylation of guanine is better correlated with the mutagenic activity of alkylating agents than is the amount of N-7 alkylation of guanine.

It is well known that the amounts of bound RNA- and DNA-carcinogen derivatives also differ as a function of a number of variables, including the dose of the carcinogen, the route, and the time at which the analyses are made. In general, loss of bound carcinogen residues begins soon after administration of the compound and is more rapid for residues bound to RNA or protein than for those bound to DNA. The fractions of these losses, which are due to normal turnover of proteins or RNA's, repair of DNA, or cell death, have not been determined but are obviously of importance in interpretation of the data. In particular, considerable attention has been directed to the "persistent binding" of carcinogen residues to DNA (e.g., Refs. 74 and 75). However, at least equally important may be those instances in which the carcinogen residue is lost from the DNA or RNA because of the chemical instability of the adduct, with the result that the nucleic acid is altered but contains no easily recognized marker.

METHODS OF REDUCING EXPOSURES OF CRITICAL TARGETS TO ULTIMATE CHEMICAL CARCINOGENS

While it is evident that our knowledge of chemical carcinogenesis is still very incomplete, it is important that consideration be given to whatever approaches may lead to the prevention or delay of chemical carcinogenesis in man. Surely the most obvious approach is to prevent or reduce the exposures of man to chemical carcinogens. This

is scarcely a new approach; it was successfully applied to the protection of chimney sweeps on the European continent just a few years
after Pott published his observation on the apparent relationship
between scrotal skin cancer and prolonged contact with coal soot (14).
However, no matter how obvious the relationship is, prevention by
avoidance of contact may not always be an easy precept to follow.
The cigarette-lung cancer problem is a case in point (5). Nevertheless, the recognition of the relationships between cancer in man and
specific exposures to chemicals (Table 1) can result in a major
reduction in the incidence of industrially induced cancers, either by
elimination of these agents from the workers' environment or by reductions of exposure. Similar preventive approaches must eventually be
used in attempts to reduce the occurrence in man of all cancers that
have important environmental elements in their etiologies. As discussed above, such action requires, as a minimum, some knowledge
of the environmental sources of the chemicals and the routes of
exposure which are important in the induction of cancer in man.
Success will require the close coordination of epidemiological studies
with research on model systems for the detection of environmental
carcinogenic agents and for studies of the interactions between various agents (chemicals, viruses, and radiations).

Knowledge of the metabolism of chemical carcinogens also offers
several possibilities for the control of these agents after their
entrance into susceptible organisms. Most of the known chemical
carcinogens, with the exception of the alkylating agents, must be
metabolically activated, and all chemical carcinogens appear to
undergo metabolic deactivation in vivo. To the extent that one could
increase the extent of deactivation, decrease the amount of activation, or increase the removal of ultimate carcinogens by noncritical
pathways, the carcinogenic response to a given chemical carcinogen
should be reduced. Some experimental models exist for each of
these three processes (reviewed in Refs. 76 and 77). However, at
the present it is not evident how these approaches could be used in a
practical way for reduction of chemical carcinogenesis in the human.

POSSIBLE GENETIC OR EPIGENETIC NATURE OF EARLY STEPS IN
CARCINOGENESIS BY VARIOUS CHEMICALS

The lack of definitive data on the nature of the critical target(s) in
any instance of chemical carcinogenesis and the difficulty of obtaining
this information have led to much speculation on the essential natures
of the carcinogenic processes and of the neoplastic tissues. These
speculations have usually been based explicitly or implicitly on the
assumption, which seems very reasonable, that the controlled growth

of normal tissues and the heritable reduction in growth control in neo-plastic tissues are functions of the composition and/or amount of specific informational molecules (i. e. , nucleic acids, proteins, or both). The ability of ultimate chemical carcinogens to attack these informational molecules in vivo suggests that some of these reactions may constitute the first steps in processes of chemical carcinogenesis. Both genetic and epigenetic mechanisms of carcinogenesis are possible (Table 2).

Table 2 lists genetic mechanisms that can give rise to heritable changes in the DNA genome (DNA's in the nucleus, mitochondria, or elsewhere in the cell). The first mechanism listed is the direct and heritable modification of the DNA genome by reaction with an ultimate chemical carcinogen. Reactions with specific proteins or RNA's could also, at least theoretically, lead to heritable changes in the DNA genome. The existence of RNA-directed DNA polymerase activity in the RNA tumor viruses and in certain apparently uninfected cells provides a means by which the misinformation in a chemically altered RNA could be transcribed to yield an abnormal DNA [78]. Likewise, chemical alteration of a protein, especially DNA polymerase, could decrease the fidelity of copying of DNA and introduce critical and heritable changes in the DNA. The precedent for this model is the high mutation frequency of certain strains of bacteriophage T4 as a consequence of the poor fidelity with which the DNA polymerase of these strains copies the phage DNA [79].

These genetic changes could thus lead to mutations in genes involved in growth control and yield daughter cells with reduced capacities to respond to messages in the host (e. g. , cell surfaces of contiguous cells, hormones, etc.) that control the growth of normal cells. This somatic mutation concept of the origin of cancer has been disputed for many years. It is attractive since carcinogenesis and mutagenesis are grossly alike in that each process leads to heritable changes in phenotype, although the time scales on which these processes operate

TABLE 2
Possible Mechanisms of Chemical Carcinogenesis

I. Genetic mechanisms — heritable changes in DNA genome via
   1. Direct modification of existing DNA
   2. Modification of RNA which is subsequently transcribed into DNA that becomes integrated into host DNA
   3. Alterations which decrease, at least temporarily, the fidelity of copying of DNA
II. Epigenetic mechanisms — nongenomic changes leading to
   1. Quasipermanent changes in the transcription of DNA (including integrated virus genomes and oncogenes)
   2. The preferential proliferation of previously existing preneo-plastic or neoplastic cells

---

appear to be widely different in most cases. The attractiveness of the somatic mutation concept of chemical carcinogenesis has been enhanced by recent work showing that chemical mutagens and chemical carcinogens have much in common (80). Thus the active forms of most, and possibly all, chemical carcinogens and of many, but not all, chemical mutagens are electrophilic reactants. The exceptions among the chemical mutagens appear to be the frame shift-inducing mutagens and the mutagenic base analogs since neither of these groups acts through electrophilic forms. Furthermore, neither of these groups of compounds has received adequate tests for carcinogenicity.

In the early studies on the mutagenicity of chemical carcinogens there were hopes that a close correlation between the mutagenic and carcinogenic properties of chemicals might indicate that mutagenic events were a part of chemical carcinogenic processes. It is now evident that it is not possible to establish this point from gross correlations, no matter how good, between mutagenicity and carcinogenicity. This conclusion follows from the ability of ultimate chemical carcinogens to react with proteins and RNA's as well as with DNA, the critical cellular target of chemical mutagens. The relationship between chemical carcinogenicity and chemical mutagenicity will remain moot until the critical target(s) of chemical carcinogens are identified and until the relationships between the two processes can be studied at the molecular level in the same cells.

Thus, while there may or may not be a causal relationship between chemical carcinogenesis and chemical mutagenesis, there is a strong formal relationship between the two processes (80). Many, perhaps all, chemical carcinogens are potential mutagens and many, but possibly not all, chemical mutagens are potential carcinogens. This relationship is of practical value in the use of mutagenesis systems to detect potential carcinogens by virtue of their mutagenicity.

The reactions of ultimate chemical carcinogens with proteins and RNA's in cells require that epigenetic mechanisms of chemical carcinogenesis also be considered (Table 2). These mechanisms are based on models of cellular differentiation in which nongenomic changes lead to quasipermanent changes in the transcription of the DNA genome. The increasing variety of expressions of fetal antigens and enzymes in chemically induced neoplasms that have been found in recent years are possible examples of the effects of chemical carcinogens on gene readout. Such changes in gene expression might cause the transcription of part or all of integrated tumor virus genomes or oncogenes (81). The second epigenetic mechanism in Table 2 is the selection of previously existing preneoplastic or neoplastic cells by effects of the chemical carcinogen on the host. Carcinogen-induced alterations in the hormonal balance or immunological capacity of the host, for example, might give proliferative advantages to such cells.

ROLES OF VIRUSES OR INTEGRATED VIRAL GENOMES
IN CHEMICAL CARCINOGENESIS

Of great interest at the present time is the roles which viruses or integrated viral genomes play in carcinogenesis by chemicals. The demonstrations by Gross, Kaplan, and Irino and their associates in the late 1950's of the presence of transmissible leukemia viruses in certain leukemias induced by irradiation of low-leukemia mice suggested that the role of the radiation was to permit the emergence of active leukemia virus (82). The subsequent demonstration of gs antigens for the murine leukemia and sarcoma viruses in lymphomas and sarcomas induced by 3-methylcholanthrene suggested that the induction of these tumors might be dependent on the derepression of integrated viral information (83, 84). Possibly more direct evidence for this point of view has developed from the experiments of Huebner and his associates (85-88) on the markedly increased efficiency of malignant transformation by polycyclic hydrocarbons, diethyl-nitrosamine, or smog extracts of murine fibroblasts which were first infected with murine leukemia virus. The possibility that the virus-infected cells also differ in some other important respect, such as the capacity to activate or deactivate the carcinogens, has apparently not been ruled out.

A somewhat similar situation has been suggested for the induction of mammary carcinomas in mice by chemicals. Thus, Bentvelzen et al. (89) believe that a repressor produced by a regulator gene controls the rate of release of genetically transferred mammary tumor virus and that this repression can be abrogated by treatment of low-mammary tumor strains with certain carcinogenic chemicals (e.g., urethane).

While definitive evidence that the induction by chemicals of sarcomas, lymphomas, or mammary carcinomas in mice in specific cases is dependent on the derepression of a part or all of integrated viral information is still lacking, such information may be available in the near future for some system. At that time, the very important question of the generality of the phenomenon will be posed. Thus, in recognizing the importance of the likelihood that some tumors may develop as a consequence of the derepression of integrated viral information on application of a chemical, we must not hastily infer that this is a general phenomenon for all tumors of one type, for all types of tumors, or for all chemicals. Thus, the ability of the ultimate carcinogenic metabolites to react with all of the informational macromolecules should alert us to the important possibility that there is not one mechanism but a series of mechanisms of tumor induction by chemicals.

ORIGIN AND IMPORTANCE OF THE TUMOR SPECIFIC
TRANSPLANTATION ANTIGENS OF CHEMICALLY INDUCED TUMORS

Their unique tumor-specific transplantation antigens are one of the most striking properties of tumors induced by chemicals in intact animals (90, 91) or in cell culture (92). Of greatest interest is the individuality of these antigens even for multiple tumors induced by a single carcinogen in the same host. Thus these antigens induce an immune state that causes rejection only of the cells of the tumor from which the antigens were derived. They differ from the transplantation antigens of virus-induced tumors, since in the latter tumors cross-reactivity is the rule, although individual antigens have been noted recently in some virus-induced tumors (93). Tumor-specific antigens have not been found in all chemically induced tumors; those induced in several rat tissues by 2-acetylaminofluorene either lack or contain only very low amounts (94). The significance of the tumor-specific antigens in carcinogenesis by chemicals is not clear. As a minimum they probably represent the effects of heritable changes in either the content or expression of the DNA genome, and they may be independent of the informational changes which are important in the initiation of the malignant transformation. For each tumor, however, the antigens may play a role in determining the growth rate of the tumor. Their individual nature seems likely to result from the variety of indiscriminate attacks of ultimate chemical carcinogens on the many vulnerable points in the informational macromolecules in cells. In view of the high probability that many tumors in the human are chemically induced, it would be of great interest to know if these tumors possess individual tumor-specific antigens. However, methodological difficulties may seriously impede progress on this point.

CONCLUSION

Each of the major topics discussed above represents a threshold of research in chemical carcinogenesis that appears poised for many further advances. In addition to providing a more coherent understanding of chemical carcinogenesis, further work in many of these areas with models of chemical carcinogenesis will certainly help in the achievement of greater control over the development of cancer in man — the overall objective of all of our studies.

REFERENCES

1. E. R. Redmond, Jr., Tobacco and cancer: The first clinical report, 1761, New Eng. J. Med., 282, 18 (1970).
2. P. Pott, Chirurgical observations relative to cancer of the scrotum. London, 1775, reprinted in Natl. Cancer Inst. Monograph, 10, 7 (1963).
3. A. L. Herbst, H. Ulfelder, and D. C. Pozkanzer, Adenocarcinoma of the vagina: association of maternal stilbestrol therapy with tumor appearance in young women, New Eng. J. Med., 284, 878 (1971).
4. J. Higginson, Present trends in cancer epidemiology, Can. Cancer Conf., 8, 40 (1969).
5. E. L. Wynder and K. Mabuchi, Etiological and preventive aspects of human cancer, Preventive Med., 1, 300 (1972).
6. W. Haenszel and M. Kurihara, Studies of Japanese migrants. I. Mortality from cancer and other diseases among Japanese in the United States, J. Nat. Cancer Inst., 40, 43 (1968).
7. M. Segi, M. Kurihara, and T. Matsuyame, Cancer Mortality for Selected Sites in 24 Countries, No. 5 (1964–1965), Sanko Printing Co., Sendai, Japan, 1969.
8. J. Kmet and E. Mahboubi, Esophageal cancer in the Caspian littoral of Iran: Initial studies, Science, 175, 846 (1972).
9. H. F. Blum, Carcinogenesis by Ultraviolet Light, Princeton Univ. Press, Princeton, N.J., 1959, p. 285.
10. F. Urbach, "Geographic Pathology of Skin Cancer," in The Biologic Effects of Ultraviolet Radiation (with Emphasis on the Skin) (F. Urbach, ed.), Pergamon, New York, 1969, p. 635.
11. J. A. Miller and E. C. Miller, Natural and synthetic chemical carcinogens in the etiology of cancer, Cancer Res., 25, 1292 (1965).
12. J. A. Miller, "Naturally-Occurring Chemicals That Can Induce Tumors," in Toxicants Occurring Naturally in Foods, National Academy of Sciences – National Research Council, Washington, D. C., 2nd ed., in press.
13. D. B. Clayson, Chemical Carcinogenesis, Little, Brown, Boston, 1962.
14. J. A. Miller, Carcinogenesis by chemicals: an overview — G. H. A. Clowes memorial lecture, Cancer Res., 30, 559 (1970).
15. J. L. Hartwell, "Survey of Compounds Which Have Been Tested for Carcinogenic Activity," Public Health Service Publ. No. 149, Washington, D. C., 2nd ed., 1951.
16. J. L. Hartwell and P. Shubik, "Survey of Compounds Which Have Been Tested for Carcinogenic Activity," Public Health Service Publ. No. 149, Supplements 1 and 2, Washington, D. C., 1957 and 1959.

17. J. I. Thompson and Co., "Survey of Compounds Which Have Been Tested for Carcinogenic Activity, " Public Health Service Publ. No. 149, 1968-1969 volume, Washington, D. C., 1972.

18. J. R. M. Innes, B. M. Ulland, M. G. Valerio, L. Petrucelli, L. Fishbein, E. R. Hart, A. J. Pallotta, R. R. Bates, H. L. Falk, J. J. Gart, M. Klein, I. Mitchell, and J. Peters, Bioassay of pesticides and industrial chemicals for tumorigenicity in mice: a preliminary note, J. Natl. Cancer Inst., 42, 1101 (1969).

19. D. Svoboda, J. Reddy, and C. Harris, Invasive tumors induced in rats with actinomycin D, Cancer Res., 30, 2271 (1970).

20. J. A. Miller and E. C. Miller, Chemical carcinogenesis: mechanisms and approaches to its control, J. Natl. Cancer Inst., 47, V (1971).

21. F. Dickens and H. E. H. Jones, Further studies on the carcinogenic action of certain lactones and related substances in the rat and mouse, Brit. J. Cancer, 19, 392 (1965).

22. B. L. Van Duuren, B. M. Goldschmidt, C. Katz, and I. Seidman, Dimethylcarbamyl chloride, a multipotential carcinogen, J. Natl. Cancer Inst., 48, 1539 (1972).

23. J. R. DeBaun, E. C. Miller, and J. A. Miller, N-Hydroxy-2-acetylaminofluorene sulfotransferase: its probable role in carcinogenesis and in protein-(methion-S-yl) binding in rat liver, Cancer Res., 30, 577 (1970).

24. V. M. Maher, E. C. Miller, J. A. Miller, and W. Szybalski, Mutations and decreases in density of transforming DNA produced by derivatives of the carcinogens 2-acetylaminofluorene and N-methyl-4-aminoazobenzene, Mol. Pharmacol., 4, 411 (1968).

25. J. R. DeBaun, J. Y. R. Smith, E. C. Miller, and J. A. Miller, Reactivity in vitro of the carcinogen N-hydroxy-2-acetylaminofluorene: Increase by sulfate ion, Science, 167, 184 (1970).

26. J. H. Weisburger, R. S. Yamamoto, G. M. Williams, P. H. Grantham, T. Matsushima, and E. K. Weisburger, On the sulfate ester of N-hydroxy-N-2-fluorenylacetamide as a key ultimate hepato-carcinogen in the rat, Cancer Res., 32, 491 (1972).

27. H. Bartsch, M. Dworkin, J. A. Miller, and E. C. Miller, Electrophilic N-acetoxyaminoarenes derived from carcinogenic N-transacetylation in liver, Biochim. Biophys. Acta, 286, 272 (1972).

28. H. Bartsch and E. Hecker, On the metabolic activation of the carcinogen N-hydroxy-2-acetylaminofluorene III. Oxidation with horseradish peroxidase to yield 2-nitrosofluorene and N-acetoxy-N-2-acetylaminofluorene, Biochim. Biophys. Acta, 237, 567 (1971).

29. E.C. Miller, P.D. Lotlikar, J.A. Miller, B.W. Butler, C.C. Irving, and J.T. Hill, Reactions in vitro of some tissue nucleophiles with the glucuronide of N-hydroxy-2-acetylaminofluorene, Mol. Pharmacol., 4, 147 (1968).
30. C.C. Irving, R.A. Veazey, and J.T. Hill, Reaction of the glucuronide of the carcinogen N-hydroxy-2-acetylaminofluorene with nucleic acids, Biochim. Biophys. Acta., 179, 189 (1969).
31. C.C. Irving and L.T. Russell, Synthesis of the O-glucuronide of N-2-fluorenylhydroxylamine. Reaction with nucleic acids and with guanosine-5'-monophosphate, Biochemistry, 9, 2471 (1970).
32. G. Stöhrer and G.B. Brown, Oncogenic purine derivatives: evidence for a possible proximate oncogen, Science, 167, 1622 (1970).
33. G. Stöhrer, E. Corbin, and G.B. Brown, Enzymatic activation of the oncogen 3-hydroxyxanthine, Cancer Res., 32, 637 (1972).
34. D.R. McCalla, Reaction of N-methyl-N'-nitro-N-nitrosoguanidine and N-methyl-N-nitroso-p-toluenesulfonamide with DNA in vitro, Biochim. Biophys. Acta, 155, 114 (1968).
35. P.N. Magee and J.M. Barnes, Carcinogenic nitroso compounds, Advan. Cancer Res., 10, 163 (1967).
36. R. Preussmann, H. Druckrey, S. Ivankovic, and A.v. Hodenberg, Chemical structure and carcinogenicity of aliphatic hydrazo, azo, and azoxy compounds and of triazenes, potential in vivo alkylating agents, Ann. N.Y. Acad. Sci., 163, 697 (1969).
37. A.R. Mattocks, Toxicity of pyrrolizidine alkaloids, Nature, 217 723 (1968).
38. A.R. Mattocks, Dihydropyrrolizine derivatives from unsaturated pyrrolizidine alkaloids, J. Chem. Soc., 1969, 1155.
39. I.N.H. White and A.R. Mattocks, Reaction of dihydropyrrolizines with deoxyribonucleic acids in vitro, Biochem. J., 128, 291 (1972).
40. J.K. Selkirk, E. Huberman, and C. Heidelberger, An epoxide is an intermediate in the microsomal metabolism of the chemical carcinogen, dibenz(a,h)anthracene, Biochem. Biophys. Res. Commun., 43, 1010 (1971).
41. P.L. Grover, A. Hewer, and P. Sims, Epoxides as microsomal metabolites of polycyclic hydrocarbons, FEBS Letters, 18, 76 (1971).
42. P.L. Grover and P. Sims, Interactions of the K-region epoxides of phenanthrene and dibenz(a,h)anthracene with nucleic acids and histones, Biochem. Pharmacol., 19, 2251 (1970).
43. T. Kuroki, E. Huberman, H. Marquardt, J.H. Selkirk, C. Heidelberger, P.L. Grover, and P. Sims, Binding of K-region epoxides and other derivatives of benz(a)anthracene and dibenz(a,h)anthracene to DNA, RNA, and proteins of transformable cells, Chem.-Biol. Interactions, 4, 389 (1971/72).

44. E. C. Miller and J. A. Miller, Low carcinogenicity of the K-region epoxides of 7-methylbenz(a)anthracene and benz(a)anthracene in the mouse and rat, Proc. Soc. Exp. Biol. Med., 124, 915 (1967).

45. B. L. Van Duuren, L. Langseth, B. M. Goldschmidt, and L. Orris, Carcinogenicity of epoxides, lactones, and peroxy compounds. VI. Structure and carcinogenic activity, J. Natl. Cancer Inst., 39, 1217 (1967).

46. E. Boyland and P. Sims, The carcinogenic activities in mice of compounds related to benz(a)anthracene, Intern. J. Cancer, 2, 500 (1967).

47. P. L. Grover, P. Sims, E. Huberman, H. Marquardt, T. Kuroki, and C. Heidelberger, In vitro transformation of rodent cells by K-region derivatives of polycyclic hydrocarbons, Proc. Nat. Acad. Sci., 68, 1098 (1971).

48. H. Marquardt, T. Kuroki, E. Huberman, J. K. Selkirk, C. Heidelberger, P. L. Grover, and P. Sims, Malignant transformation of cells derived from mouse prostate by epoxides and other derivatives of polycyclic hydrocarbons, Cancer Res., 32, 716 (1972).

49. E. Huberman, T. Kuroki, H. Marquardt, J. K. Selkirk, C. Heidelberger, P. L. Grover, and P. Sims, Transformation of hamster embryo cells by epoxides and other derivatives of polycyclic hydrocarbons, Cancer Res., 32, 1391 (1972).

50. E. Huberman, L. Aspiras, C. Heidelberger, P. L. Grover, and P. Sims, Mutagenicity to mammalian cells of epoxides and other derivatives of polycyclic hydrocarbons, Proc. Nat. Acad. Sci., 68, 3195 (1971).

51. M. J. Cookson, P. Sims, and P. L. Grover, Mutagenicity of epoxides of polycyclic hydrocarbons correlates with carcinogenicity of parent hydrocarbons, Nature New Biol., 234, 186 (1971).

52. B. N. Ames, P. Sims, and P. L. Grover, Epoxides of carcinogenic polycyclic hydrocarbons are frameshift mutagens, Science, 176, 47 (1972).

53. P. Borchert, P. G. Wislocki, J. A. Miller, and E. C. Miller, The metabolism of the naturally-occurring hepatocarcinogen safrole to 1'-hydroxysafrole and the electrophilic reactivity of 1'-acetoxysafrole, Cancer Res., 33, 575 (1973).

54. P. Borchert, J. A. Miller, E. C. Miller, and T. K. Shires, 1'-Hydroxysafrole: a proximate carcinogenic metabolite of safrole in the rat and mouse, Cancer Res., 33, 590 (1973).

55. E. C. Miller and J. A. Miller, The presence and significance of bound aminoazodyes in the livers of rats fed p-dimethyl-aminoazobenzene, Cancer Res., 7, 468 (1947).

56. S. Sorof and E. M. Young, "Soluble Cytoplasmic Macromolecules of Liver and Liver Tumor," in Methods in Cancer Research, Vol. 3 (H. Busch, ed.), Academic Press, New York, 1967, p. 467.

57. S. Sorof, V. M. Kish, and B. Sani, Purification and properties of the principal liver protein conjugate of a hepatic carcinogen, Biochem. Biophys. Res. Commun., 48, 860 (1972).
58. G. Litwack, B. Ketterer, and I. M. Arias, Ligandin: A hepatic protein which binds steroids, bilirubin, carcinogens and a number of exogenous organic anions, Nature, 234, 466 (1971).
59. T. Sugimoto and H. Terayama, The changing pattern of carcinogenic aminoazo dye-binding during the course of continuous feeding of 3'-methyl-4-dimethylaminoazobenzene, Chem.-Biol. Interactions, 2, 391 (1970).
60. P. Brookes and P. D. Lawley, Reaction of some mutagenic and carcinogenic compounds with nucleic acids, J. Cell. Comp. Physiol., 64 (Suppl. 1), 111 (1964).
61. C. Heidelberger, Studies on the molecular mechanism of hydrocarbon carcinogenesis, J. Cell. Comp. Physiol., 64 (Suppl. 1), 129 (1964).
62. L. Goshman and C. Heidelberger, Binding of tritium-labeled polycyclic hydrocarbons to DNA of mouse skin, Cancer Res., 27, 1678 (1967).
63. J. G. Tasseron, H. Diringer, N. Frohwirth, S. S. Mirvish, and C. Heidelberger, Partial purification of soluble protein from mouse skin to which carcinogenic hydrocarbons are specifically bound, Biochemistry, 9, 1636 (1970).
64. R. K. Boutwell, N. H. Colburn, and C. C. Muckerman, In vivo reactions of β-propiolactone, Ann. N. Y. Acad. Sci., 163, 751 (1969).
65. F. Marroquin and E. Farber, The binding of 2-acetylaminofluorene to rat liver ribonucleic acid in vivo, Cancer Res., 25, 1262 (1965).
66. T. Matsushima and J. H. Weisburger, Inhibitors of chemical carcinogens as probes for molecular targets: DNA as decisive receptor for metabolite from N-hydroxy-N-2-fluorenylacetamide, Chem.-Biol. Interactions, 1, 211 (1969/70).
67. E. Kriek, On the mechanism of action of carcinogenic aromatic amines. I. Binding of 2-acetylaminofluorene and N-hydroxy-2-acetylaminofluorene to rat-liver nucleic acids in vivo, Chem.-Biol. Interactions, 1, 3 (1969/70).
68. E. Kriek, On the mechanism of action of carcinogenic aromatic amines. II. Binding of N-hydroxy-N-acetyl-4-aminobiphenyl to rat-liver nucleic acids in vivo, Chem.-Biol. Interactions, 3, 19 (1971).
69. P. F. Swann and P. N. Magee, Nitrosamine-induced carcinogenesis. The alkylation of N-7 of guanine of nucleic acids of the rat by diethylnitrosamine, N-ethyl-N-nitrosourea and ethyl methanesulphonate, Biochem. J., 125, 841 (1971).

70. P. F. Swann and P. N. Magee, Nitrosamine-induced carcinogenesis. The alkylation of nucleic acids of the rat by N-methyl-N-nitrosourea, dimethylnitrosamine, dimethyl sulphate and methyl methanesulphonate, Biochem. J., 110, 39 (1968).
71. P. D. Lawley, "Some Effects of Chemical Mutagens and Carcinogens on Nucleic Acids, " in Progress in Nucleic Acid Research and Molecular Biology, Vol. 5 (J. N. Davidson and W. E. Cohn, eds.), Academic Press, New York and London, 1966, p. 89.
72. A. Loveless, Possible relevance of O-6 alkylation of deoxyguanosine to the mutagenicity and carcinogenicity of nitrosamines and nitrosamides, Nature, 223, 206, 1969.
73. P. D. Lawley and C. J. Thatcher, Methylation of deoxyribonucleic acid in cultured mammalian cells by N-methyl-N'-nitro-N-nitrosoguanidine, Biochem. J., 116, 693 (1970).
74. G. P. Warwick and J. J. Roberts, Persistent binding of butter yellow metabolites to rat liver DNA, Nature, 213, 1206 (1967).
75. D. Szafarz and J. H. Weisburger, Stability of binding of label from N-hydroxy-N-2-fluorenylacetamide to intracellular targets, particularly deoxyribonucleic acid in rat liver, Cancer Res., 29, 962 (1969).
76. E. C. Miller and J. A. Miller, "Approaches to the Mechanisms and Control of Chemical Carcinogens, " in Environment and Cancer, The University of Texas M. D. Anderson Hospital and Tumor Institute at Houston, 24th Annual Symposium on Fundamental Cancer Research, Williams and Wilkins, Baltimore, 1972, p. 5.
77. L. W. Wattenberg, "Enzymatic Reactions and Carcinogenesis, " in Environment and Cancer, The University of Texas M. D. Anderson Hospital and Tumor Institute at Houston, 24th Annual Symposium on Fundamental Cancer Research, Williams and Wilkins, Baltimore, 1972, p. 241.
78. H. M. Temin, The protovirus hypothesis: Speculations on the significance of RNA-directed DNA synthesis for normal development and for carcinogenesis, J. Natl. Cancer Inst., 46, III-VII (1971).
79. J. F. Speyer, J. D. Karam, and A. B. Lenny, On the role of DNA polymerase in base selection, Cold Spring Harbor Symp. Quant. Biol., 31, 693 (1966).
80. E. C. Miller and J. A. Miller, "The Mutagenicity of Chemical Carcinogens: Correlations, Problems, and Interpretations, " in Chemical Mutagens — Principles and Methods for Their Detection, Vol. 1 (A. Hollaender, ed.), Plenum, New York, 1971, p. 83.
81. G. J. Todaro and R. J. Huebner, The viral oncogene hypothesis: New evidence, Proc. Nat. Acad. Sci., 69, 1009 (1972).
82. H. S. Kaplan, On the natural history of the murine leukemias: Presidential address, Cancer Res., 27, 1325 (1967).

83. J. J. Igel, R. J. Huebner, H. C. Turner, P. Kotin, and H. L. Falk, Mouse leukemia virus activation by chemical carcinogens, Science, 166, 1624 (1969).

84. C. E. Whitmire, R. A. Salerno, L. S. Rabstein, R. J. Huebner, and H. C. Turner, RNA tumor-virus antigen expression in chemically induced tumors. Virus-genome-specified common antigens detected by complement fixation in mouse tumors induced by 3-methylcholanthrene, J. Nat. Cancer Inst., 47, 1255 (1971).

85. A. E. Freeman, P. J. Price, H. J. Igel, J. C. Young, J. M. Maryak, and R. J. Huebner, Morphological transformation of rat embryo cells induced by diethylnitrosamine and murine leukemia viruses, J. Nat. Cancer Inst., 44, 65 (1970).

86. P. J. Price, A. E. Freeman, W. T. Lane, and R. J. Huebner, Morphological transformation of rat embryo cells by the combined action of 3-methylcholanthrene and Rauscher leukemia virus, Nature New Biol., 230, 144 (1971).

87. J. S. Rhim, W. Vass, H. Y. Cho, and R. J. Huebner, Malignant transformation induced by 7,12-dimethylbenz(a)anthracene in rat embryo cells infected with Rauscher leukemia virus, Intern. J. Cancer, 7, 65 (1971).

88. J. S. Rhim, H. Y. Cho, L. Rabstein, R. J. Gordon, R. J. Bryan, M. B. Gardner, and R. J. Huebner, Transformation of mouse cells infected with AKR leukemia virus induced by smog extracts, Nature, 239, 103 (1972).

89. P. Bentvelzen, J. H. Daams, P. Hageman, and J. Calafat, Genetic transmission of viruses that incite mammary tumor in mice, Proc. Nat. Acad. Sci., 67, 377 (1970).

90. G. Klein, Tumor-specific transplantation antigens —G. H. A. Clowes Memorial Lecture, Cancer Res., 28, 625 (1968).

91. R. W. Baldwin, Tumour specific antigens associated with chemically induced tumours, Europ. J. Clin. Biol. Res., 15, 593 (1970).

92. S. Mondal, P. T. Iype, L. M. Griesbach, and C. Heidelberger, Antigenicity of cells derived from mouse prostate cells after malignant transformation in vitro by carcinogenic hydrocarbons, Cancer Res., 30, 1953 (1970).

93. J. Vaage, T. Kalinovsky, and R. Olson, Antigenic differences among virus-induced tumors arising in the same C3H/Crgl host, Cancer Res., 29, 1452 (1969).

94. R. W. Baldwin and M. J. Embleton, Immunology of 2-acetylaminofluorene induced rat mammary adenocarcinomas, Intern. J. Cancer, 4, 47 (1969).

Chapter 2

METABOLIC ACTIVATION OF BENZO(a)PYRENE:
SIGNIFICANCE OF THE FREE RADICAL

Cikayoshi Nagata, Yusaku Tagashira, and Masahiko Kodama

Biophysics Division
National Cancer Center Research Institute
Chuo-ku, Tokyo, Japan

INTRODUCTION

Four decades have elapsed since benzo(a)pyrene was isolated from coal tar as a pure polycondensed aromatic carcinogen. During this time, this potent carcinogen, benzo(a)pyrene, has played the leading part in the history of the study of chemical carcinogens because of its usefulness in the study of carcinogenesis mechanisms, and also of its widespread distribution in our environment.

It has been supposed that benzo(a)pyrene is converted into an active intermediate and that this intermediate binds to the tissue components during the early stage of carcinogenesis by benzo(a)-pyrene. However, the metabolic pathways of benzo(a)pyrene are extremely complicated, and its active form has remained unrevealed.

Recent in vitro experiments by Morreal et al. (1), Ts'o et al. (2-4), and Wilk and Girke (5) showed that some chemical activators such as I_2, H_2O_2, or Fenton's reagent ($H_2O_2 + FeCl_2$) accelerate the binding of benzo(a)pyrene to tissue components and opened a way to investigate the active form of benzo(a)pyrene. Further, the K-region epoxide of benzo(a)pyrene has also been identified by Grover and Sims in the incubation experiment using liver homogenates (6), and this form was assumed to be the proximate structure in the light of the fact that epoxides of aromatic hydrocarbons such as benzo(a)anthracene and dibenzo(a, h)anthracene were carcinogenic to the tissue cultured cells (7, 8).

By means of the electron spin resonance method, the present authors have found that benzo(a)pyrene was converted into a free radical by incubation with rat liver homogenates, and the structure of the free radical was identified as the 6-oxy-benzopyrene radical (9). As this free radical was unstable and chemically reactive, it was supposed that the free radical might be a candidate for the proximate form of benzo(a)pyrene.

In this communication, studies on the enzymatic formation of the 6-oxy-benzopyrene radical, on the binding of 6-hydroxybenzo(a)-pyrene, which is considered as a precursor of the radical, to nucleic acids, and on 6-hydroxybenzo(a)pyrene's carcinogenicity to mice and rats are reported; causal significance of the free radical in benzo-pyrene carcinogenesis is discussed.

ENZYMATIC FORMATION OF 6-OXY-BENZOPYRENE RADICAL

Condition for the Formation of the Free Radical

Livers (15 g) from male rats were homogenized in 3 volumes of ice-cold 1.15% (w/v) KCl in a Potter & Elvehjem type homogenizer. The homogenate was centrifuged at 0°C for 20 min at 1500 g, and the supernatant (70 ml) was mixed with equal volumes of 0.1 M phosphate buffer (pH 7.4) containing 0.88 g of niacinamide, 15 mg of NADP, and 125 mg of glucose-6-phosphate. Five milligrams of benzo(a)-pyrene dissolved in 1 ml of acetone were added to the homogenate and shaken in a water bath at 37°C. At the end of incubation, the hydro-carbon was extracted several times with 100 ml of benzene from the ice-cold reaction mixture. The benzene extract was evaporated to dryness, and the residue was dissolved in 0.5 ml of benzene for the ESR measurement. As seen in Fig. 1(a), the sample gave a strong symmetrical signal, showing that a free radical is formed by incuba-tion (9).

In order to obtain a hyperfine structure of the signal, the sample was degassed using a high-vacuum pump to the extent of 2×10^{-3} mm Hg. The hyperfine structure, composed of five lines, was observed when the modulation width was 1.6 G [Fig. 1(b)] and this signal was further split by using a smaller modulation width of 0.8 G [Fig. 1(c)].

The free radical formation was largely dependent upon the conditions used. Namely, when liver homogenate heated at 65°C for 15 min was used, the signal became extremely small compared with that of the nonheated sample [Fig. 2(a), (b)]. This clearly shows that the free radical formation was enzymatic. Co-factors were necessary for the free radical formation, and the signal was very small when the co-factors were omitted [Fig. 2(c)]. No ESR signal was observed when benzo(a)pyrene was omitted [Fig. 2(d)] or when benzo(a)pyrene in ben-zene alone was incubated [Fig. 2(e)]. Benzo(a)pyrene is sensitive to light, so care was taken to carry out all procedures in the dark.

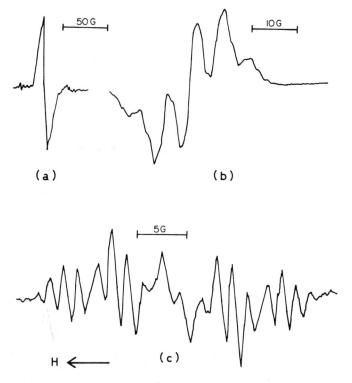

FIG. 1. ESR signal of the free radical produced by incubating benzo(a)pyrene with liver homogenate. Modulation width: (a) 4 G, (b) 1.6 G, and (c) 0.8 G.

Identification of the Free Radical

The peroxy radical, cation or anion radical, semiquinone radicals, and oxy radicals were considered as the structure of the free radical. Of these, the peroxy radical was excluded because the g-value of the radical under consideration, 2.004, is greatly different from that of peroxy radical (g = 2.015) (10). The cation radical was investigated after it was formed by dissolving benzo(a)pyrene in concentrated H_2SO_4. But its hyperfine structure was different from that of the free radical concerned [Fig. 3(a)]. The possibility of an anion radical, the hyperfine structure of which is similar to that of the cation radical, was accordingly excluded. Three types of benzo(a)-pyrene quinones were prepared by oxidizing benzo(a)pyrene with chromic acid; they were fractionated by partially deactivated alumina column chromatography. Semiquinone radicals were obtained by reducing the corresponding benzopyrene quinones with NaOH in dimethyl sulfoxide.

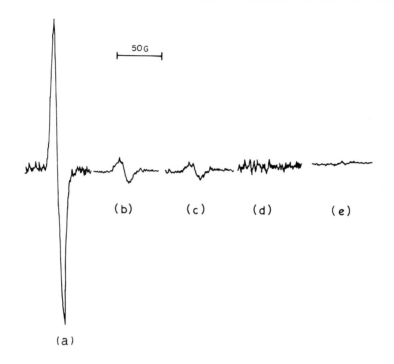

(b)   (c)   (d)   (e)

(a)

FIG. 2. ESR signal of the free radical produced by incubating
benzo(a)pyrene with liver homogenate. Modulation width: 4 G.
(a) Benzo(a)pyrene and liver homogenate with co-factors, (b) benzo-
(a)pyrene and liver homogenate heated at 65°C for 15 min, (c) benzo-
(a)pyrene and liver homogenate without co-factors, (d) liver homogenate alone, and (e) benzo(a)pyrene alone.

The hyperfine structures of the ESR signal for these semiquinone
radicals were different from that of the signal for the free radical
under study [Fig. 3(b-d)] (9).

   Finally, the possibility of an oxy-benzopyrene radical was investigated. From the viewpoint of organic chemical reactions, the most
·reactive position in benzo(a)pyrene is the 6 position. Thus, frontier
electron density, which has been proved to be a good chemical reactivity index (11-13), predicts that the 6 position is the most reactive
toward all types of reagents, electrophilic, nucleophilic, and radical
(Fig. 4) (14). Experimental results on the chemical reactivity of
benzo(a)pyrene have also shown that the 6 position is the most reactive in substitution reactions. Namely, benzo(a)pyrene is known to
be substituted exclusively in the 6 position by oxidation with lead
tetraacetate, chlorination, sulfonation, and condensation with
formanilide, and the next reactive positions were 3 and 1 (15,16).

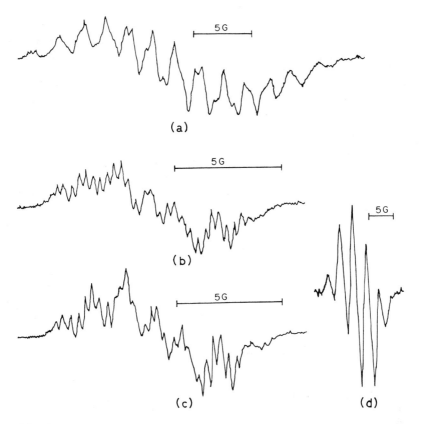

FIG. 3. Hyperfine structures of ESR signals of (a) cation radical, (b) benzopyrene-3, 6-semiquinone radical, (c) -1, 6-semiquinone radical, and (d) -6, 12-semiquinone radical. Modulation width: 0.7 G.

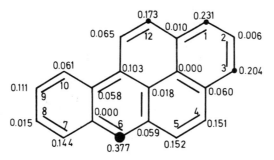

FIG. 4. Frontier electron densities for benzo(a)pyrene. The filled circles show the predicted reactive positions.

In view of these theoretical predictions and the experimental facts, attention was first paid to the reaction product at the 6 position. The 6-oxy-benzopyrene radical was formed by oxidizing 6-hydroxybenzo-(a)pyrene with ceric sulfate, and ESR spectrum was measured. As shown in Fig. 5(a), the shape of the ESR signal was exactly the same as that of the free radical produced by incubating benzo(a)pyrene with liver homogenate.

The same ESR signal was obtained by irradiating benzo(a)pyrene in benzene with visible light [Fig. 5(b)], showing that the 6-oxy-benzopyrene radical can also be produced by photoirradiation (17). This radical was converted into benzopyrene quinones by further photoirradiation; this means that the 6-oxy-benzopyrene radical is an intermediate from benzo(a)pyrene to benzopyrene quinones (17). The 6-oxy-benzopyrene radical was produced also by stirring benzo-(a)pyrene with albumin in the dark (18).

Effect of the Co-factors on the Free Radical Formation

Detailed study on the effect of the co-factors on the free radical formation showed that the co-factors used above (Fig. 2) could be substituted by NADPH without glucose-6-phosphate, NADP, and niacinamide. Both NADPH and NADH were necessary for maximal

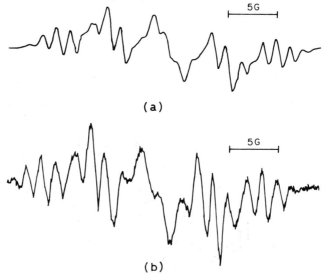

(a)

(b)

FIG. 5. ESR signal of (a) 6-oxy-benzopyrene radical produced by oxidizing 6-hydroxybenzo(a)pyrene with ceric sulfate and (b) the same radical produced by irradiating benzo(a)pyrene in benzene with visible light.

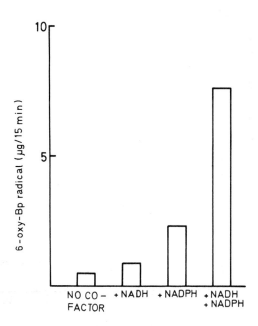

FIG. 6. The requirement of NADPH and NADH for the formation of 6-oxy-benzopyrene radical. Twenty-five grams of rat liver were used per flask. Experimental conditions were the same as described in the text, except 100 mg NADP and/or NADPH were added to the reaction mixture instead of the NADPH-generating system. The incubation time was 15 min. Amounts of 6-oxy-benzopyrene radical were determined by comparing the solution's spin density with that of a standard sample of DPPH.

activity, but NADPH alone supported relatively high activity. On the other hand, the activity was very low in the presence of NADH alone (Fig. 6).

Time Course of Enzymatic Formation of the Free Radical

The effect of incubation time was demonstrated in Fig. 7. The amount of enzymatically formed 6-oxy-benzopyrene radical reached a maximum when incubated for 20 min; it then rapidly decreased. This result suggests that the 6-oxy-benzopyrene radicals formed from benzo(a)pyrene are rapidly metabolized during the incubation.

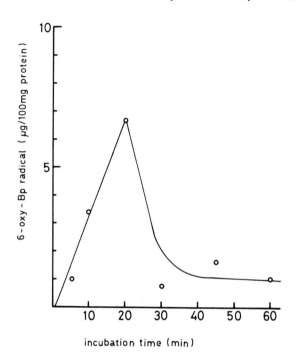

FIG. 7. The effect of incubation time on the formation of 6-oxy-benzopyrene radical. Experimental conditions were the same as in Fig. 6. NADPH (100 mg) was used as the co-factor.

Distribution of the Enzyme Capable of Converting Benzo(a)pyrene to 6-Oxy-benzopyrene Radical

Figure 8 shows the intracellular distribution of enzyme activity. Mitochondrial, microsomal, and supernatant fractions were obtained from the homogenate in isotonic sucrose solution by differential centrifugation. The nuclear fraction was prepared and purified according to the method of Matsuyama et al. (19). Microsomal and nuclear fractions showed high enzyme activity, but mitochondrial and supernatant fractions had only a trace or low activity. It should be stressed here that the enzyme activity in the nuclear fraction was unexpectedly large. This is of importance in considering the relation between the site of metabolic activation and carcinogenesis reaction.

Induction of the Enzyme by Methylcholanthrene

Since it is well known that the administration of 3-methyl-cholanthrene increases the benzopyrene hydroxylase in rat liver

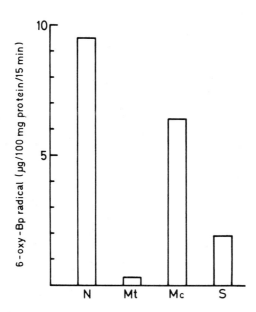

FIG. 8. The intracellular distribution of the enzyme. Each cellular fraction was suspended in KCl-phosphate buffer (0.5% KCl, 0.05 M phosphate buffer, pH 7.4) and incubated for 15 min under the same conditions as in Fig. 7. N: nuclear fraction, Mt: mitrochondrial fraction, Mc: microsomal fraction, S: supernatant fraction.

microsome (20, 21), induction of the enzyme capable of converting benzo(a)pyrene to the 6-oxy-benzopyrene radical was investigated. A single intraperitoneal injection of 3-methylcholanthrene significantly increased the enzyme activity in the homogenate as well as in the nuclear fraction (Fig. 9).

Free Radical Formation by Skin Homogenate

It may be of importance to know whether the homogenate of skin, which is a target tissue for benzo(a)pyrene, is able to produce the same free radical as the liver homogenate. Benzo(a)pyrene was incubated with mouse skin homogenate at 37°C for 60 min, and the ESR signal due to 6-oxy-benzopyrene radical was observed (Fig. 10). Rat skin homogenate was also found to give an ESR signal ascribable to the 6-oxy-benzopyrene radical. But the signal was far smaller than that obtained in the case of mouse skin homogenate, probably because of the stiff and fibrous nature of rat skin.

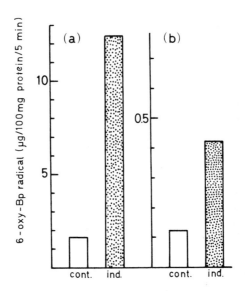

FIG. 9. Induction of the enzyme by 3-methylcholanthrene. Homogenate and nuclear fraction were prepared 24 hr after intraperitoneal injection of methylcholanthrene (2 mg/100 g body weight). Experimental conditions were the same as in Figs. 7 and/or 8. The incubation time was 5 min. (a) Homogenate (supernatant of liver homogenate centrifuged at 1500 g for 20 min); (b) nuclear fraction; cont.: control rat without induction; Ind.: induction by methylcholanthrene.

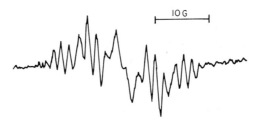

FIG. 10. ESR signal of 6-oxy-benzopyrene radical produced by incubating benzo(a)pyrene with skin homogenate.

Metabolic Pathway of Benzo(a)pyrene in Relation to the Formation of 6-Oxy-benzopyrene Radical

The calculated spin densities for the 6-oxy-benzopyrene radical are indicated in Fig. 11. The spin densities at the 1, 3, 4, and 12 positions are especially large compared with the values at other positions, and this explains well the fact that benzopyrene-1, 6-

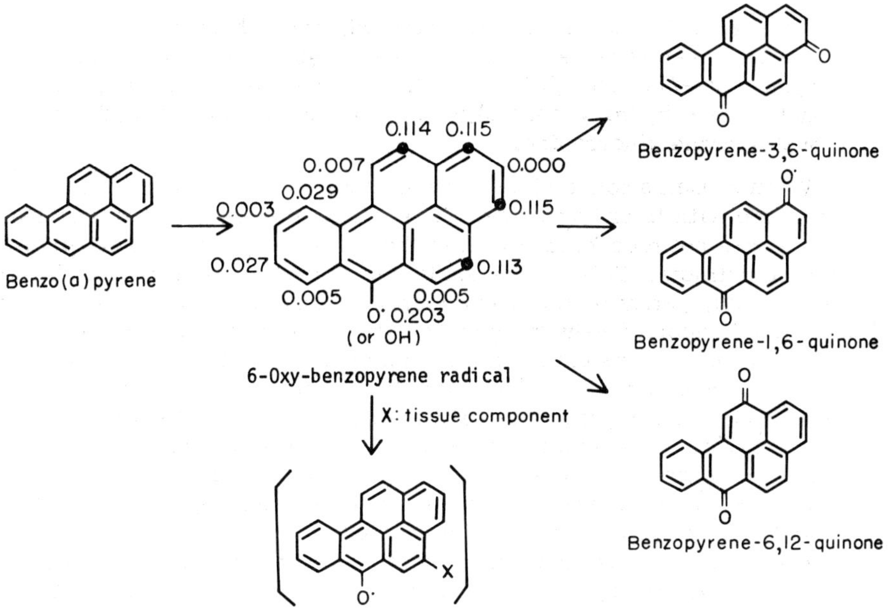

FIG. 11. Calculated spin densities for the 6-oxy-benzopyrene radical and enzymatic and photooxidation processes of benzo(a)pyrene.
The exact structure of the compound in parentheses has not yet been
determined.

quinone, -3, 6-quinone, and -6, 12-quinone were formed metabolically
as well as in the photoirradiation experiment (17). In spite of large
electron density at the 4 position, benzopyrene-4, 6-quinone has
never been detected as a metabolic product or as a photoproduct. At
present, this is difficult to explain, and probably it may be ascribed
to the instability of benzopyrene-4, 6-quinone. Otherwise, the following scheme might be involved: A greater part of the 6-oxy-benzopyrene
radicals were detoxicated through the 1, 6-, 3, 6-, and 6, 12-quinones,
but a smaller part of the molecule binds to the tissue components at
the 4 position (Fig. 11). In connection with this scheme, it is worthy
of note that the special importance of the 4 position in hydrocarbon
carcinogenesis was pointed out by Miller and Miller (22, 23).

Comparison with 3-Hydroxylated Metabolite

As described above, large amounts of 6-oxy-benzopyrene radical
were detected as a metabolite of benzo(a)pyrene. Nevertheless,
6-hydroxybenzo(a) pyrene, which is considered to be a precursor of

the free radical, has never been detected, and 3-hydroxybenzo(a)-
pyrene has been regarded exlusively as a major metabolite of benzo-
(a)pyrene (24-26), though Falk et al. (27) postulated the metabolic
formation of 6-hydroxybenzo(a)pyrene from the detected 6-hydroxy-
benzo(a)pyrene glucuronide.

When a small amount of 6-hydroxybenzo(a)pyrene (2×10^{-6} M) was
incubated with liver homogenate (0-15 min), free 6-hydroxybenzo(a)-
pyrene was not recovered from liver homogenate by benzene or ethyl
acetate extracts. This can be explained partly by the formation of the
free radical, partly by the conversion into unknown metabolites. Such
rapid conversion of 6-hydroxybenzo(a)pyrene to the free radical and
unknown metabolites explains well the reason why the former compound
has never been detected as a major metabolite. On the other hand,
3-hydroxybenzo(a)pyrene was far more stable than the 6-hydroxy compound from the standpoint of convertibility into free radical. Thus,
6-hydroxybenzo(a)pyrene easily converted into free radical even when
it was dissolved in organic solvents such as benzene, alcohol, and
dimethyl sulfoxide, but the 3-hydroxy compound was stable and gave
no ESR signal in these organic solvents. In order to get a free radical
of 3-hydroxybenzo(a)pyrene, a drastic method to abstract the hydrogen
atom of the hydroxyl group is necessary. Thus, conversion of 3-
hydroxybenzo(a)pyrene into a free radical in dimethylsulfoxide was
achieved by adding ceric sulfate under alkaline condition (Fig. 12).
Exact comparison between the amounts of the metabolically formed
3-hydroxy and 6-hydroxy compounds is difficult, but rough estimates
based on the spin density showed that almost the same amount of
6-oxy-benzopyrene radical with 3-hydroxybenzo(a)pyrene was produced by incubating benzo(a)pyrene with liver homogenate.

BINDING OF 6-HYDROXYBENZO(a)PYRENE WITH NUCLEIC ACIDS

Physical Binding with DNA

As in the case of benzo(a)pyrene, 6-hydroxybenzo(a)pyrene was
found to form a physical complex with DNA. That is, although the
compound was scarcely soluble in aqueous solution, the solubility
was remarkably increased in aqueous DNA solution, and the absorption maximum was shifted toward the longer wavelengths by 20 nm
compared with that in ethanol solution. Direct evidence of complex
formation was obtained by means of the flow dichroic method, by
which 6-hydroxybenzo(a)pyrene was proved to be oriented parallel to
the DNA bases, as in the cases of benzo(a)pyrene and other intercalat-
ing dyes (Fig. 13) (28). Using ^{3}H-labeled 6-hydroxybenzo(a)pyrene,
the binding ratio was estimated as one hydrocarbon molecule per 500
base pairs.

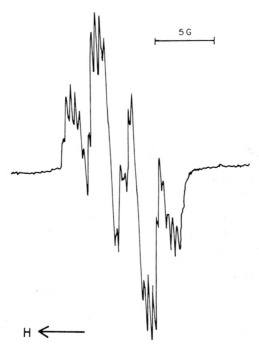

FIG. 12. ESR signal obtained by oxidizing 3-hydroxybenzo(a)-
pyrene in dimethylsulfoxide with ceric sulfate under alkaline condition.

Chemical Binding with DNA and DNA Bases

The reaction mixture (40 ml), which contained 33% ethanol, 5 mM
phosphate buffer, pH 7, 0.5 mM calf thymus DNA (heat-denatured),
and 3×10^{-5} M [^{3}H]-6-hydroxybenzo(a)pyrene (7.5 mCi/mmole), was
stirred for 24 hr at room temperature, then extracted three times with
equal volumes of chloroform, twice with 80% phenol (pH 7.5), and
once with ether; finally DNA precipitated by ethanol was dissolved
in 4 ml distilled water. The radioactivity of the 0.3 ml of DNA solution was measured by a dioxane scintillator.

Some parts of the physical complex were converted to chemically
bound states, and this is noticeable in connection with the case of
benzo(a)pyrene, in which no chemical binding occurred with DNA
under similar conditions. In Table 1, the results of the binding
experiment are indicated. Heat-denatured DNA bound twice as much
6-hydroxybenzo(a)pyrene as native, double-stranded DNA. Apyrimidinic
acid bound 40 times as much hydrocarbon as apurinic acid, indicating

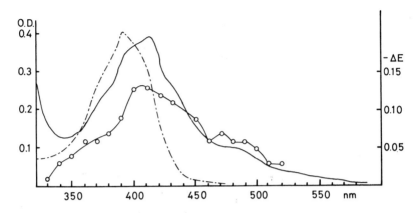

FIG. 13. Absorption and flow dichroic spectra of 6-hydroxybenzo(a)-
pyrene. Absorption spectra in ethanol (— ‑ —), in DNA aqueous solution (———), and flow dichroic spectrum in DNA aqueous solution
(—o—o—). A 20-mg portion of 6-hydroxybenzo(a)pyrene was stirred
with 10 ml of 0.5% calf thymus DNA in pure water for 40 hr at 4°C,
and after spinning off the excess hydrocarbon (15,000 rpm, 60 min),
the DNA solution was applied for the measurement of flow dichroism.
$\Delta E = E_{\parallel} - E_{\perp}$, where $E_{\parallel}$ and $E_{\perp}$ designate the optical density
parallel and perpendicular to the flow. For details, see Ref. 28.

TABLE 1

Amounts of 6-Hydroxybenzo(a)pyrene (6-OHB)
Chemically Bound to DNA

DNA	Activators or inhibitors	Bound 6-OHB (mmole) / mole of DNA
Double stranded DNA	—	0.053
Single-stranded DNA	—	0.089–0.140
Single-stranded DNA	Benzoylperoxide (4×10^{-5} M)	4.000
Single-stranded DNA	H_2O_2 (1.5×10^{-2} M)	0.657
Single-stranded DNA	$CuCl_2$ (1×10^{-5} M)	2.160
Single-stranded DNA	NaOH (10^{-2} M)	0.028
Single-stranded DNA	EDTA (10^{-3} M)	0.039
Apurinic acid	Benzoylperoxide (4×10^{-5} M)	0.099
Apyrimidinic acid	Benzoylperoxide (4×10^{-5} M)	3.710

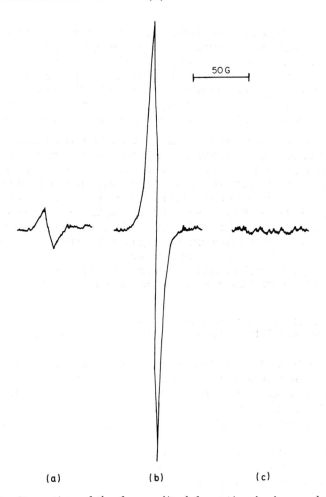

FIG. 14. Promotion of the free radical formation by benzoylperoxide. (a) 6-Hydroxybenzo(a)pyrene in ethanol (0.3 mg/ml), (b) addition of 3 mg of benzoylperoxide to (a), and (c) benzoylperoxide in ethanol (3 mg/ml).

the binding specificity in the purine bases. In the case of single-stranded DNA, the binding was accelerated by benzoylperoxide, H_2O_2, or Cu^{2+}. Thus, the binding ratio was one hydrocarbon molecule per 7000 bases in case of single-stranded DNA; this increased to one hydrocarbon per 250 bases when benzoylperoxide was added. In contrast to this, the binding ratio was diminished by addition of alkali or EDTA. Benzoylperoxide was shown to promote the formation of the 6-oxy-benzopyrene radical from 6-hydroxybenzo(a)pyrene progressively (Fig. 14). That Cu^{2+} has a similar effect has already been reported by Tagashira and Yamamoto (29). On the other hand, EDTA or alkali inhibited the formation of the 6-oxy-benzopyrene radical or accelerated the decay of the radical. These results strongly suggest that the 6-oxy-benzopyrene radical is involved in the covalent binding between 6-hydroxybenzo(a)pyrene and DNA. DNA-bound 6-hydroxy-benzo(a)pyrene showed an absorption maximum around 400 nm, suggesting that the conjugated ring structure is preserved intact.

A binding experiment was carried out using four nucleotides. In order that both the nucleotide and hydrocarbon were solubilized, a 50% ethanol solution was used and benzoylperoxide was added to accelerate the binding reaction. After complete extraction with equal volumes of chloroform (five times) and then 10 ml of ether (three times), the solution gave an absorption spectrum, the maximum of which lies around 410 nm. As seen in Fig. 15, the absorption spectrum of the reacted 6-hydroxybenzo(a)pyrene was most prominent in the case of guanylic acid. This result, together with the above-stated experimental results on apurinic and apyrimidinic acids, indicates that the guanine residue is the main site of binding in DNA.

Correlation between 6-Hydroxybenzo(a)pyrene or 6-Oxy-benzopyrene Radical and Active Forms of Benzo(a)pyrene Induced by I_2 or H_2O_2

Iodine is well known to remove one electron from an aromatic molecule, giving rise to a cation radical. This radical is very reactive so the chemical binding formed between the active form induced by I_2 and DNA or DNA bases are unambiguously considered to be responsible for the cation radical. On the other hand, the chemical structure of the active form of benzo(a)pyrene induced by H_2O_2 has not yet been identified. H_2O_2 is a source of the OH radical, whose attack on the benzo(a)pyrene probably results in the formation of hydroxylated benzo(a)pyrene. If this were the case, the active form of benzo(a)-pyrene induced by H_2O_2 is deemed to be the hydroxylated benzo(a)-pyrene or oxy-benzopyrene radical. In fact, Hoffmann et al. (3) supposed from the difference in binding behavior that the active intermediate induced by H_2O_2 was different from that induced by I_2.

In this connection it may be interesting to examine the effect of I_2 and H_2O_2 on the carcinogenicity of benzo(a)pyrene. Whereas the effect of I_2 on the carcinogenicity of benzo(a)pyrene was nil (30), H_2O_2 showed slight accelerating effect when the carcinogenicity was compared in terms of the Iball index. Acceleration was more remarkable when Fenton's reagent, which was known as a stronger source of OH radical than H_2O_2 alone, was used instead of H_2O_2 (31).

The above results do not necessarily lend support to the idea that the active form induced by H_2O_2 or Fenton's reagent is the oxy-benzopyrene radical. But it is strongly suggested that some oxygenated

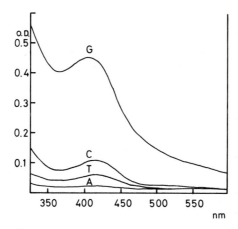

FIG. 15. Absorption spectra of 6-hydroxybenzo(a)pyrene chemically bound to the DNA bases.

benzopyrene radical is involved in the carcinogenesis mechanism of benzo(a)pyrene.

FREE RADICAL FORMATION FROM VARIOUS KINDS OF CHEMICAL CARCINOGENS

Besides benzo(a)pyrene, many chemical carcinogens were found to be converted into free radicals. Thus, 4-hydroxyaminoquinoline-1-oxide, which is considered to be a proximate form of 4-nitroquinoline-1-oxide, was converted into a free radical in organic solvents, in alkaline aqueous solution (32), or by enzymatic reaction (33). 2-Amino-1-naphthol and 1- and 2-hydroxyaminonaphthalenes, which were considered to be proximate forms of 2-naphthylamine, gave their respective free radicals (34). Further, N-methyl-N'-nitro-N-nitrosoguanidine gave an ESR signal when stirred in a buffer solution; the free radical formation depended largely upon the pH value (35). An additional example of free radical formation from the activated metabolite was given by Bartsch et al. (36, 37). They found that the proximate carcinogen, N-hydroxy-N-2-acetylaminofluorene, was oxidized enzymatically as well as chemically to yield a nitroxide radical.

The above-stated facts that proximate forms of chemical carcinogens are easily converted into free radicals are worthy of note, and the possible importance of the free radical in carcinogenesis is suggested. Although it may be premature at present to connect directly free radical formation to the genesis of tumors, the role of free radicals in chemical carcinogenesis may be worthy of study in future.

TABLE 2

Results of carcinogenicity Experiments of 6-Hydroxybenzo(a)pyrene

Animal		Solvent	Route of application	No. of applications	No. of animals	Effective no. of animals[a]	No. of animals with tumor	Duration of the experiment, days
Mouse (female)	Solvent 0.1 ml	TCR[b]	sc[c]	6	7	—	0	625
	6-OH-B 0.1 mg/0.1 ml	TCR	sc	6	8	—	0	625
	6-OH-B 0.1 mg/0.1 ml	TCR	sc	6	33	—	0	567
	6-OH-B 0.3 mg/0.1 ml	TCR	sc	1	11	—	0	497
	6-OH-B 0.06 mg/0.02 ml	TCR	ic[d]	1	10	—	0	466
	6-OH-B[e] 0.5 mg/0.25 ml	Acetone	Painting	33	10	—	0	420
	Solvent 0.1 ml	Benzene	sc	1	30	—	0	466
	6-OH-B 0.3 mg/0.1 ml	Benzene	Painting	52	33	—	0	507
	6-OH-B 0.3 mg/0.1 ml	Benzene	sc	1	30	30	1[f]	466
	6-OH-B 0.06 mg/0.02 ml	Benzene	ic	1	10	10	1[f]	466
Rat (female)	6-OH-BP 0.5 mg/0.1 ml	TCR	sc	6	6	6	5	533

[a]The number of mice surviving at the time of appearance of the first tumor.
[b]TCR, tricaprylin.   [c]sc, subcutaneous injection.   [d]ic, intracutaneous injection.
[e]Single application of DMBA (125 μg/0.25 ml) was given before the treatments of 6-OH-B.
[f]See Ref. 30

CARCINOGENIC ACTIVITY OF 6-HYDROXYBENZO(a)PYRENE

Because the 6-oxy-benzopyrene radical was proven to be a true metabolic product of benzo(a)pyrene and to bind to DNA in vitro, carcinogenicity experiments on 6-hyroxybenzo(a)pyrene, which is considered to be a precursor of the 6-oxy-benzopyrene radical, were undertaken.

In order to know the dependence of the carcinogenicity on the solvent, on route of application, and on species of animal, several preliminary experiments were carried out (Table 2). No tumor was observed in mice when tricaprylin was used as a solvent. Painting of acetone solution was also noneffective even after single application of 125 μg of dimethylbenz(a)anthracene. However, one of 30 mice and one of 10 mice developed tumors by subcutaneous and intracutaneous injections, respectively, when benzene was used as a solvent, although no tumor was observed from the painting experiment. These tumors were all malignant and histologically fibrosarcoma (Fig. 16).

Rats were more sensitive to 6-hydroxybenzo(a)pyrene than mice. Thus, by injection of the compound in tricaprylin, five of 10 rats developed malignant tumors, all of them were histologically fibrosarcoma (Fig. 17). It is noticeable that almost all those rats that survived for about one year developed tumors (Fig. 18). Experiments using various kinds of solvents are under way in our laboratory.

6-Hydroxybenzo(a)pyrene was proven to be carcinogenic to experimental animals, especially to rats; nonetheless its carcinogenicity was far lower than that of benzo(a)pyrene. This seemed to throw some doubts on the supposition that 6-hydroxybenzo(a)pyrene or 6-oxy-benzopyrene radical is a proximate form of benzo(a)pyrene. However, it is not necessarily true that an active form of a carcinogen is more carcinogenic than its parent compound, especially when the active intermediate is unstable. Thus, as was pointed out by Dipple et al. (38), the relationship between the site of production of the active metabolite within the cell and the location of the essential cellular receptor is a factor of great importance. In this connection, our finding that considerable amounts of enzyme capable of converting benzo(a)pyrene into the 6-oxy-benzopyrene radical were located in the nuclear fraction should be kept in mind. Benzo(a)pyrene molecules are considered to reach the nuclei in an intact state and to be metabolized by the enzyme within the nuclei to active intermediates. On the other hand, active intermediates generated outside the nuclei are considered to react with cellular components before penetrating to the nuclei. The difficulty inherent in the experiment on test animals might be overcome partly by in vitro experiments using tissue cultured cells, which are under study by our group.

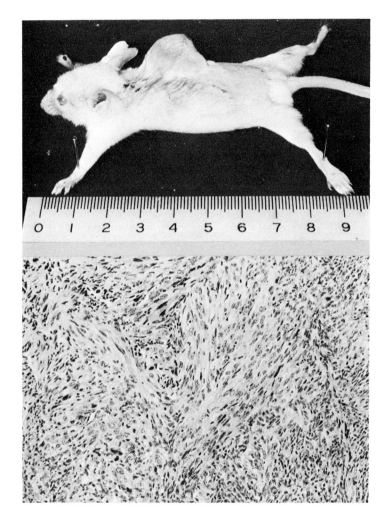

FIG. 16. Fibrosarcoma produced in mice by subcutaneous injection
of 6-hydroxybenzo(a)pyrene in benzene.

SUMMARY

1. A free radical was produced enzymatically by incubating benzo(a)-
pyrene with rat liver homogenate at 37°C, and it was identified as
the 6-oxy-benzopyrene radical. The enzyme was distributed mainly
in the microsomal and nuclear fractions, to a lesser extent in the

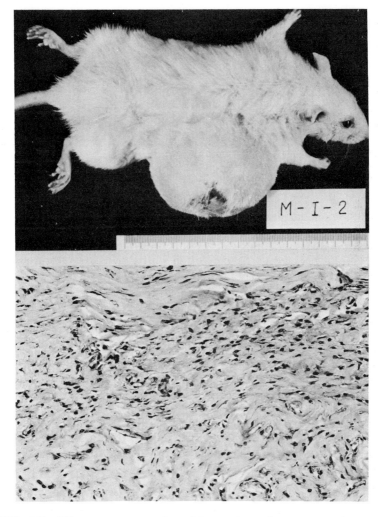

FIG. 17. Fibrosarcoma produced in rat by subcutaneous injection of 6-hydroxybenzo(a)pyrene in tricaprylin.

supernatant fraction, and only a small amount in mitochondria. Induction of the enzyme by methylcholanthrene was observed as in the case of 3-hydroxybenzo(a)pyrene.

2. The 6-oxy-benzopyrene radical was produced enzymatically by incubating benzo(a)pyrene with rat or mouse skin homogenate which is the target tissue of benzopyrene carcinogenesis.

3. 6-Hydroxybenzo(a)pyrene, which was assumed to be a precursor

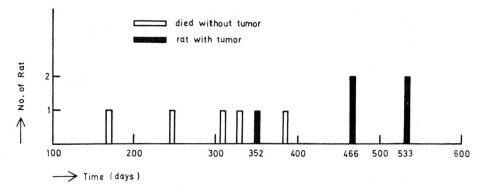

FIG. 18. Tumor production in 10 rats (Donryu strain) treated with
6-hydroxybenzo(a)pyrene.

of the 6-oxy-benzopyrene radical, was found to form a physical
complex with DNA. This complex was slowly converted into a
chemically bound form without addition of any activator. Under
the same conditions, no chemical binding occurred between
benzo(a)pyrene and DNA. Single-stranded DNA was more likely
to bind to 6-hydroxybenzo(a)pyrene than was double-stranded
DNA. Binding to the single-stranded DNA was accelerated by
benzoylperoxide, H_2O_2, or Cu^{2+}, whereas binding was diminished
by alkali or EDTA. Binding of 6-hydroxybenzo(a)pyrene to
apyrimidinic acid was 40 times as great as the binding to apurinic
acid, showing that purine bases are the main site of binding. The
experiment on the binding between 6-hydroxybenzo(a)pyrene and
DNA bases proved that the guanine residue is the preferred binding
site.

4. 6-Hydroxybenzo(a)pyrene was proven to have feeble carcinogen-
    icity in mice, but rather potent carcinogenicity was found in rats.
    Carcinogenicity depended largely upon the conditions used: that
    is, as a solvent, benzene was more effective than tricaprylin in
    the case of mice, and subcutaneous or intracutaneous injection
    was more favorable than painting to the skin.

ACKNOWLEDGMENTS

The authors thank Dr. Waro Nakahara for his encouragement
throughout this work and Dr. Shoichi Oboshi for the histological
preparation and diagnosis. The authors also thank Dr. Harry V.
Gelboin for his kindness in supplying 3-hydroxybenzo(a)pyrene.
This work was supported in part by a Grant-in-Aid for Scientific
Research from the Ministry of Education.

REFERENCES

1. C. E. Morreal, T. L. Dao, K. Eskins, C. L. King, and J. Dienstag, Peroxide induced binding of hydrocarbons to DNA, Biochim. Biophys. Acta, 169, 224 (1968).
2. P. O. P. Ts'o, S. A. Lesko, and R. S. Umans, "The Physical Binding and the Chemical Linkage of Benzopyrene to Nucleotides, Nucleic Acids and Nucleohistone," Physicochemical Mechanisms of Carcinogenesis (E. D. Bergmann and B. Pullman, eds.), Israel Academy of Science and Humanities, Jerusalem, 1969, p. 106.
3. H. D. Hoffmann, S. A. Lesko, Jr., and P. O. P. Ts'o, Chemical linkage of polycyclic hydrocarbons to deoxyribonucleic acids and polynucleotides in aqueous solution and in a buffer-ethanol solvent system, Biochemistry, 9, 2594 (1970).
4. S. A. Lesko, Jr., P. O. P. Ts'o, and R. S. Umans, Interaction of nucleic acids, V. Chemical linkage of 3, 4-benzopyrene to deoxyribonucleic acid in aqueous solution, Biochemistry, 8, 2291 (1969).
5. M. Wilk and W. Girke, "Radical Cations of Carcinogenic Alternant Hydrocarbons, Amines, and Azo Dyes, and Their Relations with Nucleobases," Physicochemical Mechanisms of Carcinogenesis (E. D. Bergmann and B. Pullman, eds.), Israel Academy of Science and Humanities, Jerusalem, 1969, p. 91.
6. P. L. Grover and P. Sims, Metabolic formation of a K-region epoxide of benzo(a)pyrene, Proc. Amer. Cancer Assoc., 13, 25 (1972).
7. P. L. Grover, P. Sims, E. Huberman, H. Marquardt, T. Kuroki, and C. Heidelberger, In vitro transformation of rodent cells by K-region derivatives of polycyclic hydrocarbons, Proc. Nat. Acad. Sci., 68, 1098 (1971).
8. H. Marquardt, T. Kuroki, E. Huberman, J. K. Selkirk, C. Heidelberger, P. L. Grover, and P. Sims, Malignant transformation of cells derived from mouse prostate by epoxide and other derivatives of polycyclic hydrocarbons, Cancer Res., 32, 716 (1972).
9. C. Nagata, M. Inomata, M. Kodama, and Y. Tagashira, Electron spin resonance study on the interaction between the chemical carcinogens and tissue components. III. Determination of the structure of the free radical produced either by stirring 3, 4-benzopyrene with albumin or incubating it with liver homogenates, Gann, 59, 289 (1968).
10. R. W. Fessenden and R. H. Schuler, Electron spin resonance studies of transient alkyl radicals, J. Chem. Phys., 39, 2147 (1963).
11. K. Fukui, T. Yonezawa, and H. Shingu, A molecular orbital theory of reactivity in aromatic hydrocarbons, J. Chem. Phys., 20, 722 (1952).

12. K. Fukui, T. Yonezawa, C. Nagata, and H. Shingu, Molecular orbital theory of orientation in aromatic, heteroaromatic, and other conjugated molecules, J. Chem. Phys., 22, 1433 (1954).
13. K. Fukui, T. Yonezawa, and C. Nagata, Interrelations of quantum-mechanical quantities concerning chemical reactivity of conjugated molecules, J. Chem. Phys., 26, 831 (1957).
14. C. Nagata, K. Fukui, T. Yonezawa, and Y. Tagashira, Electronic structure and carcinogenic activity of aromatic compounds. 1. Condensed aromatic hydrocarbons, Cancer Res., 15, 233 (1955).
15. L. F. Fieser and E. B. Hershberg, Oxidation of methylcholanthrene and 3, 4-benzopyrene with lead tetraacetate: further derivatives of 3, 4-benzopyrene, J. Amer. Chem. Soc., 60, 2542 (1938).
16. A. Windaus and S. Rennhak, Some derivatives of 3, 4-benzopyrene, Z. Physiol. Chem., 249, 256 (1937).
17. M. Inomata and C. Nagata, Photoinduced phenoxy radical of 3, 4-benzopyrene, Gann, 63, 119 (1972).
18. C. Nagata, Y. Tagashira, and M. Kodama, Electron spin resonance study on the interaction between chemical carcinogens and tissue components. II. Free radical produced by stirring aromatic hydrocarbons with tissue components such as skin homogenates or proteins, Gann, 58, 498 (1967).
19. A. Matsuyama, Y. Tagashira, and C. Nagata, A circular dichroism study on the conformation of DNA in rat liver chromatin, Biochim. Biophys. Acta, 240, 184 (1971).
20. A. H. Conney, E. C. Miller, and J. A. Miller, Substrate-induced synthesis and other properties of benzopyrene hydroxylase in rat liver, J. Biol. Chem., 228, 753 (1957).
21. H. V. Gelboin, Carcinogens, enzyme induction and gene action, Advan. Cancer Res., 10, 1 (1967).
22. E. C. Miller and J. A. Miller, The carcinogenicity of fluoro derivatives of 10-methyl-1, 2-benzanthracene, 1, 3- and 4'-monofluoro derivatives, Cancer Res., 20, 133 (1960).
23. J. A. Miller and E. C. Miller, The carcinogenicities of fluoro derivatives of 10-methyl-1, 2-benzanthracene. II. Substitution of the K region and the 3'-, 6-, and 7 positions, Cancer Res., 23, 229 (1963).
24. I. Berenblum and R. Schoental, The metabolism of 3, 4-benzpyrene in mice and rats. I. The isolation of hydroxy and a quinone derivatives, and a consideration of their biological significance, Cancer Res., 3, 145 (1943).
25. I. Berenblum, D. Crowfoot, E. R. Holiday, and R. Schoental, The metabolism of 3, 4-benzpyrene in mice and rats. II. The identification of the isolated products as 8-hydroxy-3, 4-benzpyrene and 3, 4-benzpyrene-5, 8-quinone, Cancer Res., 3, 151 (1943).

26. K. H. Harper, The intermediary metabolism of 3, 4-benzpyrene, Brit. J. Cancer, 12, 121 (1958); The intermediary metabolism of 3, 4-benzpyrene: The biosynthesis and identification of the X_1 and X_2 metabolites, ibid., 12, 645 (1958).

27. H. L. Falk, P. Kotin, S. Lee, and A. Nathan, Intermediary metabolism of benzo(a)pyrene in the rat, J. Natl. Cancer Inst., 28, 699 (1962).

28. C. Nagata, M. Kodama, Y. Tagashira, and A. Imamura, Interaction of polynuclear aromatic hydrocarbons, 4-nitroquinoline 1-oxides and various dyes with DNA, Biopolymers, 4, 409 (1966).

29. Y. Tagashira and N. Yamamota, Interaction of the two hydroxylated forms of benzo(a)pyrene with bacterial and phage genomes, to be published.

30. C. Nagata, Y. Tagashira, M. Inomata, and M. Kodama, Effect of iodine on the carcinogenicity of 3, 4-benzopyrene, Gann, 62, 309 (1971).

31. C. Nagata, Y. Tagashira, M. Kodama, Y. Ioki, and S. Oboshi, Effect of hydrogen peroxide, Fenton's reagent and Fe ions on the carcinogenicity of 3, 4-benzopyrene, Gann, 64, 277 (1973).

32. C. Nagata, N. Kataoka, A. Imamura, Y. Kawazoe, and G. Chihara, Electron spin resonance study on the free radical produced from 4-hydroxyaminoquinoline 1-oxide and its significance in carcinogenesis, Gann, 57, 323 (1966).

33. A. Matsuyama and C. Nagata, "Detection of the Unstable Intermediate, 4-Nitrosoquinoline 1-oxide," Topics in Chemical Carcinogenesis (W. Nakahara, S. Takayama, T. Sugimura, and S. Odashima, eds.), Univ. of Tokyo Press, 1972, p. 35.

34. C. Nagata, Y. Ioki, M. Inomata, and A. Imamura, Electron spin resonance study on the free radicals produced from carcinogenic aminonaphthols and N-hydroxy-aminonaphthalenes, Gann, 60, 509 (1969).

35. C. Nagata, M. Nakadate, Y. Ioki, and A. Imamura, Electron spin resonance study on the free radical production from N-methyl-N'-nitro-N-nitrosoguanidine, Gann, 63, 471 (1972).

36. H. Bartsch, M. Traut, and E. Hecker, On the metabolic activation of N-hydroxy-N-2-acetylaminofluorene. II. Simultaneous formation of 2-nitrosofluorene and N-acetoxy-N-2-acetylaminofluorene from N-hydroxy-N-2-acetylaminofluorene via a free radical intermediate, Biochim. Biophys. Acta, 237, 556 (1971).

37. H. Bartsch and E. Hecker, On the metabolic activation of the carcinogen N-hydroxy-N-2-acetylaminofluorene. III. Oxidation with horseradish peroxidase to yield 2-nitrosofluorene and N-acetoxy-N-2-acetylaminofluorene, Biochim. Biophys. Acta, 237, 567 (1971).

38. A. Dipple, P. D. Lawley, and P. Brookes, Theory of tumour initiation by chemical carcinogens: Dependence of activity on structure of ultimate carcinogen, Eur. J. Cancer, 4, 493 (1968).

Chapter 3

BASIC MECHANISMS IN POLYCYCLIC HYDROCARBON CARCINOGENESIS

P. O. P. Ts'o, W. J. Caspary, B. I. Cohen,* J. C. Leavitt,
S. A. Lesko, Jr., R. J. Lorentzen, and L. M. Schechtman

Division of Biophysics
Department of Biochemical and Biophysical Sciences
The Johns Hopkins University
Baltimore, Maryland

INTRODUCTION AND OBJECTIVES

Research on chemical carcinogenesis in our laboratory was guided by the following principles: (1) The interaction of polycyclic hydrocarbons with nucleic acids should have serious biological consequences, although carcinogenesis perhaps could also be initiated by interaction of these hydrocarbons with other cellular macromolecules. (2) Both reversible and irreversible interactions of polycyclic hydrocarbons with nucleic acids may be important for the manifestation of their biological activity and therefore should be investigated. (3) It is an enormous task to isolate and characterize the products resulting from the interaction of polycyclic hydrocarbons with nucleic acid in vivo. Therefore, the main objective of our investigation is to find an informative model system with conditions sufficiently similar to those existing in cells and tissues; this model should also exhibit a correlation between carcinogenicity and the extent of interaction of polycyclic hydrocarbons with nucleic acid, especially with DNA.

Such an investigation on the covalent linkage of these carcinogens with DNA requires us to search for suitable methods of activating the inert polycyclic hydrocarbons under mild and essentially physiological conditions, and of chemically synthesizing the presumed biologically activated intermediates which can react with the DNA. The physical, chemical, biochemical, and biologic properties of the product(s)

---

*Present address: Department of Lipid Research, Public Health Institute, New York, New York

resulting from the interaction of DNA and carcinogenic hydrocarbons should be investigated to provide information pertinent to the carcinogenic process at the molecular level. At the end, we should also ponder the basic, biologic mechanism of carcinogenesis and envisage how the chemical investigation can be made relevant to the understanding of this biologic process.

PHYSICAL BINDING OF THE POLYCYCLIC HYDROCARBON TO NUCLEIC ACID

Native and denatured DNA in equilibrium with a saturated aqueous solution of benzo(a)pyrene [B(a)P] physically bind the hydrocarbon to the extent of about one B(a)P per 1000-3000 nucleotides with binding constants ranging from 2 to 6×10^4 M^{-1} and with an apparent free energy change of 5.5 to 6 kcal in the binding process (1). Conclusive proof of the existence of a physical complex was obtained by sucrose density gradient centrifugation and density gradient electrophoresis studies. In these experiments, the DNA (measured by absorbance at 260 nm) and the [^{3}H]B(a)P were shown to move together as a single band in a centrifugal or electric field. Spectral studies demonstrated that the mode of interaction of B(a)P with DNA was by intercalation of the hydrocarbon between the base stacks in the nucleic acid. Binding studies with the homopolynucleotides showed that poly G, helical poly A (in acidic pH), and poly G·poly C complex, bind B(a)P with a much greater affinity than poly U, poly C, and neutral poly A. This observation indicates that the purine polynucleotides and polynucleotides possessing a high degree of secondary structure have a much larger affinity for the B(a)P (1, 22). The physical interaction between the polycyclic hydrocarbons with the DNA and polynucleotides show no specificity as related to the biologic properties of these compounds, i.e., the noncarcinogenic benzo(e)pyrene [B(e)P] and dibenz(a, c)-anthracene are bound to the same extent as their carcinogenic isomers, B(a)P and dibenz(a, h)anthracene. Binding of B(a)P to calf thymus nucleohistone has also been observed and confirmed by the sucrose gradient centrifugation and gradient electrophoresis (1). The extent of the binding of B(a)P to the nucleohistone is about 60% of that to the native DNA.

In conclusion, the large affinity between the polycyclic hydrocarbons [such as B(a)P] and the DNA and nucleohistone has been clearly demonstrated. In such a physical interaction, the hydrocarbons are in close contact with the planar bases (face-to-face) due to the hydrophobic-stacking properties of the bases in nucleic acid. The physical binding process, however, is not correlated to the carcinogenicity of these polycyclic hydrocarbons.

CHEMICAL LINKAGE OF THE POLYCYCLIC HYDROCARBON
TO NUCLEIC ACID

Chemical complexes of polycyclic hydrocarbons with DNA and RNA have been found in animal systems (2-7) and in cell culture systems (8-12). The available data indicate that the carcinogenic potency of these compounds can be correlated with the extent of their chemical linkage with nucleic acid (3, 9, 11). B(a)P has been covalently linked to DNA through the action of a microsomal enzyme system involving NADPH (13, 14). Since the amount of adduct formed in these biological systems is very small, it is necessary to find an in vitro model system to provide larger quantities for chemical study. Our first attempt to establish such a model system involved the use of radiation energy, the second was by chemical activation, and the third involved the chemical synthesis of an active metabolitic intermediate.

PROCEDURE FOR THE ESTABLISHMENT OF A COVALENT LINKAGE
BETWEEN DNA AND POLYCYCLIC HYDROCARBONS

When DNA is precipitated by ethanol from an aqueous solution containing a $[^3H]B(a)P$-DNA physical complex, and the precipitate is washed repeatedly with ethanol, about 99.7% of the physically bound hydrocarbon can be extracted (15, 16). However, when $[^3H]B(a)P$ is covalently linked to DNA, it can no longer be removed by precipitation and extraction with organic solvent (16). The possibility of a mere exchange of tritium between the $[^3H]$-hydrocarbon and DNA can be excluded when no radioactivity is found in the DNA extracted from a reaction mixture containing $[^3H]$-water instead of $[^3H]B(a)P$ (17).

In order to show that the chemical complex is not contaminated by any $[^3H]B(a)P$ reaction products that are insoluble in organic solvents, solutions of washed chemical complex are analyzed by physicochemical techniques. It can be demonstrated that under the influence of a force field (electrical or centrifugal), or in a system of molecular-sieve chromatography, the movement of $[^3H]B(a)P$ is coincident with the movement of DNA. These findings provide a strong argument that the $[^3H]B(a)P$ assayed after the washing procedure is actually attached to DNA.

Finally the $[^3H]B(a)P$-DNA chemical complex can be enzymatically hydrolyzed and examined by sucrose gradient electrophoresis and other chromatographic techniques. However, we do not exclude the possibility that attachment of polycyclic hydrocarbons to DNA will

inhibit complete enzymatic degradation. Demonstrating that electrophoretic migration of [^{3}H]B(a)P results from attachment to the hydrolytic products of DNA provides conclusive proof of a covalent linkage.

FORMATION OF [^{3}H]B(a)P-DNA COMPLEX WITH RADIATION ENERGY

Photoirradiation of [^{3}H]B(a)P-DNA physical complexes under nitrogen at wavelengths above 340 nm, where nucleic acid absorbs very
little photo energy, induces the formation of a chemical complex with
little damage to DNA as indicated by sedimentation analyses (15).
Under our experimental conditions, 30% of the [^{3}H]B(a)P-DNA physical
complexes are converted to chemical complexes after one hour and the
conversion reaches a maximal value of about 50% in 3 to 4 hr. Since
most of the DNA in higher organisms is in the form of nucleohistone
complexes, the formation of [^{3}H]B(a)P-nucleohistone chemical complexes as induced by photoirradiation was investigated. When
[^{3}H]B(a)P-nucleohistone physical complexes were photoirradiated for
1 hr, about 25 to 30% of the hydrocarbon became covalently linked
to the nucleohistone. About 10% of the bound radioactivity was
chemically linked to isolated histones and about 10% of the bound
radioactivity was chemically linked to DNA free of protein, while
most of the bound radioactivity (60-80%) was linked chemically to a
small fraction containing both DNA and protein. The data suggest
that photoirradiation caused a cross-link between DNA and protein
mediated in some manner through B(a)P. Upon X-ray irradiation (250 kV,
dose rate from 100 to 2500 rad/min) with dosages of 20 and 40 krad,
4-15% and 10-30%, respectively, of [^{3}H]B(a)P-DNA physical complexes were converted to chemical complexes (17). This conversion
was accompanied by degradation of DNA caused by irradiation, as
shown by the loss of viscosity and by the decrease in sedimentation
coefficient.

Preliminary experiments have been done to investigate the specificity of the photoirradiation reaction. For the same dosage of irradiation at wavelengths above 300 nm, the percentage of conversion from
physical complex to chemical complex with DNA revealed no clear-cut
specificity for carcinogenic compounds over noncarcinogenic hydrocarbons.

FORMATION OF POLYCYCLIC HYDROCARBON-DNA
CHEMICAL COMPLEXES BY CHEMICAL ACTIVATION

The success in the X-ray experiments suggested that the covalent
linkage between [^{3}H]B(a)P and DNA may be mediated by hydroxyl

radicals formed during X-ray irradiation. Rochlitz in 1967 (18) reported that B(a)P could be linked to pyridine via activation by iodine. He proposed that the reaction mechanism involves the cationic radical of B(a)P and that the product was a 6-benzo(a)pyrenyl pyridinium salt. Boyland, Kimura, and Sims in 1964 (19) have compared the reaction products of several polycyclic hydrocarbons obtained in a rat liver microsomal enzyme system with those obtained in the model hydroxylation system of Udenfriend et al. (20). The similarity of products obtained in the two systems prompted us to test the ability of the model hydroxylating system to link polycyclic hydrocarbons to DNA. Thus, the H_2O_2 system (for hydroxyl radicals), the iodine system [for the cationic B(a)P radicals], and the model hydroxylating system were the activation systems used in our chemical reactions.

Table 1 shows the specificity of chemical complex formation and the influence of the conformational states of DNA when hydrocarbons were activated with I_2 and H_2O_2. Both reactions are specific in two respects: Carcinogenic B(a)P reacts with DNA to a much greater extent than noncarcinogenic B(e)P; with B(a)P, the extent of the reaction is much higher for denatured DNA than for native DNA (16). This correlation between the specificity of the chemical reaction and the carcinogenicity of the compounds was also found in the model hydroxylating system. When a physical complex of [^{3}H]B(a)P–denatured DNA was placed in the model hydroxylating system [6.8 × 10^{-3} M EDTA, 1.4×10^{-3} M $FeSO_4$, 1.5×10^{-2} M ascorbic acid (20)] for 24 hr, there was a 42% conversion to a chemical complex. The reaction is specific with 32% of the physically bound [^{3}H]B(a)P being covalently linked after 7 hr while only 7% of the [^{3}H]B(e)P is linked in the same time period. The [^{3}H]B(a)P–DNA chemical complexes induced by iodine and H_2O_2 were also characterized by sucrose gradient electrophoresis and gel filtration chromatography before and after enzymic degradation as described in our earlier reports (16).

The extent of DNA degradation produced by these chemical reactions has been examined. No diminution in sedimentation coefficient of DNA was found after the iodine reaction. However, CsCl density gradient sedimentation as well as ultraviolet hyperchromicity studies on heat- or alkaline-denatured B(a)P–DNA revealed that a considerable portion of the DNA (up to 40%) became cross-linked upon reaction with the B(a)P in the iodine-induced reaction (21). On the other hand, there was a reduction in the sedimentation coefficient of DNA after reaction with B(a)P in a H_2O_2–$FeCl_2$ system or in the model hydroxylating system. The data suggested the occurrence of chain scission of DNA by the hydroxyl or perhydroxyl radicals (see references in 16).

We have been able to improve the reaction yield of the iodine system by conducting the reaction in a solution composed of 0.01 M

phosphate buffer (pH 6.8)-ethanol (1:1 v/v), where the concentration
of I_2 and B(a)P can be substantially increased. The kinetics of the
reaction indicate that the [³H]B(a)P becomes depleted within an hour;
therefore, the reaction yield can also be increased by adding more
[³H]B(a)P at hourly intervals during the course of a 4-hr reaction.
Finally, the DNA-[³H]B(a)P adduct can be isolated and then reacted
again under identical conditions. With a combination of these approaches and after two reaction sequences, about 3.2 molecules of
[³H]B(a)P have been linked per 10^3 bases of mouse DNA. The specificity of the iodine-induced covalent linkage of polycyclic hydrocarbons to DNA is maintained in the ethanol-phosphate buffer system,
i.e., the carcinogenic hydrocarbons [B(a)P, 7,12-dimethyl-benz(a)-
anthracene, 3-methylcholanthrene] are manyfold (4- to 14-fold) more
reactive than their noncarcinogenic analogs [B(e)P and benz(a)-
anthracene]. The extraction procedure has also been improved. The
new procedure involves the removal of iodine by chloroform extraction, the removal of the unbound hydrocarbons by phenol extraction,
and the removal of water-soluble tritium by dialysis.

BASE SPECIFICITY OF THE CHEMICALLY INDUCED COVALENT LINKAGE

The base specificity of the chemically induced covalent linkage of
polycyclic hydrocarbons to nucleic acids has been examined using

TABLE 1

Percentage of Physically Bound [³H]B(a)P and B(e)P That
Becomes Chemically Linked to DNA in Reactions Induced
by Iodine (1×10^{-4} M, 2 hr, room temperature) and
by H_2O_2 (1.5×10^{-2} M, 37°, 24 hr) in HMP [a]

	Iodine	H_2O_2	
		1×10^{-2} M citrate	1×10^{-3} M FeCl$_2$
Native DNA			
Benzo(a)pyrene	10.5	4.5	15.5
Benzo(e)pyrene	1.0	2.0	3.0
Denatured DNA			
Benzo(a)pyrene	31.5	15.0	40.0
Benzo(e)pyrene	1.0	1.0	2.0

[a] HMP — 1×10^{-2} M phosphate buffer, pH 6.8

homopolynucleotides and their double-stranded complexes as model systems (22). The reaction with [³H]B(a)P is indeed base specific with poly G being more reactive than the other polynucleotides in the iodine system. This is true even when poly G is complexed with poly C in a double helical conformation. When [³H]B(a)P is activated in a H_2O_2/Fe^{2+} system, the hydrocarbon is bound preferentially to purine polynucleotides with poly G still being the most reactive. The specificity is the same in both solvent systems, viz., 1×10^{-2} M phosphate buffer or buffer-ethanol (1:1).

In order to exclude the possibility of tritium exchange between [³H]B(a)P and poly G and to further substantiate the existence of a covalent linkage, the following experiment was performed (22). Poly G was reacted with B(a)P containing a mixture of [³H]- and [¹⁴C]-labeled hydrocarbons in a ratio of 18:1. After precipitation and washing, the isolated B(a)P-poly G complex was found to contain radioactivity with a [³H]/[¹⁴C] ratio of 15:1. This finding completely excludes the possibility that the radioactivity associated with nucleic acids, in experiments using only [³H]B(a)P, could have originated from tritium exchange. The reduction of [³H]/[¹⁴C] ratio is equivalent to a loss of about 16% of the tritium of [³H]B(a)P in reacting with poly G. Formation of a covalent bond between [³H]B(a)P and poly G should remove at least one hydrogen atom (therefore, also the corresponding amount of tritium) from the hydrocarbon. If the [³H]B(a)P is labeled randomly with the tritium, the loss of tritium should be 8.3%. Further oxidation or nonrandom labeling can lead to a greater percentage of loss as observed.

MECHANISM OF IODINE ACTIVATION OF POLYCYCLIC HYDROCARBONS

The radical cation of B(a)P has been proposed as the intermediate in the reaction of B(a)P with pyridine or nucleic acid bases in a solid phase system activated by I_2 vapor (18, 23). The 6-benzo(a)pyrenyl-pyridinium adduct reported by Rochlitz in the solid phase system (18) was also found by us in our B(a)P-pyridine-I_2-aqueous system (22). The chemical mechanism for the reaction induced by hydroxyl radicals in the H_2O_2-Fe^{2+} system does not appear to be identical to that induced by I_2 (22).

Electron spin resonance studies in our laboratory have shown the presence of B(a)P radicals (Fig. 1) induced by I_2 at 25° and measured in frozen solutions of benzene, methanol, and cyclohexane (24). The steady-state concentration of B(a)P radicals in benzene was reached rapidly (within 1 min) upon addition of I_2 and remained constant for at least 2 hr. The maintenance of constant steady-state radical

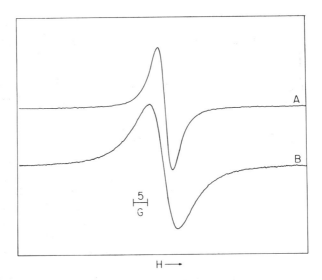

FIG. 1. EPR spectra of B(a)P (A) and MCA (B) when mixed with I_2 in benzene and quick frozen in liquid nitrogen. Spectra taken at −25° using hydrocarbon concentration of 5×10^{-4} M and I_2 concentration of 5×10^{-3} M. Modulation amplitude, 1.66 G; microwave power, 5 mW.

concentrations was also observed with other hydrocarbons in this system. The highest steady-state concentration of radicals found in the solution of B(a)P was about 10% and the formation of the radical was critically dependent on I_2 concentration (Table 2). The difference in radical concentration in the various solvents at similar I_2 concentration appears to be a result of complex formation between I_2 and benzene as well as different reaction rates of the radicals in methanol.

The steady-state radical concentration of the B(a)P radicals in benzene was not reduced by the introduction of methanol, isopropanol, acetaldehyde, and water, or by bubbling nitrogen gas through the system. The B(a)P radical concentration, however, was drastically reduced upon introduction of substituted adenosine or guanosine (substituted at the ribose hydroxyl groups to increase solubility in benzene). Table 3 shows that many nitrogenous compounds, such as imidazole, purine, pyrimidine, pyridine, aniline, and nucleosides, can quench the B(a)P radicals in methanol. The extent of quenching was proportional to the nucleoside concentration; at low nucleoside concentration, adenosine was slightly more effective as a quencher than guanosine.

The steady-state radical concentration of 14 hydrocarbons formed in the presence of I_2 have been investigated by EPR (Table 4). In

TABLE 2

Formation of B(a)P Radicals in
Different Solvents and Iodine Concentrations[a]

Iodine Concentration, M	Benzene, $-25°$		Cyclohexane, $-25°$		Methanol, $-120°$	
	Radical[b] conc, 10^{-6} M	Per cent radical[c]	Radical[b] conc, 10^{-6} M	Per cent radical[c]	Radical[b] conc, 10^{-6} M	Per cent radical[c]
2.5×10^{-1}	20	10	—	—	—	—
5×10^{-2}	19	9.5	—	—	18	9
2.5×10^{-2}	20	10	20	10	18	9
5×10^{-3}	3	1.5	17	8.5	15	7.5
2.5×10^{-3}	0	0	19	9.5	6	3
5×10^{-4}	0	0	11	5.5	0	0
2.5×10^{-4}	—	—	6	3	—	—
2×10^{-4}	—	—	7	3.5	—	—

[a] B(a)P conc at 2×10^{-4} M.

[b] Accuracy $\pm 10\%$.

[c] (Radical conc/B(a)P conc) $\times 100$.

general, the carcinogenic compounds such as B(a)P, 7,12-dimethyl-benz(a)anthracene (DMBA), 3-methylcholanthrene (MCA), and dibenzo(a,h)pyrene have a much higher concentration of radicals than the noncarcinogenic compounds, such as B(e)P, benz(a)anthracene, pyrene, anthracene, picene, dibenz(a,c)anthracene, naphthalene, and naphthacene, etc. The steady-state radical concentrations of these compounds do not correlate well with their ionization potentials, though the compounds having low ionization potentials do tend to yield higher concentrations of radicals (Table 4).

The difference in the I_2-induced steady-state radical concentration produced by carcinogenic B(a)P and noncarcinogenic B(e)P under identical conditions was found to be dependent on the concentration of I_2 and hydrocarbon in the system. Under conditions favorable for radical formation (high I_2 and hydrocarbon concentrations), the difference in radical concentrations of these two hydrocarbons is only several fold; under unfavorable conditions (low I_2 and hydrocarbon

TABLE 3

Quenching Effect of Various Compounds on B(a)P Radicals
Activated by Iodine in Methanol Solution[a]

Compound	% reduction of radical concentration	
	1 min after	2 hr after
Imidazole	66	95
Nitroimidazole	31	100
Phenol	0	0
N'-Methyl-cytosine	100	100
N^3-Methyl-uracil	71	99
Purine	100	100
N^9-Methyl-adenine	100	100
2',3'-Isopropylidene adenosine	100	100
2',3'-Isopropylene guanosine	80	84
5'-mmtr-(2',3')-ipr- Adenosine	100	100
5'-mmtr-(2',3')-ipr- Guanosine	96	100
Aniline[b]	99	—
N,N-Dimethyl-aniline[b]	99	—
Pyridine[b]	99	—
Pyrimidine[b]	99	—

[a] The compound/B(a)P ratio was 10:1. B(a)P concentration, 2×10^{-4} M; I_2 concentration, 2.5×10^{-2} M. Four minutes after mixing the B(a)P and I_2, the compound was added, and the solution was allowed to stand at room temperature for periods of 1 min and 2 hr before assaying at liquid nitrogen temperature of $-130°$.

[b] The compound/B(a)P ratio was 8:1. B(a)P concentration, 1.25×10^{-3} M; I_2 concentration, 1.6×10^{-2} M.

TABLE 4

Comparison of Ionization Potential (IP) and Steady-State Radical Concentration of Various Hydrocarbons after Mixing 5×10^{-2} M Iodine and 2×10^{-4} M Hydrocarbon

IP (Spectroscopy)	Structure	Name	Per cent of hydrocarbons found as radical		
			Benzene	Benzene–methanol mixture (v/v, 4:1)	Benzene–water mixture (v/v: 99:1)
8.12–8.16		Naphthalene	0	—	—
7.62–7.75		Picene	0	—	—
7.60–7.73		Benzo(e)-pyrene	2.5 ± 1.0	—	2.3
7.58–7.72		Pyrene	2.7	—	—
7.43–7.6		Dibenz(a,c)-anthracene	0.2	—	—

TABLE 4 (Contd)

IP (Spectroscopy)	Structure	Name	Per cent of hydrocarbons found as radical		
			Benzene	Benzene-methanol mixture (v/v, 4:1)	Benzene-water mixture (v/v, 99:1)
7.42–7.58		Dibenz(a,h)-anthracene (weakly carcinogenic)	0	—	—
7.35–7.53		Benz(a) anthracene	0.5	—	—
7.23–7.43		Anthracene	0	—	—
7.15–7.37		Benzo(a) pyrene (carcinogenic)	11 ± 1	7.6	11
6.83–7.11		Perylene	7.4	11.9	8.7

Compound				
Dibenz(a,h)-pyrene (carcinogenic)	6.75–7.04	12.5	11.3	11.7
Naphthacene[a]	6.64–6.95	3.0	—	—
7,12-dimethyl-benz(a)anthracene[b] (carcinogenic)		9.0	—	3.5–7.0
3-methyl-cholanthrene (carcinogenic)		17	13.3	19.1

[a] Recrystallized

[b] It was found that the steady-state radical concentration of DMBA is sensitive to temperature and to atmosphere, contrary to the B(a)P.

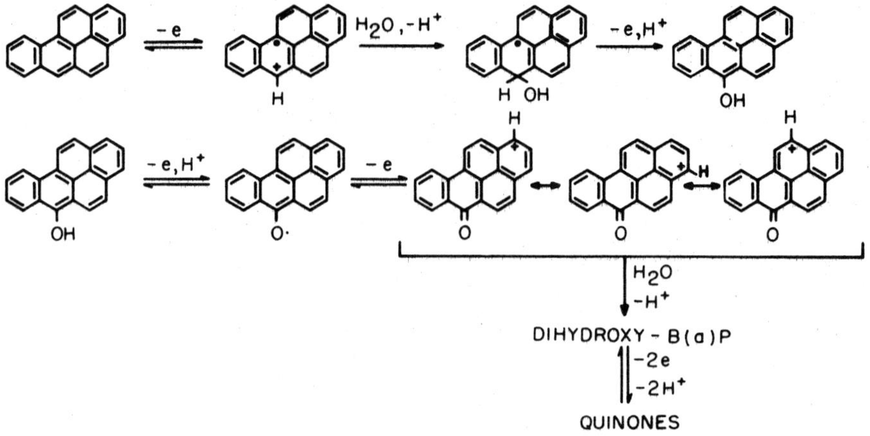

FIG. 2. General reaction scheme for electrochemical oxidation of B(a)P proposed by Jeftic and Adams (25).

concentrations), the decrease in the radical production from B(e)P is much larger, resulting in a ratio which is 10- to 100-fold in favor of B(a)P over B(e)P.

In the previous section, we described the extensive and specific chemical reaction of the carcinogens B(a)P, MCA, and DMBA with DNA and polynucleotides when induced by I_2 in an aqueous system or aqueous-ethanol system. The results in this section provide strong support for the hypothesis that the chemical reaction of these carcinogens with nucleic acid induced by I_2 proceeds via a radical intermediate(s). The formation, stabilities, and reactivities of these hydrocarbon radicals indicate that these radicals can be the active intermediates of these chemical reactions.

As for the mechanism of the formation of B(a)P radicals, the general reaction scheme (Fig. 2) proposed by Jeftic and Adams (25) and based on an electrochemical oxidation study on B(a)P appears to be applicable. In this scheme (Fig. 2) the oxidation of B(a)P can be conveniently thought to occur in two steps: the first step begins with formation of the radical cation, then the hydrated neutral radical, and finally results in 6-hydroxy B(a)P; the second step begins with the formation of a neutral oxo radical, which is then further oxidized to a carbonium ion, and finally ends with dihydroxyl-B(a)P. The dihydroxyl-B(a)P can be further oxidized to the quinone. All these radicals and the electrophilic carbonium ion species can potentially participate in chemical reactions with nucleic acids.

It is not unexpected that the steady-state concentrations of radicals produced by the 12 hydrocarbons so far investigated are not correlated with the ionization potentials of these compounds (Table 4). Since the radical concentration measured is governed by the balance between rate of formation and rate of decay, a compound such as naphthacene, which has the lowest ionization potential, may not yield the highest steady-state concentration of radicals if the radical also has a high rate of decay. On the whole, however, the hydrocarbons that have low ionization potentials and therefore greater ease in surrendering an electron, tend to yield a higher steady-state radical concentration in the I_2 oxidative system. One may expect, however, that if the initiation process in hydrocarbon carcinogenesis is related to the chemical reaction with these radicals, then the hydrocarbon that yields a high steady-state concentration of radicals will have carcinogenic activity, especially when this radical is chemically reactive to biologically active substances (such as nitrogenous compounds) but is stable in aqueous medium. By and large, this expectation is verified, though not with perfect correlation, among the 14 compounds so far investigated. Among the exceptions is the compound perylene, which is not a carcinogen but yields a relatively high steady-state concentration of radicals. This radical may be, however, less ractive toward the nucleosides. When an adenosine/hydrocarbon ratio of 0. 5 was used in a quenching experiment, B(a)P and MCA radicals were quenched by 50-60%, but the perylene radical concentration remained unchanged; with an adenosine/hydrocarbon ratio of 2, the B(a)P and MCA radicals were quenched completely while perylene radicals were quenched to about 80%. The other exception is the weak carcinogen dibenz(a, h)anthracene which does not yield any radicals. These exceptions indicate the need for further investigation and possibly the limitation of this model system of chemical oxidation of hydrocarbons. Hopefully, this study may lead to a convenient and reliable procedure for screening the carcinogenic potential of polycyclic hydrocarbons.

BIOLOGIC AND BIOCHEMICAL CONSEQUENCES OF THE COVALENT LINKAGE OF POLYCYCLIC HYDROCARBONS TO DNA

Procedures have been described earlier in this communication for obtaining a relatively high number of polycyclic hydrocarbons covalently linked to DNA, thus providing one with the material necessary to examine directly the following problems concerning the effect of the covalent linkage of carcinogenic hydrocarbons to DNA in model systems (22): (1) survival of biological activity of such DNA necessary to carry out genetic transformation, (2) the induction of forward mutation, (3) evidence for repair of damage by cellular enzymes, (4) ability of M. luteus RNA polymerase to transcribe such DNA.

The biological study was based on an in vitro transforming DNA mutation system of B. subtilis (26). The presence of chemically linked B(a)P or DMBA on the donor DNA (base/hydrocarbon ratio about 100-200) resulted in a loss of the ability of the DNA to transform the recipient strain to tryptophane-independence (21). Such reacted DNA retained only 6 to 20% of the original transforming ability (some of the loss was due to the physical handling of the DNA), while unreacted DNA containing one hydrocarbon physically bound per 100 bases retained all its original transforming activity. The DNA linked with hydrocarbons exhibited a much lower level (three- to six-fold) of biologic activity when given to the uvr⁻ or hcr⁻ strains than that obtained from the wild type. In these repair-deficient mutants, the enzyme system responsible for repair of ultraviolet light-induced lesions in DNA has been deleted or damaged. Evidence that carcinogen-induced lesions on DNA were being recognized specifically came from the fact that DNA that had a loss of transforming activity due to physical damage did not exhibit a lowering of transforming ability when assayed with the repair-deficient mutant (uvr⁻ strain). Thus, the increase in the transforming activity when assayed with the wild type (the uvr⁺ strain) instead of the uvr⁻ mutant, was due to the specific action of the enzyme system, which can repair the damage in the DNA caused by the chemical reaction with the hydrocarbon.

The covalent linkage of B(a)P and DMBA to B. subtilis SB19 transforming DNA (base/hydrocarbon ratio about 100-200) resulted in an increase (8- to 12-fold) in the frequency of forward mutation. This increase in mutation was directly correlated with the loss of transforming activity of the treated DNA (21). Unreacted DNA containing physically bound B(a)P exhibited no increase in mutation; however, I_2 alone (5×10^{-3} M) without B(a)P did cause a slight increase in mutation (three-fold). The majority of these hydrocarbon-induced mutations (89%) were not able to revert spontaneously, thus indicating that they were probably not caused by simple base-pair changes.

Covalent linkage of B(a)P on calf thymus DNA (base/hydrocarbon ratio about 330) caused up to an 80% inhibition of in vitro transcription of DNA by highly purified M. luteus RNA polymerase under template saturation conditions as compared with untreated DNA (21). A portion of this inhibition (about 30%) was due to physical damage in processing the DNA during the chemical reaction. When control DNA and B(a)P-DNA were used as templates for poly A synthesis with ATP as substrate in the RNA polymerase system, no difference was observed (21). This observation suggests that the hydrocarbon adduct on the template impaired the relative movement of the enzyme along the DNA strand rather than the enzymic polymerization of the nucleoside triphosphate. This suggestion is based on the knowledge that poly A synthesis on a

DNA template is from a reiterative copying of one base by a stationary polymerase, whereas RNA synthesis is from a transcription of the DNA base sequence along the template by a moving enzyme. Such impairment of enzyme movement should result in premature termination of the RNA synthesis.

PROPERTIES OF 6-HYDROXYBENZO(a)PYRENE [6—OH—B(a)P]

A logical step following our previous study on chemical activation of B(a)P is to search for a proximate carcinogen that may be generated inside the cell through the metabolism of B(a)P. Falk et al. (27) reported in 1962 that the first metabolite detected in the bile of rat after intravenous injection of [^{14}C]B(a)P was 6-OH-B(a)P glucuronide. Casu et al (28) and Pihar and Spaleny (29) also have identified 6-OH-B(a)P as a metabolite of B(a)P.

Chemical studies indicated that position six of the B(a)P nucleus is the most nucleophilic site on the molecule (30) and is also the primary site of attack in ordinary chemical oxidation (31) and electrochemical oxidation (25). In 1971, our laboratory reported the chemical linkage of DNA and poly G with [^{3}H]6-OH-B(a)P in a buffer-ethanol solvent system (32). Independently, this observation was also made by Nagata et al. (see Nagata et al., Chap. 4). The chemical synthesis of 6-OH-B(a)P was achieved using a modified procedure of Fieser and Hershberg (31). [^{3}H]6-OH-B(a)P with a specific activity of 3.3 × 10^{7} cpm/mmole was synthesized from [^{3}H]B(a)P to study the covalent linkage of 6-OH-B(a)P to nucleic acids.

6-OH-B(a)P is reactive and is easily oxidized to mixtures of the 1, 6; 3, 6; and 6, 12 quinones of B(a)P. Even in the solid state, when exposed to the atmosphere, this process takes place slowly and it seems to be particularly sensitive to moisture. In solution, the oxidation can take place rapidly. The difference in UV-visible spectral characteristics between 6-OH-B(a)P and the quinone products allow kinetics of the oxidation process to be followed. Absorbance at 470 nm reflects the concentration of quinones and absorbance at 390 nm reflects the concentration of 6-OH-B(a)P. Though other absorbing species are also generated during the oxidation process, these compounds apparently do not significantly affect the measurement at 390 and at 470 nm. In a solution of 0.02 M phosphate buffer — 95% ethanol (1:1 mixture), pH 7.0, at room temperature, and in the presence of polyadenylic acid, the optical data yielded pseudo first-order reaction kinetics for the oxidation process with a half-life for the reaction of about 80 min. The rate of this oxidation process is enhanced somewhat in the presence of laboratory light and in the

absence of the polynucleotides, which appear to protect the 6-OH-
B(a)P from exposure to the solvent. While the results are still preliminary, laboratory light appears to affect both the rate of formation
and the relative amounts of various oxidation products. The oxidation
process is also pH dependent with an increasing rate of oxidation at
higher pH. In organic solvents, the oxidation rate is slower in benzene, ethanol, and ether but is rather rapid in acetone and dimethylsulfoxide. Spectral analyses indicated the presence of a species which
is rather long-lived; in fact the lifetime of this species during the auto-
oxidation process is similar to the lifetime of the 6-oxy-B(a)P radicals
to be described below.

In benzene or in a 0.02 M phosphate buffer/ethanol mixture,
6-OH-B(a)P forms a radical spontaneously. This radical affords a
characteristic multiplet ESR spectrum centered at g = 2.004 (Fig. 3),
and has been identified by Nagata and co-workers (33) as the 6-oxy-
B(a)P radical (see Chap. 4). The radical is formed rapidly in buffer-
ethanol mixture, and its concentration continues to increase during
the first 100 min and then decays slowly (8-20 hr) to yield a stable
but unidentified singlet (g = 2.004). The maximal amount of radicals
formed is larger at pH 7.8 than at 6.3 (by about 2.5-fold) and is also
larger in the presence of poly A (by about 40%) than in its absence.
Laboratory light has a dramatic quenching effect on the radical concentration at the late stage of the decay process. At the very beginning
of the oxidation, exposure of the sample briefly to light has little
effect on the radical concentration. At this stage, presumably, the
formation of the radical is predominant. The results so far obtained
lead us to the conclusion that light mostly affects the stability of
the radical itself rather than its formation, since at various stages
of the reaction the light-quenched solution will give rise to more
radicals if placed in the dark. In benzene solution the radical is
much more stable than in buffer-ethanol mixture. While much more
work is needed, so far we have no direct evidence to indicate that
the 6-oxy-B(a)P radical is the immediate precursor of the quinones in
the auto-oxidation process of our experiment as would be the case in
the electrochemical oxidation process proposed by Jeftic and Adams
(25). The rate of production of quinones is more rapid than the decay
of radicals. However, a quantitative evaluation of the radical concentration as well as an understanding of the singlet radical is needed
before this question can be answered with greater certainty.

As described in the subsequent section, 6-OH-B(a)P reacts spontaneously with nucleic acid; Fig. 4 shows the kinetics of the chemical linkage of 6-OH-B(a)P to poly A, together with the kinetics of the
formation and the decay of the radicals. A certain degree of correlation results from this data that suggests that the radical could be the
species that reacts with the poly A.

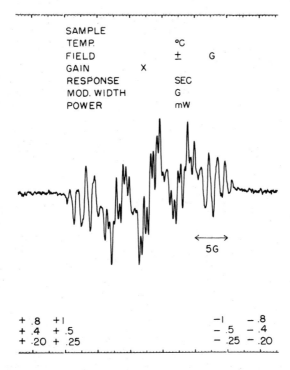

SAMPLE
TEMP.   °C
FIELD   ±   G
GAIN   X
RESPONSE   SEC
MOD. WIDTH   G
POWER   mW

5G

```
+ .8   +1                      −1      − .8
+ .4   + .5                    − .5    − .4
+ .20  + .25                   − .25   − .20
```

FIG. 3. EPR spectrum of 6-oxy-B(a)P radical in ethanol-Na phosphate buffer (1:1, pH 7.0). Modulation amplitude, 0.2 G; time constant, 1 sec; microwave power, 10 mW; room temperature.

REACTION BETWEEN 6-OH-B(a)P AND DNA

To study the chemical reactions of 6-OH-B(a)P with nucleic acids, a solvent system is needed that would dissolve moderate amounts of hydrocarbon as well as high molecular weight DNA in native form at physiological pH. The solvent systems chosen were 2×10^{-2} M Ma phosphate buffer-ethanol (1:1, pH between 7 and 8) and 5×10^{-2} M Tris-ethanol (1:1, pH 7.9). When B. subtilis transforming DNA and [³H]6-OH-B(a)P were dissolved in the phosphate buffer-ethanol system and incubated for 40 hr at room temperature (Table 5), a small portion of 6-OH-B(a)P became covalently linked to the DNA with a concomitant decay of most of the 6-OH-B(a)P to a mixture of quinones as indicated by efficiency of conversion [DNA-linked B(a)P versus quinones].

As shown in Table 5, the reaction of 6-OH-B(a)P with denatured DNA was much more extensive than with the native DNA. A reaction

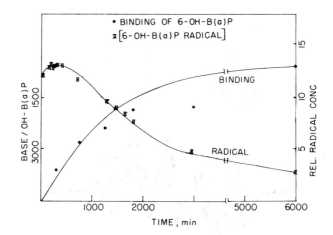

FIG. 4. Comparison of the kinetics of the 6-oxy-B(a)P radical and of the covalent binding of [³H]6-OH-B(a)P to poly A at room temperature in ethanol-Na phosphate buffer (1:1, pH 7). Hydrocarbon/base, 1:1, poly A concentration, 5×10^{-4} M in nucleotide. Radical concentration is measured by comparing the peak heights of the 6-oxy radical and a standard. After 3000 min, the 6-oxy radical concentration has diminished to zero, and the radical observed shows a singlet spectrum whose peak height is measured and included in the graph. Between 2000 and 3000 min a combination of singlet and 6-oxy radical multiplet is observed.

TABLE 5

Extent and Efficiency of Adduct Formation upon Incubation of 6-OH-B(a)P with SB 19 Transforming DNA in 1×10^{-2} Na Phosphate-Ethanol Buffer (1:1, pH 7.5) at Room Temperature[a]

Hours incubation	Base/B(a)P	Efficiency of conversion
	Native DNA	
16	13,000	1/2500
40	10,000	1/2000
	Denatured DNA	
16	2,600	1/500
40	1,550	1/300

[a] Hydrocarbon/base, 1:5; DNA concentration, 3.8×10^{-4} M in nucleotide.

with poly A and poly G (both at 4×10^{-4} M concentration) was carried out with a ratio of 6-OH-B(a)P/base of 1.6 under the same conditions as those shown in Table 5. The amount of 6-OH-B(a)P reacted was the same for both poly A and poly G: 1 B(a)P per 450 bases with an efficiency of conversion of one adduct formed per 880 quinones produced.

In these reactions, the quinones and other possible byproducts are removed from the nucleic acid by repeated extraction with phenol (previously saturated with buffer) and then with ether to remove the phenol, a procedure similar to that described for iodine reaction. The nucleic acid is then dialyzed against 1×10^{-2} M Na phosphate buffer (pH 7) to remove water-soluble radioactive contaminants. Covalent attachment has been proved by enzymic degradation of the DNA-[³H]6-OH-B(a)P and by demonstration that electrophoretic migration of hydrocarbon (measured by radioactivity) resulted from attachment to hydrolytic products of DNA as described earlier.

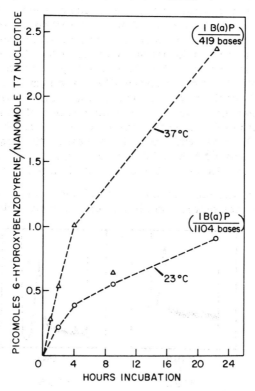

FIG. 5. Kinetics of covalent binding of [³H]6-OH-B(a)P to T7 DNA in 2×10^{-2} M Tris buffer-ethanol (1:1, pH 7.9). Hydrocarbon/base, 2.9:1; DNA concentration, 6.5×10^{-4} M in nucleotide.

Native T7 DNA also was reacted with 6–OH–B(a)P at both 23° and 37°C and with an input ratio of 6–OH–B(a)P/base of 2.9. As shown in Fig. 5, after 23 hr at 37°, one 6–OH–B(a)P was linked to about 420 bases in the T7 DNA. The yield was higher at 37° than at 23°. Introduction of higher DNA concentration (from 20 to 85 μg/0.1 ml) in the reaction mixture for a given concentration of 6–OH–B(a)P (50 μg/0.1 ml) decreased the ratio of B(a)P/base of the product as expected, but not proportionally. The increase in DNA concentration also increased the efficiency of binding of 6–OH–B(a)P to DNA versus its conversion to quinones from 1/1000 to 2.5/1000.

Incubation of T7 DNA with 6–OH–B(a)P under the conditions described above to obtain a B(a)P–DNA adduct with a B(a)P/base ratio of 1:400 resulted in considerable degradation of the DNA (three to nine double-strand breaks per genome). B(a)P–DNA adducts with lower B(a)P/base ratios (1:2000–4000) still had 10–20 single-strand breaks per genome as measured by alkaline sedimentation. Recently, we have found that addition of EDTA (0.01-1 mM) to the reaction mixture completely inhibits the production of single-strand breaks in DNA, but it also inhibits adduct formation by about 90%. Figure 6 shows that the T7 DNA sample treated with 6-OH-B(a)P together with EDTA (6B) and the control sample (6A) treated physically in the same manner without exposure to 6-OH-B(a)P, have identical sedimentation profiles in alkaline. Since the presence of such a low concentration of EDTA which does not alter the course of 6-OH-B(a)P autooxidation, but inhibits both the reaction of 6-OH-B(a)P with the DNA as well as the degradation, we tentatively conclude that the DNA degradation observed is due directly to the chemical reaction of 6-OH-B(a)P with DNA and not to other factors.

To observe the biochemical effect of the reaction of 6–OH–B(a)P with T7 DNA, templates containing various frequencies of adduct

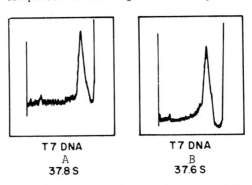

T7 DNA
A
37.8 S

T7 DNA
B
37.6 S

FIG. 6. Analytical ultracentrifugation of control T7 DNA (A) and T7 DNA (B) exposed to 6-OH-B(a)P in the presence of EDTA. The band sedimentation was conducted in 0.9 M NaCl, 0.1 M NaOH at 25,980 rpm (20°C) following the procedure described by Studier (36).

were assayed for activity with E. coli DNA-dependent RNA polymerase (holo enzyme). In this experiment, rifampicin was added at the time of initiation of transcription; addition of this drug prevented the initiation of RNA transcription at any site other than the true promotion site of T7 DNA (34, 35). Furthermore, results from the hybridization of the RNA product from this reaction to the two separated strands of T7 DNA ensured that the transcription under this condition was completely asymmetric. As compared with the control (Fig. 7), the reaction of 6-OH-B(a)P with T7 DNA dramatically inhibited its template activity with respect to RNA polymerase. At a dosage of 1 adduct per 1241 nucleotides (or 621 base pairs), total transcription was reduced more than 70%. The experiment in Fig. 8 shows that reduction in template activity was primarily due to a blockage of chain elongation. A dosage of 1 B(a)P adduct per 1241 nucleotides resulted in the reduction of the size of the RNA product from greater than 25S to approximately 8S.

It should be noted that both 6-OH-B(a)P and its synthetic precursor, 6-acetoxy-B(a)P, are very toxic to mammalian cells in culture. The 6-acetoxy-B(a)P can be hydrolyzed by an esterase such as chymotrypsin to 6-OH-B(a)P. At the concentration of 10 μg/ml of either 6-OH-B(a)P or 6-acetoxy-B(a)P, 55-66% of the Syrian hamster embryonic cells in culture were killed after a 40-hr incubation, and 87-89% killed after a 64-hr incubation. With this concentration of B(a)P, there was little effect on the growth of the hamster cells. Similar toxic effects on human neonatal cells have been observed by Dr. V. Maher (unpublished data). With 1 μg/ml concentration of 6-OH-B(a)P or 6-acetoxy-B(a)P, all human cells in culture were killed after 12 days of incubation. Again, with B(a)P at a concentration of 2.5 μg/ml, no effect on human cell growth was observed. Thus, as far as toxicity to cell growth is concerned, 6-OH-B(a)P is clearly more reactive than B(a)P.

MECHANISM OF CHEMICAL CARCINOGENESIS

In the preceding sections, various model systems have been described through which the carcinogenic hydrocarbon can form a covalent linkage with nucleic acid. Regardless of the exact mechanism of this reaction, it is known that such linkage indeed occurs inside the cell. The central question remains — How is the linkage of carcinogenic hydrocarbon to nucleic acid related to carcinogenesis? In this section, we briefly consider this problem, one that we must constantly be aware of when we conduct our in vitro experiments.

In this consideration, we adopt the phenomenon of cell transformation in vitro as a model system for in vivo carcinogenesis. Basically,

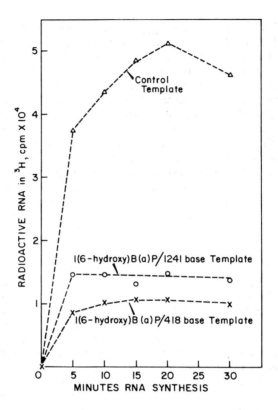

FIG. 7. The effect of 6-OH-B(a)P on the template activity of T7 DNA. Template activity was determined by the ability of T7 DNA, modified by the 6-OH-B(a)P reaction, to support DNA-dependent RNA polymerase in RNA synthesis. RNA polymerase holoenzyme was purified by the procedure of Berg, Barrett, and Chamberlin (37). RNA synthesis in the presence of rifampicin was measured as described by Dausse et al. (34). RNA polymerase (4 μg) was first preincubated with T7 DNA (2 μg) for 20 min at 23°C, and then RNA synthesis was initiated by the simultaneous addition of 5 μg/ml rifampicin and the four ribonucleoside triphosphates containing [^{3}H]UTP (0.62 μCi/nmole UTP) and further incubation at 35° for the times indicated. The following symbols represent the extent of RNA synthesis on different T7 DNA templates: Δ‐‐Δ, T7 DNA control [not exposed to 6-OH-B(a)P]; ∘‐‐∘, T7 DNA that contains one covalent 6-OH-B(a)P residue per 1241 nucleotides; x‐‐x, T7 DNA that contains one covalent 6-OH-B(a)P residue per 418 nucleotides.

this has been the approach of this volume. In the discussion of this model system, we temporarily ignore the important in vivo effects on

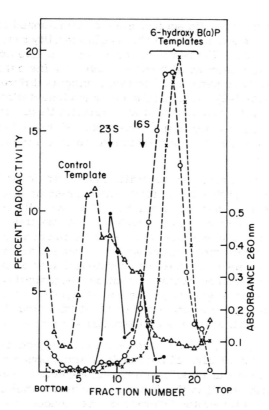

FIG. 8. Determination of the size of the RNA product synthesized with T7 DNA templates altered by the 6-OH-B(a)P reaction. RNA synthesis was described in the legend to Fig. 7. Reaction mixtures were terminated by addition of 0.5% SDS and 200 μg E. coli ribosomes. Sucrose gradient analysis of the phenol-extracted [³H]RNA synthesized is described by Leavitt, Moldave, and Nakada (38).

carcinogenesis such as hormonal control, immune response, metastasis, vascularization of the tumors, and other environmental factors. Attention is focused on this problem as a cellular event.

The characteristics of the transformed cell have been amply described in other chapters. For the present purpose, it would be useful to mention three such properties in particular. (a) The transformed cells tend to lose their sensitivity to environmental controls, e.g., decrease in sensitivity to hormones, serum factors, and cell contact inhibition; they may even lose their ability to form inducible enzymes as in the case of hydrocarbon hydroxylase induction. (b) The membrane properties of the transformed cells are different from those of nontransformed cells (39-41). One indication of cell surface

differences is the specific agglutination of transformed cells by concanavalin A. The acquisition of this agglutinability requires at least
one cell generation. The nontransformed cell can also acquire this
property through treatment with trypsin (39). (c) The cells in neoplastic tissues have patterns of protein synthesis different from those
of normal tissues (42). An indication of this characteristic is the
appearance of embryonic antigens in neoplastic tissue as described
by Coggin in his chapter in the second part of this volume. Apparently,
these three characteristics of transformed cells are interrelated at the
molecular level.

There are other characteristic traits of the transformation process
worth mentioning at this time. First, the expression of the transformation event depends upon the completion of a new cell cycle. This has
been recognized generally by the reviewers of this field. Pierce stated
that "mitotic activity is a prerequisite for carcinogenesis" (43).
Becker noted mitotic proliferation as a requirement of malignant alteration (42). Ryser observed that "cell proliferation is a fundamental
requirement for carcinogenesis. Promotion mechanism(s) (such as
phorbol esters) are essentially based on stimulation of cell proliferation" (44). Finally, Prescott concluded that "the breakdown in the
control of cell proliferation is an essential element in neoplasia" (45).

Another important characteristic related to the process of transformation is the individuality of the resulting transformed cells. This
question has been examined from different aspects by various laboratories. (a) With regard to the variation in chromosomal aberration,
Mitelman et al. (46) wrote: "Fibrosarcomas induced in Chinese
hamsters and rats by Rous sarcoma virus and DMBA are associated
with nonrandom chromosomal variation. Although histologically indistinguishable, the tumors induced by the virus or chemical in each
host species are characterized by completely different karyotypic
patterns. If the chromosomal changes are indicators of the underlying
variation in the genic material on the molecular level, it appears that
with different oncogenic agents essentially different pathways must
be involved. " (b) Concerning the variation in antigenicity of the
transformed cell, Mondal et al. (47) wrote: "Individual clones of
mouse prostate cells transformed to malignancy in vitro with MCA are
antigenic. . . . That two malignant clones within the same dish were
noncross-reactive is quite analogous to the situation in vivo, where
two tumors in the same mouse induced by the same hydrocarbon have
distinctly different antigens. . . . In the experiments on the cloned
cells, no cross-reactivity was detected in six pairs of clones derived
from the same dishes. Nor was cross-reactivity found when three
pairs of clones from different dishes were studied. . . . Our in vitro
experiments are in good accord with the vast in vivo experience that,
by and large, chemically induced sarcomas in mice are not cross-
reactive; . . . the subsequent experiments of **Vaage** and Vaage et al.

. . . found nonvirus-specific transplantation antigens in spontaneous virus-induced mouse mammary carcinomas. Some of these antigens were noncross-reactive. '' (c) With respect to the variation in response to contact inhibition of the transformed cell, Borek and Sachs (48) reported that "hamster cells transformed by polyoma virus (PV) were not inhibited by other hamster or rat cells transformed by PV; that mouse cells transformed by simian virus 40 (SV40) were not inhibited by other mouse or hamster cells transformed by SV40; but that cells transformed by PV were able to inhibit and be inhibited by cells transformed by SV40. . . . Cells transformed by X-irradiation or carcinogenic hydrocarbons did not inhibit transformed cells from the same cell line. However, two cell lines independently transformed by X-irradiation inhibited one another; a line transformed by BP inhibited a line transformed by MCA; and cells doubly transformed by X-irradiation and PV were inhibited by cells of both parental types. ''

The final characteristic of the transformation process to be considered is the relatively high scoring of transformation relative to the frequency of mutational events in cell culture. In this consideration, we should bear in mind that the precise mechanism in these in vitro mammalian cell mutation experiments has not always been firmly established (see other chapters on this subject). Nevertheless, the mutation frequencies induced by hydrocarbon carcinogens, as measured by 8-azaguanine resistance among survivors at a 50-90% survival level, are about $1/10^4$ (49); however, the transformation frequencies caused by these carcinogenic hydrocarbons vary from 1/100 to 1/10 (50, 51). The question may arise as to the validity of such a comparison between these different assay systems. Huberman, Donovan, and DiPaolo reported recently (52) that N-2-fluorenylacetamide, N-hydroxy-N-2-fluorenylacetamide, and N-acetoxy-N-2-fluorenylacetamide were studied in two cell systems: (a) Chinese hamster cells for toxicity and mutagenicity, and (b) Syrian hamster cells for toxicity and transformation. In this study, a dosage of 2 µg/ml of N-acetoxy-N-2-fluorenyl-acetamide caused about 30-40% death in Chinese hamster cells and about 0.08% mutation as scored by 8-azaguanine resistance assay; this same dose caused about 50% death in Syrian hamster cells and 2% transformation. Thus, in this particular case, a transformation frequency-mutation frequency ratio of 25 was obtained. This observation suggests that the genetic target size for transformation appears to be considerably larger (25- to 50-fold) than that for mutation. This ratio appears to be much greater if spontaneous reversion rates are taken into consideration, which for a given mammalian cell marker is about 10^{-5}-10^{-6}. On the other hand, transformed cells can have a much higher "reversion" rate. This phenomenon is especially well illustrated by the studies of Sachs and his associates (53, 54) on the reversion of the hamster cells transformed by polyoma virus. The culture of transformed cells at low cell density without a feeder layer reverted to a state in which some of the characteristics of transformation are lost. The reversion rate was found to be as much as 50% as assayed by the criterion of growth at 41°; however, this occurred without the loss of the viral genome. This culture condition also induces a change in chromosome number from diploid to aneuploid. The percentage of revertants formed under these conditions was related to the percentage of aneuploid cells, which may have a chromosomal constitution favorable for the "reverted state" and unfavorable for the "transformed state."

The above description of the characteristics of transformed cells and of the transformation process provides the background for a discussion of the mechanism of transformation. Scheme A outlines cellular events associated with the process of transformation. The lesion in the genetic apparatus resulting from an attack by the carcinogen can only be expressed after cell division(s), an event which naturally occurs in stem cells, but one which requires a promotion or a stimulation to occur in mature cells. After cell division, the genetic lesion alters the cell in such a way as to become a "mutated embryonic" cell rather than a "normal embryonic" cell, which usually goes on to differentiation and maturity (Scheme A). Instead, the "mutated embryonic" cell continues to replicate with a short G_1 phase in its life cycle and is unresponsive to environmental regulation. In vivo, such cells can become tumorigenic. Under certain conditions, these "mutated embryonic" cells go through a repair process of the genetic apparatus. This process leads to the formation of a "repaired embryonic" cell which can then proceed to differentiation.

Our model is dependent upon certain generally accepted cell properties, which include (1) stimuli receptors on the cell surface; (2) stimuli transmitters and response transmitters in the cytoplasm; and (3) regulatory machinery in the nucleus for control of the replication event and for control of the responses to stimuli. The entire stimuli-response-regulation system is certainly under the control of the genetic apparatus. The number of genes involved in this control machinery may be large, say 50 as suggested by the ratio of transformation frequency/mutation frequency described above. After cell division, the absence of a proper gene product (or the presence of an improper gene product) due to the genetic lesion caused by the carcinogenic attack, may cause a disruption of the stimuli-response-regulation process leading to the formation of a neoplastic cell. The reversion of the transformed cell due to the repair of the damaged process in this multi-channel network, can be achieved by (a) restoration of the original path, (b) bypassing the damaged step in the original path, or (c) building of a totally new path. The reverted cell,

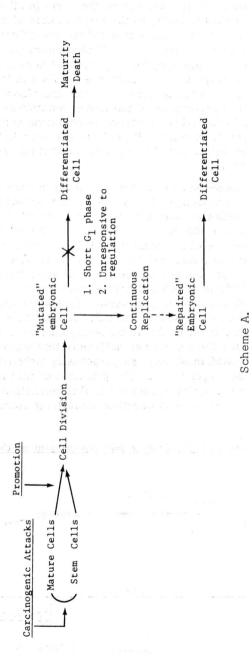

Scheme A.

while functioning normally, may not be the same in all respects as the original cell. Similarly, owing to the large number of genes vulnerable as targets, the transformed cells themselves are different in molecular details though they have similar overall physiological processes. Indeed, Scheme A and the hypothesis presented here can account for the characteristic properties of transformed cells and for the characteristics of the transformation process. This transformation hypothesis emphasizes the importance of the proper functioning of the entire battery of genes in the stimuli-response-regulation system and not any one particular "oncogene." It predicts that any disturbance of the genetic apparatus controlling regulatory function can trigger the neoplastic process.

What type of model system in cell culture is needed to test the above hypothesis critically? The model system suitable for this task should have the following characteristic, as presented in Scheme B, i.e., the ontogeny of the cell in culture should repeat the ontogeny of the tissue or even the whole organism. It is of great interest to know whether embryonic antigens can be found in cells immediately following division in a synchronous culture, and whether the expression of proteins characteristic of the differentiated state soon follows. With such a system (Scheme B) we can perhaps follow the transformation process of different cells at the molecular level. We may be able to locate the disturbance(s) in the stimuli-response-regulation system that short-circuited the growth and differentiation processes and that maintained the transformed cells as perpetually embryonic and in a state of unregulated replication. The principle of this ideal model is to reduce the more complex processes of differentiation and coordination of a metazoan to the less complex unicellular process of

Does ontogeny of the cell in culture repeat the ontogeny of the whole organism?

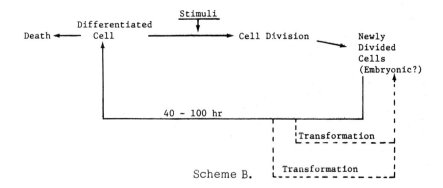

Scheme B.

macromolecular synthesis at the protozoan level. Such a simplification is necessary in that the present concepts of molecular biology are limited to phenomena related to intracellular events and do not adequately describe those at an intercellular level.

ACKNOWLEDGMENT

This research is supported in part by National Cancer Institute Grant No. CA 13370-01 and by Atomic Energy Commission Contract No. AT(11-1)-3280. W.J. Caspary is a special fellow of the National Cancer Institute, 1972. B.I. Cohen was a postdoctoral fellow of the American Cancer Society, 1970-1972. J.C. Leavitt is a postdoctoral fellow of the National Cancer Institute, 1972.

REFERENCES

1. S.A. Lesko, A. Smith, P.O.P. Ts'o, and R.S. Umans, Interaction of nucleic acids. IV. The physical binding of 3, 4-benzpyrene to nucleosides, nucleotides, nucleic acids, and nucleoprotein, Biochemistry, 7, 434 (1968).
2. P. Brookes and C. Heidelberger, Isolation and degradation of DNA from cells treated with tritium labeled 7, 12-dimethylbenz-(a)anthracene: Studies on the nature of the binding of this carcinogen to DNA, Cancer Res., 29, 157 (1969).
3. P. Brookes and P.D. Lawley, Evidence for the binding of poly-nuclear aromatic hydrocarbons to the nucleic acids of mouse skin: Relation between carcinogenic power of hydrocarbons and their binding to deoxyribonucleic acid, Nature, 202, 781 (1964).
4. L.M. Goshman and C. Heidelberger, Binding of tritium labelled polycyclic hydrocarbons to DNA of mouse skin, Cancer Res., 27, 1678 (1967).
5. F.C. Carlassare, C. Antonello, F. Baccichetti, and P. Malfer, On the binding of benz(a)pyrene to DNA in vivo, Naturforsch., 27b, 200 (1972).
6. D.H. Janss, R.C. Moon, and C.C. Irving, The binding of 7, 12-dimethylbenz(a)anthracene to mammary parenchyma DNA and protein in vivo, Cancer Res., 32, 254 (1972).
7. R.S. Zeiger, R. Salomon, N. Kinoshita, and A.C. Peacock, The binding of 9, 10-dimethyl-1, 2, -benzanthracene to mouse epidermal satellite DNA in vivo, Cancer Res., 32, 643 (1972).
8. S.H. Yuspa, S.D.A. Eaton, D.L. Morgan, and R.P. Bates, The binding of 7, 12-dimethylbenz(a)anthracene to replicating and non-replicating DNA in cell cultures, Chem.-Biol. Interactions, 1, 223 (1969/70).

9. M. Ducan, P. Brookes, and A. Dipple, Metabolism and binding to cellular macromolecules of a series of hydrocarbons by mouse embryo cells in culture, Intern. J. Cancer, 4, 813 (1969).

10. M. Ducan and P. Brookes, The relation of metabolism to macromolecular binding of the carcinogen benzo(a)pyrene by mouse embryo cells in culture, Intern. J. Cancer, 6, 496 (1970).

11. M. Ducan and P. Brookes, Metabolism and macromolecular binding of dibenz(a, c)anthracene and dibenz(a, h)anthracene by mouse embryo cells in culture, Intern. J. Cancer, 9, 349 (1972).

12. T. Kuroki and C. Heidelberger, The binding of polycyclic aromatic hydrocarbons to the DNA, RNA, and proteins of transformable cells in culture, Cancer Res., 31, 2168 (1971).

13. P. L. Grover and P. Sims, Enzyme-catalyzed reactions of polycyclic hydrocarbons with deoxyribonucleic acid and protein in vitro, Biochem. J., 110, 159 (1968).

14. H. V. Gelboin, A microsome-dependent binding of benzo(a)pyrene to DNA, Cancer Res., 29, 1272 (1969).

15. P. O. P. Ts'o and P. Lu, Interaction of nucleic acids. II. Chemical linkage of the carcinogen 3, 4-benzpyrene to DNA induced by photoirradiation, Proc. Nat. Acad. Sci., 51, 272 (1964).

16. S. A. Lesko, P. O. P. Ts'o, and R. S. Umans, Interaction of nucleic acids. V. Chemical linkage of 3, 4-benzpyrene to deoxyribonucleic acid in aqueous solution, Biochemistry, 8, 2291 (1969).

17. S. A. Rapaport and P. O. P. Ts'o, Interaction of nucleic acids. III. Chemical linkage of the carcinogen 3, 4-benpyrene to DNA induced by X-ray irradiation, Proc. Nat. Acad. Sci., 55, 381 (1966).

18. J. Rochlitz, Neue raktionen der carcinogenen kohlenwasserstoffe. II, Tetrahedron, 23, 3043 (1967).

19. E. Boyland, M. Kimura, and P. Sims, The hydroxylation of some aromatic hydrocarbons by the ascorbic acid model hydroxylating system and by rat-liver microsomes, Biochem. J., 92, 631 (1964).

20. S. Udenfriend, C. T. Clark, J. Axelrod, and B. Brodie, Ascorbic acid in aromatic hydroxylation. I. A model system for aromatic hydroxylation, J. Biol. Chem., 208, 731 (1954).

21. V. M. Maher, S. A. Lesko, Jr., P. A. Straat, and P. O. P. Ts'o, Mutagenic action, loss of transforming activity and inhibition of DNA template activity in vitro caused by the chemical linkage of carcinogenic polycyclic hydrocarbons to DNA, J. Bacteriol., 108, 202 (1971).

22. H. D. Hoffmann, S. A. Lesko, Jr., and P. O. P. Ts'o, Chemical linkage of polycyclic hydrocarbons to DNA and polynucleotides in aqueous solution and in a buffer-ethanol solvent system, Biochemistry, 9, 2594 (1970).

23. M. Wilk and W. Girke, "Radical Cations of Carcinogenic Alternant Hydrocarbons, Amines and Azo Dyes, and Their Reactions with Nucleo Bases, Physicochemical Mechanisms of Carcinogenesis, Vol. 1 (E. D. Bergmann and B. Pullman, eds.), Israel Academy of Sciences and Humanity, Jerusalem, 1969, p. 91.

24. W. Caspary, B. Cohen, S. A. Lesko, Jr., and P. O. P. Ts'o, Electron paramagnetic resonance study on iodine induced radicals of benzo(a)pyrene and other polycyclic hydrocarbons, Biochemistry, 12, 2649 (1973).

25. L. Jeftic and R. N. Adams, Electrochemical oxidation pathways of benzo(a)pyrene, J. Amer. Chem. Soc., 92, 1332 (1970).

26. E. Freese and H. B. Strack, Induction of mutations in transforming DNA by hydroxylamine, Proc. Nat. Acad. Sci., 48, 1796 (1972).

27. H. L. Falk, P. Kotin, S. Lee, and A. Nathan, Intermediary metabolism of benzo(a)pyrene in the rat, J. Nat. Cancer Inst., 28, 699 (1962).

28. B. Casu, A. Dansi, A. Garzia, E. Morelli, M. Reggiani, and F. Sant-Elia, Esperimenti sull'azione del fegato in vitro sopro it 3, 4-benzopirene, Tumori, 37, 527 (1951).

29. O. Pihar and V. Spaleny, Bioxidation studies. VI. 6-hydroxybenzo-(a)pyrene, a new metabolite of benzo(a)pyrene. Chem. listy, 50, 296 (1956).

30. E. Caralieri and M. Calvin, Molecular characteristics of some carcinogenic hydrocarbons, Proc. Nat. Acad. Sci., 68, 1251 (1971).

31. L. F. Fieser and E. B. Hershberg, The orientation of 3. 4-benzpyrene in substitution reactions, J. Amer. Chem. Soc., 61, 4565 (1939).

32. S. A. Lesko, Jr., H. D. Hoffmann, P. O. P. Ts'o, and V. M. Maher, "Interaction and Linkage of Polycyclic Hydrocarbons to Nucleic Acids, " in Progress in Molecular and Subcellular Biology, Vol. 2, Springer-Verlag, Heidelberg, 1971, p. 348.

33. C. Nagata, M. Inomata, M. Kodama, and Y. Tagashira, Electron spin resonance study on the interaction between the chemical carcinogens and tissue components. III. Determination of the structure of the free radical produced either by stirring 3, 4-benzpyrene with albumin or incubating it with liver homogenates, Gann, 58, 289 (1968).

34. J.-P. Dausse, A. Sentenac, and P. Fromageot, Interaction of RNA polymerase from E. coli with DNA, Europ. J. Biochem., 26, 43 (1972).

35. A. M. Wu, S. Ghosh, H. Schols, and W. G. Spiegelman, Repression by the cI protein of λ phage, J. Mol. Biol., 67, 407 (1972).

36. F. W. Studier, Sedimentation studies of the size and shape of DNA, J. Mol. Biol., 11, 373 (1965).

37. D. Berg, K. Barrett, and M. Chamberlin, "Purification of Two Forms of E. coli RNA Polymerase and Sigma Component, " in Methods in Enzymology, Vol. XXI D, Academic Press, New York, 1971, p. 506.

38. J. C. Leavitt, K. Moldave, and D. Nakada, Stimulation of in vitro RNA synthesis by ribosomes and ribosomal proteins, J. Mol. Biol., 70, 15 (1972).

39. M. Inbar and L. Sachs, Interaction of the carbohydrate-binding protein concanavalin A with normal and transformed cells, Proc. Nat. Acad. Sci., 63, 1419 (1969).

40. M. Inbar, H. Ben-Bassat, and L. Sachs, Membrane changes associated with malignancy, Nature New Biol., 236, 3 (1972).

41. L. Mallucci, Binding of concanavalin A to normal and transformed cells as detected by immunofluorescence, Nature New Biol., 233, 241 (1971).

42. F. F. Becker, Cell function: its importance in chemical carcinogenesis, Fed. Proc., Fed. Amer. Soc. Exp. Biol., 30, 1736 (1971).

43. G. B. Pierce, Differentiation of normal and malignant cells, Fed. Proc., Fed. Amer. Soc. Exp. Biol., 29, 1248 (1970).

44. H. J.-P. Ryser, Chemical carcinogenesis, New Eng. J. Med., 285, 721 (1971).

45. D. M. Prescott, CA: Cancer J. Clinicians, 22 (4), 262 (1972).

46. F. Mitelman, J. Mark, G. Levan, and A. Levan, Tumor etiology and chromosome pattern, Science, 176, 1340 (1972).

47. S. Mondal, P. T. Iype, L. M. Griesbach, and C. Heidelberger. Antigenicity of cells derived from mouse prostate cells after malignant transformation in vitro by carcinogenic hydrocarbons, Cancer Res., 30, 1593 (1970).

48. C. Borek and L. Sachs, The difference in contact inhibition of cell replication between normal cells and cells transformed by different carcinogens, Proc. Nat. Acad. Sci., 56, 1705 (1966).

49. E. Huberman, L. Aspiras, C. Heidelberger, P. L. Grover, and P. Sims, Mutagenicity to mammalian cells of epoxides and other derivatives of polycyclic hydrocarbons, Proc. Nat. Acad. Sci., 68, 3195 (1971).

50. P. L. Grover, P. Sims, and E. Huberman, In vitro transformation of rodent cells by K-region derivatives of polycyclic hydrocarbons, Proc. Nat. Acad. Sci., 68, 1098 (1971).

51. J. A. DiPaolo, P. J. Donovan, and R. L. Nelson, Quantitative studies of in vitro transformation by chemical carcinogens, J. Nat. Cancer Inst., 42, 867 (1969).

52. E. Huberman, P. J. Donovan, and J. A. DiPaolo, Mutation and transformation of cultured mammalian cells by N-acetoxy-N-2-fluorenylacetamide, J. Nat. Cancer Inst., 48, 837 (1972).

53. Z. Rabinowitz and L. Sachs, Control of the reversion of properties in transformed cells, <u>Nature</u>, <u>225</u>, 136 (1970).
54. N. Bloch-Shtacher, Z. Rabinowitz, and L. Sachs, Chromosomal mechanism for the induction of reversion in transformed cells, <u>Intern. J. Cancer</u>, <u>9</u>, 632 (1972).

Chapter 4

INTERACTION OF THE CARCINOGEN
7-METHYLBENZ(a)ANTHRACENE
WITH DNA OF MAMMALIAN CELLS

Peter Brookes, William M. Baird, and Anthony Dipple

Chemical Carcinogenesis Division
Chester Beatty Research Institute
Institute of Cancer Research: Royal Cancer Hospital
Fulham Road, London

Polycyclic hydrocarbons probably comprise the most extensively studied class of chemical carcinogens, but the molecular basis of their action still remains in doubt. The nature of the essential cellular receptor is still a matter of conjecture. Professor Heidelberger's group has produced evidence suggesting the involvement of protein binding (1, 2); we were impressed by a positive correlation between carcinogenic potency of a series of hydrocarbons and the extent to which they were bound to the DNA of mouse skin following topical application (3). Subsequent studies (4, 5) with other classes of chemical carcinogens revealed similar correlations between tumor-initiating ability and DNA binding, while such was not found for RNA or protein binding.

While some classes of chemical carcinogens, such as the alkylating agents, react directly with cellular macromolecules, others, including the hydrocarbons, require in vivo activation to become reactive species.

The use of rodent embryo cells in culture allowed hydrocarbon metabolism to be studied quantitatively and enabled the relationship between binding and metabolism to be assessed (6-8). The general conclusions from such studies are summarized in Table 1. It was found that on the basis of the binding index, hydrocarbons could be divided into two groups as shown in Table 2. Those compounds with index values of binding to DNA greater than 10 are generally considered to be potent carcinogens while those with values less than 1 are usually considered to have little or no initiating activity. It

149

TABLE 1
Summary of Data on Hydrocarbon Metabolism
by Mammalian Cells in Culture

1. Some cells in culture can metabolize hydrocarbons, some cannot (6).

2. Hydrocarbons are only toxic to those cells which metabolize the hydrocarbon (11, 25).

3. In the absence of metabolism, no binding of hydrocarbons to cellular macromolecules occurs (23).

4. The sensitivity of cells to hydrocarbon toxicity may be lost on prolonged growth in culture (24).

5. Carcinogenic and noncarcinogenic hydrocarbons are metabolized equally well by mammalian cells (7).

6. Only in the case of carcinogenic hydrocarbons does metabolism lead to significant binding to cellular macromolecules (7, 8).

should perhaps be emphasized that all the hydrocarbons tested were readily metabolized by the mouse embryo cells, but in the case of the weak initiators this did not lead to appreciable nucleic acid binding. This could result either from the rapid breakdown of any reactive intermediate or from the failure of the metabolism to yield such a species.

The results summarized in Tables 1 and 2 do not resolve the problem of the mechanism of the DNA-hydrocarbon interaction. Two overlapping approaches to this problem seem possible. The study of the pathways and products of hydrocarbon metabolism might reveal the nature of the ultimate carcinogen and this approach has been followed by several groups (9-11). Alternatively the DNA with hydrocarbon bound in vivo could be analyzed in an attempt to determine the nature of the DNA-bound products and hence deduce the nature of the reactive species involved in their formation. The work described below relates to this second method of attacking the problem in relation to the carcinogen 7-methylbenz(a)anthracene (7 MBA) (Fig. 1).

Initially the DNA with bound hydrocarbon was obtained from mouse skin, but the use of rodent embryo cells in culture provided a much more convenient source of larger quantities of DNA.

Preliminary experiments (12) indicated a number of problems inherent in the analytical approach. The main difficulty concerned the extent of hydrocarbon-DNA binding, which, using the mouse embryo

TABLE 2
Binding Index of Hydrocarbons to Cellular Macromolecules
of Mouse Embryo Cells[a]

Hydrocarbon	Binding Index		
	μmole/mole P divided by nmole/ml metabolized		μmole/100 g divided by nmole/ml metabolized
	DNA	RNA	Protein
Benz(a)anthracene	0.8	1.6	5.4
Benzo(e)pyrene	0.6	0.6	1.8
Dibenz(a, c)anthracene	1.0	1.6	7.0
Benzo(a)pyrene	13	17	11
Dibenz(a, h)anthracene	14	18	26
7-Methylbenz(a)anthracene	16	23	17
3-Methylcholanthrene	44	30	10
7, 12-Dimethylbenz(a) anthracene	170	130	22

[a]To monolayer cultures of mouse embryo cells, the appropriate [^{3}H]-labeled hydrocarbon was added so that the concentration in the medium was 0.1-1.0 μM. The metabolism and extent of macromolecular binding was measured after various times (7, 8). The binding index was calculated as the extent of reaction of the hydrocarbon with the particular macromolecule resulting from the metabolism of 1 nmole of hydrocarbon per milliliter of medium to which the cells were exposed.

cell system, was of the order of 30 μmole of 7MBA per mole phosphorus. A possible way to overcome this difficulty seemed to be the synthesis of model compounds that might mimic the in vivo reactive species, and allow larger quantities of material to be obtained by in vitro reaction.

Theoretical studies (13) had suggested that the ultimate carcinogen might be a cationic species, although the molecular orbital calculations used would apply equally well to analogous radicals. In the case

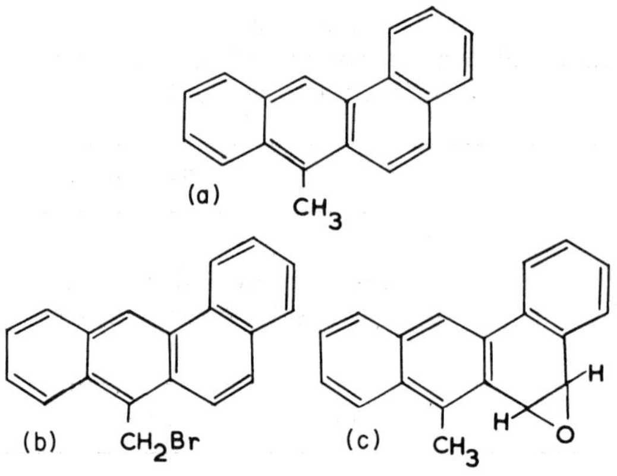

FIG. 1. Structure of hydrocarbons used in DNA binding studies.
(a) 7-methylbenz(a)anthracene; (b) 7-bromomethylbenz(a)anthracene;
(c) 7-methylbenz(a)anthracene-5, 6-oxide (K-region epoxide).

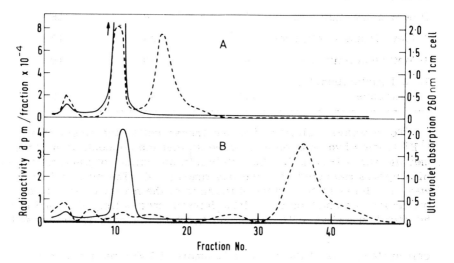

FIG. 2. (a) DNA isolated from mouse embryo cells which had been
treated with [^{3}H]7MBA or (b) DNA treated in vitro with [^{3}H]7BrMBA
was enzymatically degraded to nucleotides and chromatographed on a
column of DEAE-cellulose in 7 M urea using a 0-0.3 M sodium chloride
gradient as described by Brookes and Heidelberger (12). The UV absorption at 260 nm and the radioactivity of each fraction (6 ml) was
determined. The solid line shows the UV absorption and the dotted
line the tritium radioactivity.

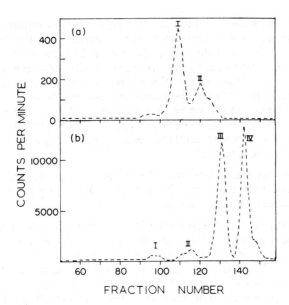

FIG. 3. (a) DNA isolated from mouse embryo cells which had been treated with [³H]7MBA or (b) salmon sperm DNA treated in vitro with [³H]7MBA-5, 6-oxide, i.e., K-region epoxide was degraded to nucleosides with DNase, snake venom diesterase, and bacterial alkaline phosphatase. The resulting solution was applied to a column (80×1.5 cm) of LH20 Sephadex packed in a 3:7 methanol to water mixture. The column was developed with a 30-100% methanol gradient and 4.5 ml fractions were collected. The dotted lines show the radioactivity in 1.0 ml samples of each fraction. (For full details of this procedure see Baird and Brookes, Cancer Res., 33, 2398 (1973).

of 7MBA the cation was predicted to result from metabolism at the methyl group, as previously suggested by Miller and Miller (14) and Boyland and Sims (15).

This reasoning led to the synthesis of 7-bromomethylbenz(a)-anthracene (7BrMBA; Fig. 1) and a study of its reaction with polynucleotides including DNA (16).

Methods for the isolation of hydrocarbon products had to take account of the fact that such moieties were usually irreversibly absorbed by materials normally employed in the fractionation of nucleic acid degradation products. Some success was achieved by the use of DEAE-cellulose in 7 M urea and a gradient of sodium chloride. The elution profiles obtained after degradation to nucleotides of DNA having in vivo bound [³H]7MBA and DNA reacted in vitro with

[^{3}H]7BrMBA are shown in Fig. 2. Although the fractionation achieved was not perfect, it was obvious that the products of the 7BrMBA reaction were not those obtained from DNA with in vivo bound 7MBA, and this finding has been confirmed using the better fractionation methods described below. It is beyond the scope of the present paper to review the published data (17) on the chemistry and biologic properties of bromomethylbenz(a)anthracene derivatives, but it is worth noting that in bacterial cells and in mammalian cells, 7BrMBA reacts in vitro with nucleic acids at the extranuclear amino groups of guanine, adenine, and probably cytosine (16).

The DEAE-cellulose system did not completely separate the 7MBA-DNA products from unreacted deoxynucleotides, and the presence of 7 M urea created recovery problems.

The introduction of LH20 Sephadex and methanol elution proved very valuable in the isolation of the 7BrMBA-DNA products as deoxy-nucleosides, but this system still failed to give complete separation of the 7MBA-DNA products. However, a satisfactory fractionation was achieved using water:methanol gradient elution on LH20 Sephadex [Fig. 3(a)]. In this system the four normal deoxynucleosides elute in the first 50 fractions while the 7MBA-DNA products elute after fraction 100. With this improved system it was possible to show by reisolation and subsequent column and paper chromatography that almost 50% of the tritium activity in the DNA was present in the normal deoxynucleosides. The mechanism by which this occurs is not yet understood.

That epoxides might be intermediates in the metabolism of hydrocarbons was suggested by Boyland in 1950 (18). Interest in this view has been revived by the work of other authors in this volume, and the reader is referred to their chapters for a review of the recent work with these compounds. We were naturally interested in 7MBA-5,6-oxide (i.e., the K-region epoxide of 7MBA, Fig. 1) as a model for the reaction of 7MBA in vivo, and we are indebted to our colleagues, Dr. P. Sims and Dr. P.L. Grover, for providing a tritium-labeled sample of this material. Reaction of the epoxide with DNA in vitro, subsequent degradation to deoxynucleosides, and fractionation as described gave the elution profile seen in Fig. 3(b). Comparison with the profile for 7MBA-DNA [Fig. 3(a)] suggested that the only possible overlap was with one of the minor epoxide-DNA products. To resolve this question, DNA was reacted extensively with unlabeled 7MBA-epoxide by Dr. Sims and Dr. Grover. After degradation and fractionation as described above, UV markers of the epoxide products were obtained. These markers and the radioactive products from [^{3}H]7MBA-DNA [Fig. 3(a) peaks I and II] were cochromatographed using the LH20 gradient system. The conclusion reached from these studies was that if any in vitro epoxide-DNA product was formed by in vivo 7MBA-DNA binding, it could not represent more than 1% of the products of reaction.

Mouse embryo cells in culture were now treated for 4 or 24 hr with [³H]7MBA-epoxide under similar conditions to those used with [³H]-7 MBA, and the DNA isolated. Enzymatic degradation and LH20 Sephadex fractionation showed the presence of the two major products, as seen in the elution profile of in vitro reacted DNA [Fig. 3(b), III and IV]. In addition, two small peaks were seen which eluted earlier and in the same positions as the 7MBA-DNA products [Fig. 3(a), I and II]. Subsequent rechromatography of each of these early in vivo epoxide products mixed with the appropriate [³H]7MBA-DNA peaks failed to resolve them, even when a very shallow water:methanol gradient was used. Experience with this column fractionation technique has indicated its powers of resolution (e. g., it resolves the cis and trans forms of 7-methylbenz(a)anthracene-5, 6-diol) and would suggest that in vivo, the epoxide and 7MBA products that are not separable by this procedure must be very similar if not identical.* Further work is necessary to decide between these alternatives, but the fact that the major 7MBA epoxide-DNA products, both in vitro and in vivo are not seen in the profile obtained with 7MBA bound to DNA in vivo must raise some questions as to the role of the K-region epoxide as the species responsible for in vivo binding of this hydrocarbon to DNA.

An alternative method for inducing the hydrocarbon-DNA reaction in aqueous solution was developed by Ts'o and his colleagues (19) following their own earlier work with X-ray induced binding (20), and that of Rochlitz (21) and Wilk (22) with iodine activation of hydrocarbons. Treatment of an aqueous-ethanol solution of DNA with iodine plus [³H]7MBA, as described by Ts'o (19) for benz(a)pyrene and 3-methylcholanthrene, gave an extent of reaction of 40 μmoles of hydrocarbon per mole DNA phosphorus. Enzymatic degradation and LH20 Sephadex fractionation of this DNA resulted in a complex elution pattern that included a peak eluting in the region of the major 7MBA-DNA product [Fig. 3(a), I]. Much more work with this system of activation is required before its relevance to the in vivo binding of hydrocarbons can be evaluated.

In summary it would seem that metabolism is required for the binding of carcinogenic hydrocarbons to cellular macromolecules. The relevance of this binding to the initiation of carcinogenesis and the nature of the essential cellular receptors still provokes controversy. It is hoped that the method being developed for the isolation of the products of hydrocarbon-DNA reaction and the development of model systems to reproduce these products in vitro will eventually result in their complete identification and perhaps a better understanding of the process of chemical carcinogenesis at the molecular level.

---

*For resolution of this problem see Baird et al., Cancer Res., 33, 2386 (1973).

ACKNOWLEDGMENTS

This investigation has been supported by grants to the Chester
Beatty Research Institute, Institute of Cancer Research: Royal Cancer
Hospital, from the Medical Research Council and the Cancer Research
Campaign. During the course of this investigation Dr. William M.
Baird was supported by a Damon Runyon Cancer Research Fellowship.

REFERENCES

1. C. Heidelberger, Studies on the molecular mechanism of hydro-
    carbon carcinogenesis, J. Cell. Comp. Physiol. (Suppl. 1), 64,
    129 (1964).
2. C. W. Abell and C. Heidelberger, Binding of tritium-labelled
    hydrocarbons to the soluble proteins of mouse skin, Cancer Res.,
    22, 931 (1962).
3. P. Brookes and P. D. Lawley, Evidence for the binding of poly-
    nuclear aromatic hydrocarbons to the nucleic acids of mouse skin:
    Relation between carcinogenic power of hydrocarbons and their
    binding to DNA, Nature, 202, 781 (1964).
4. M. D. Sporn and C. W. Dingman, 2-Acetylaminofluorene and 3-
    methylcholanthrene: Differences in binding to rat liver DNA in
    vivo, Nature, 210, 531 (1966).
5. N. H. Colburn and R. K. Boutwell, The binding of β-propiolactone
    and some related alkylating agents to DNA, RNA and protein of
    mouse skin: Relation between tumour-initiating power of alkyl-
    ating agents and their binding to DNA, Cancer Res., 28, 653
    (1968).
6. L. N. Andrianov, G. A. Belitsky, D. J. Ivanov, A. Y. Khesina,
    S. S. Khitrovo, L. M. Shabad and J. M. Vasiliev, Metabolic
    degradation of 3:4-benzpyrene in the cultures of normal and neo-
    plastic fibroblasts, Brit. J. Cancer, 21, 566 (1967).
7. M. Duncan, P. Brookes and A. Dipple, Metabolism and binding
    to cellular macromolecules of a series of hydrocarbons by mouse
    embryo cells in culture, Intern. J. Cancer, 4, 813 (1969).
8. M. Duncan and P. Brookes, The relation of metabolism to macro-
    molecular binding of the carcinogen benzo[a]pyrene, by mouse
    embryo cells in culture, Intern. J. Cancer, 6, 496 (1970); also
    see Metabolism and macromolecular binding of dibenz[a, c]-
    anthracene by mouse embryo cells in culture, ibid., 9, 349 (1972).
9. E. Boyland, "The Biochemistry of Aromatic Hydrocarbons, Amines
    and Urethane," Physicochemical Mechanisms of Carcinogenesis
    (F. D. Bergmann and B. Pullman, eds.), Israel Academy of Sciences
    and Humanities, Jerusalem, 1969, p. 25.

10. H. V. Gelboin, A microsome-dependent binding of benzo[a]-pyrene to DNA, Cancer Res., 29, 1272 (1969).

11. L. Diamond, C. Sardet and C. H. Rothblat, The metabolism of 7, 12-dimethylbenz[a]anthracene in cell cultures, Intern. J. Cancer, 3, 838 (1968).

12. P. Brookes and C. Heidelberger, Isolation and degradation of DNA from cells treated with tritium-labelled 7, 12-dimethylbenz-[a]anthracene. Studies on the nature of the binding of this carcinogen to DNA, Cancer Res., 29, 157 (1969).

13. A. Dipple, P. D. Lawley and P. Brookes, Theory of tumour initiation by chemical carcinogens: Dependence of activity on structure of ultimate carcinogen, Europ. J. Cancer, 4, 493 (1968).

14. E. C. Miller and J. A. Miller, Low carcinogenicity of the K-region epoxides of 7-methylbenz[a]anthracene and benz[a]anthracene in the mouse and rat, Proc. Soc. Exp. Biol. N. Y., 124, 915 (1967).

15. E. Boyland and P. Sims, The metabolism of 7, 12-dimethylbenz[a]-anthracene by rat-liver homogenates, Biochem. J., 95, 780 (1965).

16. A. Dipple, P. Brookes, D. S. Mackintosh and M. P. Rayman, Reaction of 7-bromomethylbenz[a]anthracene with nucleic acids, polynucleotides, and nucleosides, Biochemistry, 10, 4323 (1971).

17. A. Dipple and T. A. Slade, Reactivity and carcinogenicity of 7-bromomethylbenz[a]anthracene and 7-bromomethyl-12-methyl-benz[a]anthracene, Europ. J. Cancer, 6, 417 (1970); see also Studies of variously substituted 7-bromomethylbenz[a]anthracenes, ibid., 7, 473 (1971).

18. E. Boyland, The biological significance of metabolism of polycyclic compounds, Biochem. Soc. Symp., 5, 40 (1950).

19. H. D. Hoffmann, S. A. Lesko and P. O. P. Ts'o, Chemical linkage of polycyclic hydrocarbons to DNA and polynucleotides in aqueous solution and in a buffer-ethanol solvent system, Biochemistry, 9, 2594 (1970).

20. S. A. Rapaport and P. O. P. Ts'o, Chemical linkage of the carcinogen, 3, 4-benzpyrene to DNA induced by X-ray irradiation, Proc. Nat. Acad. Sci., 55, 381 (1966).

21. J. Rochlitz, Neue reaktionen der carcinogen kochlenwasserstoffe, Tetrahedron, 23, 3043 (1967).

22. M. Wilk and W. Girke, Radical cations of carcinogenic alternant hydrocarbons, amines and azo-dyes, and their reactions with nucleobases, Physicochemical Mechanisms of Carcinogenesis (E. D. Bergmann and B. Pullman, eds.), Israel Academy of Sciences and Humanities, Jerusalem, 1969, p. 91.

23. M. E. Duncan, unpublished results.

24. L. Diamond, V. Defendi and P. Brookes, The development of resistance to carcinogen-induced cytotoxicity in hamster embryo cultures, Exp. Cell Res., 52, 180 (1968).

25. L. Diamond, Metabolism of polycyclic hydrocarbons in mammalian cell cultures, Intern. J. Cancer, 8, 451 (1971).

Chapter 5

ACTION OF HALOGENOMETHYL HYDROCARBON DERIVATIVES ON
IN VITRO DNA AND RNA SYNTHESIS, AND ON tRNA PROPERTIES.
RELATIONSHIP WITH CARCINOGENIC POTENCY OF
METHYL PARENT HYDROCARBONS

Nguyen P. Buu-Hoi, Martine Croisy-Delcey, and Pierre Jacquignon

Institut de Chimie des Substances Naturelles
Centre National de la Recherche scientifique
91190 Gif-sur-Yvette, France

Cyril Chayet, Pascaline Daudel, Françoise Gachelin, Anne Jacquier,
Ghislaine Lataillade, and Jacques Moreau

Laboratoire Curie
Fondation Curie – Institut du Radium
Paris 5e, France

During the Jerusalem Symposia on Quantum Chemistry and Biochemistry (1968), Brookes and Dipple said (1) "An alternative candidate for the role of ultimate carcinogen is therefore required . . . two
new types of reactive species for the hydrocarbons were proposed.
These were aralkylating species of the general type I for unsubstituted
hydrocarbons and of the general type II (Fig. 1) for methyl substituted
hydrocarbons. Further it was shown that a positive correlation existed
between the calculated stabilities of such carbonium ions and the
carcinogenic potencies of the parent compounds." Such an hypothesis
is attractive because it is in agreement with Miller's idea (2), which
assumes that a cation would be involved in the main step of chemical
carcinogenesis.

Halogenomethyl derivatives are usually considered to be able to
easily generate cations of type II. Brookes and Dipple studied (1) the
reaction of two bromomethyl hydrocarbon derivatives with DNA, nucleosides, and nucleotides to test their hypothesis. To gather further
information on this interesting problem, we decided to follow some
perturbations produced on the cell machinery by halogenomethyl derivatives as a function of the carcinogenic power of the parent compounds.

159

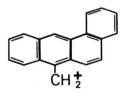

FIG. 1. A candidate for the role of ultimate carcinogen, following Brookes and Dipple (1).

We report here the effect of various halogenomethyl derivatives on the in vitro synthesis of DNA and RNA analogs and on tRNA properties.

MATERIAL AND METHODS

Halogenated Methyl Polynuclear Hydrocarbons

Bromomethyl Derivatives

Preparation of 9-bromomethylanthracene, 9-methyl 10-bromomethylanthracene, 7-bromomethylbenz(a)anthracene, 7,12-dibromomethylbenz(a)anthracene, 12-bromomethylbenz(a)acridine, and 7-bromomethylbenz(c)acridine has been described previously (3).

7-Bromomethyl 12-methylbenz(a)anthracene. 12-Methylbenz(a)-anthracene is formylated, and the aldehyde is then reduced with LiAlH$_4$ and treated with phosphorus tribromide in anhydrous benzene and refluxed for one hour. Excess PBr$_3$ is destroyed with CH$_3$OH and after several washings the organic phase is dried over sodium sulfate. Slow evaporation allows bromomethyl to crystallize in small yellow prisms (m. p. 152°, literature 140°)(4).

Analysis for C$_{20}$H$_{15}$Br

	C	H	Br
calculated	71.64	4.50	23.86
found	70.01	4.53	23.71

12-Bromomethyl 7-methylbenz(a)anthracene. A similar method is used, in which bromination is carried out in chloroform instead of benzene (m. p. 145°).

Analysis for C$_{20}$H$_{15}$Br

	C	H	Br
calculated	71.64	4.5	23.86
found	71.68	4.69	23.15

Chloromethyl Derivatives

7-Chloromethyl 12-methylbenz(a)anthracene, 7-chloromethyl--benz(a)anthracene, 9-chloromethyl 10-methylanthracene, 9-10 di-chloromethylanthracene, and 9-chloromethyl-10-methylphenanthrene were given us by Dr. Peck.

Acetoxymethyl Polynuclear Hydrocarbons

7-Acetoxymethylbenz(a)anthracene. This compound was prepared by oxidation of 7-methylbenz(a)anthracene with lead tetraacetate in acetic acid, and chromatographically purified on a silica gel column with benzene-cyclohexane (1:1) as eluant. Crystallization from alcohol yields pale yellow needles (m. p. 151-152°, literature 148-149°) (5).

Analysis for $C_{21}H_{16}O_2$

	C	H	O
calculated	83.98	5.37	10.65
found	84.02	5.19	10.70

7-Acetoxymethyl 12-acetoxybenz(a)anthracene. This compound was a by-product in the previous preparation; it appeared as pale yellow needles, m. p. 153-154°.

Analysis for $C_{23}H_{18}O_4$

	C	H	O
calculated	77.05	5.06	17.86
found	76.81	5.17	17.63

Bromo and acetoxy polynuclear hydrocarbon derivative structures were checked with NMR, and for acetoxy compounds, mass spectroscopy was employed.

Preparation of Deoxyribonucleoproteins (DNP) from Rat Liver Cells

Wistar rats were killed by decapitation and the livers perfused in situ with 0.14 M NaCl. The livers were then homogenized in 10 volumes of 0.25 M sucrose, 0.0015 M $CaCl_2$ in a mortar equipped with a Teflon pestle. The nuclei were then extracted in hypertonic sucrose media following the principle of Chauveau et al. (6); the homogenate was centrifuged 10 min at 1000 g. The resulting pellet was homogenized in 2.2 M sucrose, the suspension layered on 2.2 M sucrose, and centrifuged 60 min at 35,000 g (7). That pellet was then suspended

TABLE 1
Optical Properties of DNP

	$\dfrac{E\ 320}{E\ 260}$	$\dfrac{E\ 260}{E\ 280}$	$\dfrac{E\ 260}{E\ 240}$		$\dfrac{E\ 260}{E\ 280}$	$\dfrac{E\ 260}{E\ 230}$
DNP, unsheared	0.10	1.57	1.40	DNA	1.87	2.41
DNP, sheared	0.04	1.60	1.44			
Values calculated from the results of Manushige and Bonner	0.09	1.67	1.27			

in 0.075 M NaCl, 0.024 M EDTA pH 6.2 by the method of Dingman and Sporn (8) and centrifuged 10 min at 1000 g. The precipitate was washed by resuspension in hypotonic solution (0.2 mM EDTA pH 7.1) and homogenized with a glass mortar and Teflon pestle. Finally, sodium deoxycholate was added to the suspension to give a final concentration of 0.12%; the whole solution was layered on 1.7 M sucrose and centrifuged 120 min at 54,000 g by the method of Marushige and Bonner (9).

The nucleoprotein gel obtained is soluble in 0.2 mM EDTA; to prevent any precipitation of these materials in the DNA-dependent RNA polymerase system (as a consequence of increasing ionic force), the DNP were treated in a virtis (30 sec at 40,000 rpm).

In Table 1 the optical properties of such DNP are summarized and compared with the results of Marushige and Bonner (9).

DNA, RNA, and proteins were evaluated by the methods of Munro and Fleck for the nucleic acids (10) and Lowry et al. for proteins (11).

Preparation of Enzyme Fractions

1. DNA-dependent RNA polymerase was obtained by the method of Nakamoto et al. (12).

2. DNA-dependent DNA polymerase was prepared following Zimmerman (13). In both cases we used the fractions called V.

3. tRNA aminoacyl synthetase was prepared by the method of Wood and Berg (14).

Assays of DNA Properties after Treatment with Halogenated Methyl
Polynuclear Hydrocarbons, or Acetoxy Derivatives

RNA Polymerase System[*] (12)

Tris HCl 100, pH 7.5; $MnCl_2$, 2.5; spermidine, 1.6; DNA (calf
thymus), 0.05; GTP, UTP, CTP, 0.8, each; $[^{14}C]ATP$, 0.4 (specific
activity 2.5 $\mu Ci/\mu mole$); enzymatic fraction 20 μg proteins. Incubation
time 10 min at 30°. When DNP were used (2 to 8 μg), spermidine was
omitted, $MgCl_2$, 2 was added instead of $MnCl_2$ and mercaptoethanol
5. Incubation time, 20 min at 30°.

DNA Polymerase System (13)

Tris HCl 66, pH 7.5; $MgCl_2$, 3.3; mercaptoethanol, 1; DNA (calf
thymus), 0.1; enzymatic fraction, 18 μg; dCTP, dGTP, dATP 0.033
each; $[^{3}H]dTTP$, 0.013 (specific activity 50 $\mu Ci/\mu mole$). Incubation
time 30 min at 37°.

Assay of tRNA Properties after Treatment with 7-Bromo-
methylbenz(a)anthracene or 9-Bromomethylanthracene

Nirenberg System (15)

Tris 52, pH 7.8; thiovanol, 24; NH_4Cl, 70; ATP, 1; GTP, 0.28;
PEP, 4.3; pyruvate kinase, 16 μg; Mg acetate, 10; amino acid, 0.04
each one of them ^{14}C-labeled (specific activity 20 $\mu Ci/\mu mole$); ribo-
polynucleotide (poly A, 60 μg or poly U, 120 μg); 30S fraction, 3.6 mg
protein, incubation time 45 min at 37 °C.

Assay of Amino Acid Acceptance Capacity of tRNA (14)

Tris HCl 50, pH 7.4; $MgCl_2$, 6; PEP Na, 2.5; ATP, 2; GSH, 4;
pyruvate kinase, 20 μg; enzymatic fraction, 800 μg protein; 1 amino
acid $[^{14}C]$-labeled 20 nmoles (specific activity 20 $\mu Ci/\mu mole$). Incubation time 45 min at 37°.

Determination of Radioactivity

In all cases, at the end of incubation time, the reaction mixture
was cooled in ice, and the acid insoluble material collected on a
glass fiber filter, washed, and dried. Radioactivity was evaluated
with a Packard Tricarb Liquid Scintillation Counter.

---

[*]Concentrations, unless otherwise indicated, are given in
$\mu mole/ml$.

TABLE 2

Concentrations of Nucleic Acids and Halogenomethyl Derivatives in the Different Reactions Studied

Concentrations	RNA synthesis		DNA synthesis	Polypeptide synthesis and amino acid acceptance test
	Using DNA	Using DNP		
Halogenomethyl hydrocarbons ($\mathscr{H}$)	1.2×10^{-5}	1.4×10^{-5}	4.3×10^{-6}	1.5×10^{-3}
DNA (expressed as nucleotide residues)	16×10^{-5}	8.6×10^{-5}	16.6×10^{-5}	
tRNA (expressed as nucleotide residues)				4.5×10^{-3}
Respective evaluation of both reagents	# 7 $\mathscr{H}$ for 100 nucleotides	# 16 $\mathscr{H}$ for 100 nucleotides	# 2.5 $\mathscr{H}$ for 100 nucleotides	# 33 $\mathscr{H}$ for 100 nucleotides

Treatment of Nucleic Acids, or Deoxyribonucleoproteins with
Halogenomethyl Polynuclear Hydrocarbon or Acetoxy Derivatives

DNA and DNP Used in RNA Polymerase System (RNA synthesis)

A solution containing Tris, DNA, $MnCl_2$, and spermidine (used
further in the system) was treated for 3 min at 30° with halogenomethyl
hydrocarbon in acetone[*] (for the respective final concentrations of
hydrocarbon derivatives and DNA see Table 2). Still at 30°, the
enzymatic fraction and nucleotides (with [^{14}C]ATP) were added. A DNP
solution (140 μl EDTA 0.07 mM, pH 7 containing 1.93 nM P) was
treated with either 7-bromomethylbenz(a)anthracene or 9-bromomethyl-
anthracene in methylsulfoxide (1.25 μl). For final concentrations see
Table 2.

DNA Used in Zimmerman's System (DNA synthesis)

A solution containing the whole system except enzymatic fraction
and [^{3}H]dTTP was treated for 3 min at 37° with hydrocarbon derivatives
in acetone. See Table 2 for final concentrations.

tRNA

tRNA treatment was carried out using the method of Fink et al. (16).
An 8 ml sample of E. coli tRNA in Tris HCl 0.1 M, pH 7.8, Mg acetate
5×10^{-3} M (1.5 mg/ml) was treated two times successively with 0.4 ml
of an acetonic solution of a bromomethyl compound (see Table 2 for
final concentrations). After 5 min at 30°, excess aromatic derivatives
were extracted three times with an equal volume of ether. The aqueous
phase was then adjusted to 0.1 M with sodium acetate (pH 4.3) and
tRNA was twice precipitated in ethanol at -20°. tRNA was finally
suspended in Tris HCl 0.1 M, pH 7.8, Mg acetate 5×10^{-3} M and
adjusted to a concentration of 1.4 mg/ml.

In all cases, control samples of DNA, DNP or tRNA were identically
treated but in the absence of aromatic derivatives.

Treatment of Egg White Lysozyme with
7-Bromomethylbenz(a)anthracene

Egg white lysozyme (10 μg/ml) in Tris 5×10^{-2} M, pH 7.8, was
treated with 10 μl of an acetonic solution of 7-bromomethylbenz(a)-
anthracene (3 mg/ml) for 5 min at 25°.

Then 200 μl of this solution was added to 2 ml of Tris 5×10^{-2} M
suspension of E. coli B[E] (sensibilized with $CHCl_3$) and incubated 10

---

[*]Five microliters for 720 μl of DNA mixture.

TABLE 3
Effect of an Aqueous Solution of 7-Bromomethylbenz(a)anthracene
on Incorporation of [^{3}H]dTMP in Zimmerman's system
(expressed in cpm)

	Incubation time of the system, min			
	5	10	20	30
Control system	1930	3650	6580	9480
System treated with 7-bromomethylbenz(a)anthracene	1830	3350	6150	9500

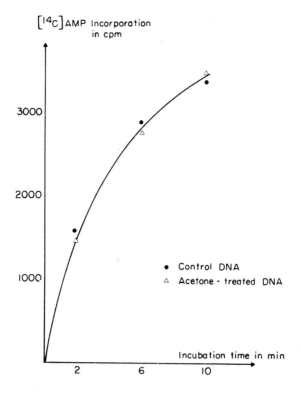

FIG. 2. Template activities of control DNA and acetone-treated
DNA in an RNA polymerase system.

min at 25°. Optical density at 450 nm was followed during 10 min and compared with a sample containing nontreated lysozyme (17).

RESULTS

Effect of Halogenated Methyl Aromatic Hydrocarbons on in Vitro Synthesis of RNA and DNA

First we check that such compounds have no effect on DNA or RNA synthesis when they are first introduced in an aqueous medium and then later on brought in contact with a DNA matrix or system.

Table 3 shows, in a study with 7-bromomethylbenz(a)anthracene, the incorporation of $[^3H]dTMP$ in acid-insoluble material in Zimmerman's system.

We also observed that acetone itself (in which halogeno aromatic derivatives are dissolved before reacting with DNA) has no effect on further properties of DNA. Figure 2 shows the incorporation of $[^{14}C]$-AMP in two different RNA polymerase systems, one working with control DNA and the other one with acetone-treated DNA.

Until now we have studied 14 halogenated polynuclear hydrocarbons from the point of view of their actions on DNA template activity in a DNA-dependent RNA polymerase system (Fig. 3). We compared the inhibitory effect of these halogenated derivatives on RNA synthesis (in test tube) with the carcinogenic potencies of the corresponding non-halogenated hydrocarbons (18). It turns out that there exists a perfect correlation between the two phenomena. While studying the effect of bromomethyl derivatives on in vitro DNA synthesis in Zimmerman's system, we also found a good correlation between the inhibitory effect that these compounds produce on $[^3H]$-dTMP incorporation and the carcinogenicity of their corresponding parent hydrocarbons with one exception: 7-bromomethylbenz(c)acridine, which is a well-known carcinogen and has no inhibitory effect (Fig. 4).

Effect on Nucleoproteins

The effect of 7-bromomethylbenz(a)anthracene and 9-bromomethyl-anthracene on template activity of nucleoproteins has been studied (Fig. 5). The four-ring compound (related to the carcinogenic non-halogenated parent) provokes an important inhibition of $[^{14}C]$-AMP incorporation in newly synthesized RNA chains, although the bromo-methylanthracene derivative (related to the noncarcinogen 9-methyl-anthracene) has almost no inhibitory effect.

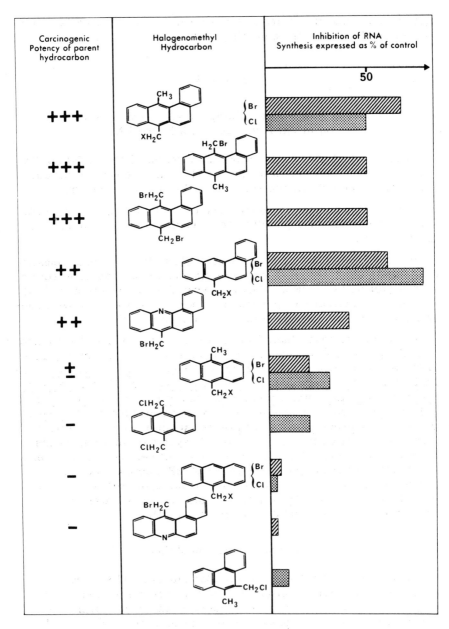

FIG. 3. Inhibition of template activity of DNA (in an RNA polymerase system) due to reaction of the nucleic acid with halogenomethyl hydrocarbon derivatives.

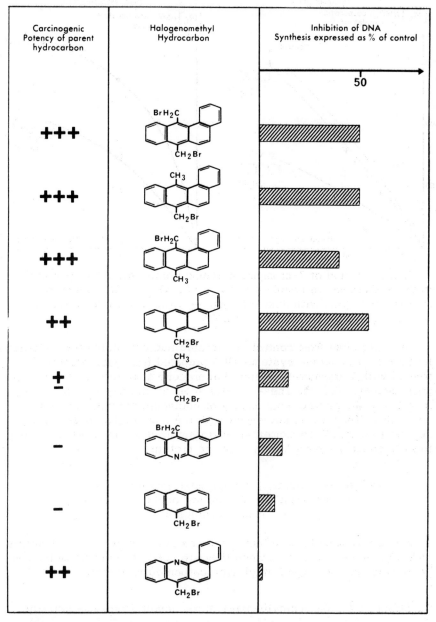

FIG. 4. Action of bromomethyl hydrocarbon derivatives on DNA synthesis.

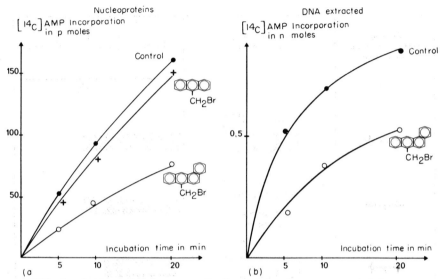

FIG. 5. Action of 7-bromomethylbenz(a)anthracene and 9-bromo-methylanthracene on template activity of DNP. (a) RNA polymerase system is working with desoxyribonucleoprotein; (b) the system is working with DNA extracted from DNP.

DNA extracted from control and treated nucleoproteins were studied in the RNA polymerase system. DNA prepared from nucleoprotein treated with 7-bromomethylbenz(a)anthracene still appears to be a poor template (Fig. 5). These results seem to indicate a preferential reaction of the nucleic acid moiety of nucleoprotein with the bromo derivative. They are in agreement with the observation of Venitt and Shooter (19) that 7-bromomethylbenz(a)anthracene binds preferentially to T7 bacteriophage DNA than to phage proteins.

Effect of 7-Acetoxy methylbenz(a)anthracene and 7-Acetoxymethyl-12-acetoxybenz(a)anthracene on DNA Synthesis

It is interesting to note that these products are absolutely inactive on DNA synthesis (at least when they are used at the same molar concentrations as the bromomethyl hydrocarbon derivatives).

Effect of 7-Bromomethylbenz(a)anthracene on Lysozyme Activity

Under the conditions described in the section on "Materials and Methods," 7-bromomethylbenz(a)anthracene-treated egg white lyso-

TABLE 4

Effect of Bromomethyl Hydrocarbon on tRNA Properties

tRNA treatment	Inhibition of polypeptide synthesis in Nirenberg's system (with treated tRNA), expressed as % of control		Inhibition of amino acid acceptance capacity of treated tRNA, expressed as % of control					
	Poly A → polylysine	Poly U → polyphenylalanine	Lysine	Phenyl-alanine	Thyrosine	Valine	Glutamic acid	Serine
7-Bromomethyl-benz(a)anthracene	48 ± 12	44 ± 13	29 ± 7	31 ± 8	11 ± 6	14 ± 11	22 ± 1	25 ± 2
9-Bromomethyl-anthracene	21 ± 13	20 ± 9	16 ± 5	14 ± 7	6 ± 3	3 ± 3	20 ± 2	22 ± 4

TABLE 5
Effect of Dose of 7-bromomethylbenz(a)anthracene
on DNA Lysine Acceptance Capacity of tRNA

Final concentration of 7-bromomethylbenz(a)-anthracene	Inhibition
1.5×10^{-3} M	40
0.75×10^{-3} M	28
0.375×10^{-3} M	12

zyme has the same lysis activity regarding E. coli B as nontreated lysozyme. This result confirms the low reactivity of such a compound with regard to protein.

Action of 7-Bromomethylbenz(a)anthracene and 9-Bromomethylanthracene on tRNA Properties

tRNA Used in Nirenberg's System

Treated tRNA was first used in a crude polypeptide synthesis system such as Nirenberg's, using either poly U or poly A to code for polypeptide synthesis. Both bromomethyl compounds have an inhibitory effect on the synthesis of either polylysine or polyphenylalanine, and the effect of 7-bromomethylbenz(a)anthracene seems slightly greater than the effect of 9-bromomethylanthracene (Table 4).

Amino Acid Acceptance Capacity of Treated tRNA

As in experiments carried out by Fink et al., who studied the action of N-acetoxyacetylaminofluorene on tRNA, we limited tRNA concentration in order to measure total acceptance capacity.

The inhibitory effects on amino acid acceptance capacity using tRNA treated by different concentrations of 7-bromomethyl aromatic hydrocarbons are reported in Table 5; the results point out a dose-dependent action.

At a concentration of 1.5×10^{-3} M we compare the effect of the two bromo derivatives. Results are summarized in Table 4.

It turns out that among the amino acid acceptance capacities we studied, a slight selectivity appears; the least selective case corresponds to tyrosine.

The four-ring compound seems to be twice as active as the three-ring compound in the test of crude polypeptide polynucleotide-directed synthesis. The differences are not so large in other tests.

DISCUSSION

The correlation that we observed between the inhibitory power of the halogenomethyl hydrocarbon derivatives on the RNA synthesis and the carcinogenic potencies of the parent compounds is very good. The probability that such a correlation is fortuitous is very small. S. S. Sung, using classical statistical methods, has shown that in fact, the probability is less than 1%.

The simplest way to interpret that relationship is to assume that an important step of the carcinogenic effect of methylaromatic hydro-carbons is the formation of a cation of type II (at least as a part of a transition state), as suggested by Brookes and Dipple, and an inhibitory effect by that ultimate cation on the nucleic acid synthesis.

Many observations which support such an interpretation can be listed.

Flesher and Sydnor (20) carried out a series of experiments [based on the findings of Boyland and Sims (21)] which led the authors to the following conclusions:

1. The first step in carcinogenesis of DMBA is the hydroxylation of the 7-methyl group.

2. The second is the formation of a derivative (e. g., sulfate ester) which would be expected to be a good leaving group and which would generate a highly reactive carbonium ion.

Furthermore, Paul (22) and Alexandrov, Vendrely, and Vendrely (23) found that various carcinogenic hydrocarbons (including 7, 12-dimethyl-benz(a)anthracene), either injected i. p. or applied topically to mouse skin, caused a preliminary decrease in the rate of RNA synthesis. The early inhibitory effects were not observed with a noncarcinogenic compound.

Also, Maher et al. (24) and Chan and Ball (25) observed an inhibition of deoxyribonucleic acid template activity in vitro caused by chemical linkage of carcinogenic polycyclic hydrocarbons to DNA.

Therefore, the simple interpretation presented here of our proposed relationship seems possible. But, obviously other interpretations could easily be found and the problem is open for more investigation.

To end, let us remark that the concentrations of halogenomethyl hydrocarbon derivatives that produced significant perturbations of tRNA properties are much more important than those which produce a significant inhibition effect on DNA or RNA synthesis.

ACKNOWLEDGMENTS

We thank F. Lutcher and J. F. Grunstein for their technical assistance, Dr. A. Mathieu and Dr. Dufour for the IR and NMR analyses of hydrocarbons derivatives which they kindly carried out for us, Dr. Eckert for helpful discussions, and Dr. Peck for his generous gift of chloro derivatives.

This investigation has been supported by grants from the "Departement de Biology" du Commissariat à l'Energie Atomique, to enable us to obtain labeled nucleotides.

Cyril Chayet is Visiting Scientist from the University of Chile, supported by a travel fellowship of "Gouvernement Français."

Ghislaine Lataillade and Jacques Moreau are holders of fellowships from "La Ligue Nationale Française contre le cancer."

REFERENCES

1. P. Brookes and A. Dipple, Physicochemical Mechanisms of Carcinogenesis, Israeli Academy of Science and Humanities, Jerusalem, 1969, p. 139.
2. See, for example, J. A. Miller and E. C. Miller, Physicochemical Mechanisms of Carcinogenesis, Israeli Academy of Science and Humanities, Jerusalem, 1969, p. 237; J. Miller, Cancer Res., 30, 559 (1970); J. A. Miller and E. C. Miller, J. Nat. Cancer Inst., 47, V (1971).
3. P. Daudel, F. Gachelin, M. Croisy-Delcey, P. Jacquignon, and N. P. Buu Hoi, Chem. Biol. Interactions, 4, 223 (1971/1972).
4. J. Pataki, R. Wlos, and Y. JaCho, J. Med. Chem., 11, 1083 (1968).
5. G. M. Badger and J. W. Cook, J. Chem. Soc., 1939, 802.
6. J. Chauveau, Y. Moulé, and C. Rouillier, Exp. Cell. Res., 11, 317 (1956).
7. R. Maggio, P. Sieckevitz, and G. E. Palade, J. Cell. Biol., 18, 267 (1963).
8. C. W. Dingman and M. B. Sporn, J. Biol. Chem., 239, 3483 (1964).
9. K. Marushige and J. Bonner, J. Mol. Biol., 15, 160 (1966).
10. H. N. Munro and A. Fleck, Methods of Biochemical Analysis, Vol. XIV, Wiley, New York, p. 159.

11. O. H. Lowry, N. J. Rosebrough, A. L. Fan, and R. J. Randall, J. Biol. Chem., 193, 265 (1951).
12. T. Nakamoto, C. F. Fox, and S. B. Weiss, J. Biol. Chem., 239, 167 (1964).
13. B. K. Zimmerman, J. Biol. Chem., 241, 2035 (1966).
14. W. B. Wood and P. Berg, Proc. Nat. Acad. Sci., 48, 94 (1962).
15. J. H. Matthaei and M. W. Nirenberg, Proc. Nat. Acad. Sci., 47, 1580 (1961).
16. L. M. Fink, S. Nishimura, and I. B. Weinstein, Biochemistry, 9, 496 (1970).
17. M. Sekiguchi and S. S. Cohen, J. Mol. Biol., 8, 638 (1964).
18. P. Shubik and J. Hartwell, Survey of compounds which have been tested for carcinogenic activity, Public Health Service Publication No. 149.
19. S. Venitt and K. V. Shooter, Biochim. Biophys. Acta, 277, 479 (1972).
20. J. W. Flesher and K. L. Sydnor, Cancer Res., 31, 1951 (1971).
21. E. Boyland and P. Sims, Intern. J. Can., 2, 500 (1967).
22. D. Paul, Cancer Res., 29, 12, 18 (1969).
23. K. Alexandrov, C. Vendrely, and R. Vendrely, Cancer Res., 30, 1192 (1970).
24. V. M. Maher, S. A. Lesko, P. A. Straat, and P. O. P. Ts'o, J. Bacteriol., 108, 202 (1971).
25. E. W. Chan and J. K. Ball, Biochim. Biophys. Acta, 238, 46 (1971).

Chapter 6

HYPOTHESIS CONCERNING THE CARCINOGENIC
ACTIVITY OF BENZ(a)ANTHRACENES

Melvin S. Newman

Regents Professor of Chemistry
The Ohio State University
Columbus, Ohio

The research in the field of chemical carcinogenesis that has been done by my group at the Ohio State University has been concerned mainly with attempts to find out how cancer is initiated by 7-methylbenz(a)anthracene [1].

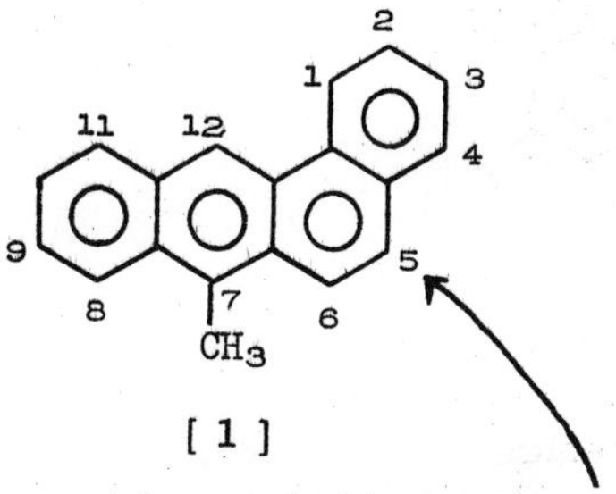

[1]

position probably involved
in carcinogenic metabolism

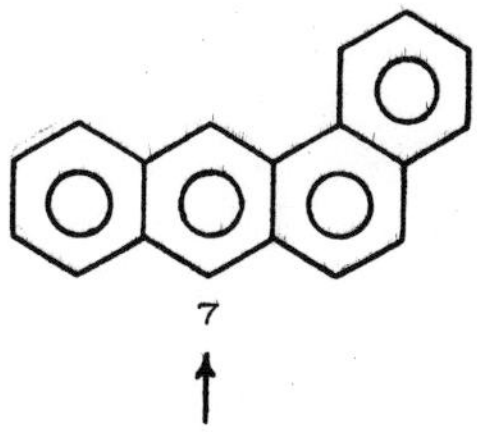

position of maximum chemical
reactivity. Also position probably involved in noncarcinogenic metabolism

At the start (about 1950), we prepared a sufficient amount of each of the monomethylbenz(a)anthracenes (1) so that any investigator who wished might be able to test all of the compounds by the same method. The results of this testing by different groups (2-6) showed that 7-methylbenz(a)anthracene is the only monomethylbenz(a)-anthracene that can be classed as a potent carcinogen. The 6-, 8-, and 12-methyl compounds have carcinogenic activity and the other derivatives are of no, or very low, activity.

177

The fact that [1] was the only potent carcinogen took on added significance when it was realized that the 7-position in benz(a)-anthracene is the one most easily attacked by a variety of chemical reagents (7). In a conversation with Dr. James A. Miller (McArdle Research Laboratory, University of Wisconsin) the following research program was initiated. My group was to prepare the 11-monofluoro-7-methylbenzanthracenes to be tested for activity by Dr. Miller. The idea was that if a fluorine atom were substituted for a hydrogen at a spot involved in the metabolic process leading to cancer then that compound would have no carcinogenic activity. If, however, the substitution of a hydrogen by fluorine yielded a compound that was appreciably carcinogenic, then the position involved would not be important in the carcinogenic mechanism.

When the compounds were made (8-13) and tested (14, 15) the result was that only 5-fluoro-7-methylbenz(a)anthracene [2] was not carcinogenic. The others (with the exceptions of the 11-fluoro and 12-fluoro compounds, which have not been tested) all proved appreciably carcinogenic (6). It thus appears that the 5-position is the important position in the metabolism leading to cancer.

[2]

noncarcinogenic

As a result of this work, the following hypothesis can be made concerning the role of benz(a)anthracenes in initiating cancer. Benz-(a)anthracenes may be metabolized in two ways in the body: (a) metabolism at position 7 results in a reaction series that leads to non-carcinogenic processes; and (b) metabolism at position 5 results in a reaction series that leads to cancer. In the parent hydrocarbon, the metabolism leading to deactivation (from the carcinogenic point of view) at position 7 must be considerably more rapid than the interaction at position 5, which leads to the production of cancer. Similarly, in other benz(a)anthracenes in which the 7-position is available for attack, one can argue that the metabolism leading to deactivation is more rapid than that leading to the production of cancer.

To assess the accuracy of the above hypotheses, the following facts should be noted.

1. 7-Methylbenzanthracene is the only monomethylbenz(a)-
    anthracene that is highly carcinogenic.

2. 6, 8-Dimethylbenz(a)anthracene [3], the only potent carcino-
    genic dimethylbenz(a)anthracene that does not have one
    methyl in the 7-position, is active because the steric effect
    of the methyl groups in the 6- and 8-positions blocks reaction
    at the 7-position (16).

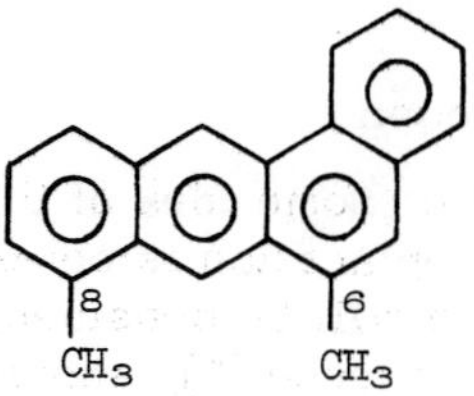

[3]

potent carcinogen

3. 5-Methyl-, 5-hydroxymethyl-, and 5-methylmercaptobenz-
    (a)anthracenes have been found to be inactive (6, 17). Hence
    groups other than fluorine in the 5-position also produce
    inactive compounds.

4. The inactivity of 5-fluoro-6, 8-dimethylbenz(a)anthracene [4]
    can be explained in the same way as the inactivity of 5-
    fluoro-7-methylbenz(a)anthracene, namely, that the metabol-
    ism that must occur at position 5 to lead to cancer is blocked.

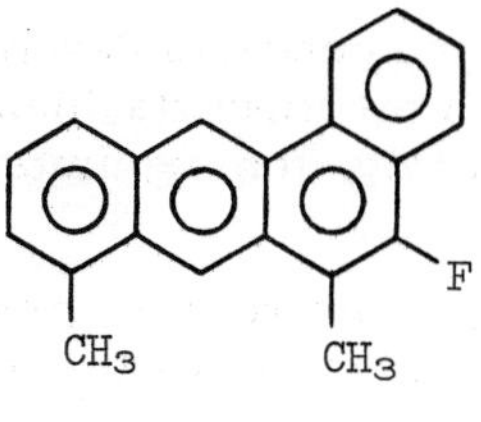

[4]

noncarcinogenic

A few words may be added in explanation of the fact that 7, 12-
dimethylbenz(a) anthracene [5] and 6, 8, 12-trimethylbenzanthracene
[6] are appreciably more active than 7-methyl- and 6, 8-dimethylbenz-
(a)anthracenes, respectively. I believe this is due to the steric effect
of the 12-methyl group. The crowding caused by this methyl group
causes the whole molecule to be strained and hence more reactive

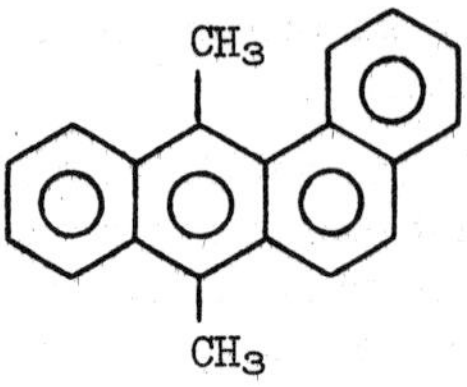

[5]

potent carcinogen

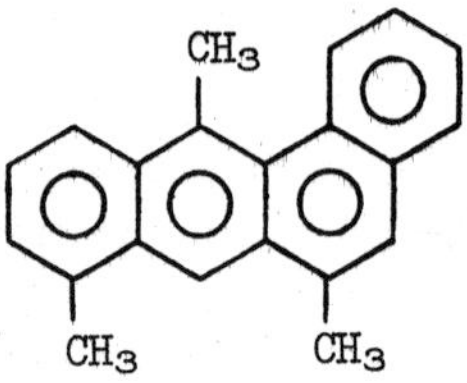

[6]

potent carcinogen

toward external reactants. Some idea of the amount of strain can be estimated (18). If this explanation is correct, then 1, 7, 12-trimethyl-benz(a)anthracene, which will be considerably more strained than 7, 12-dimethylbenz(a)anthracene [7], should be the most active carcinogen in the benz(a)anthracene series (19).

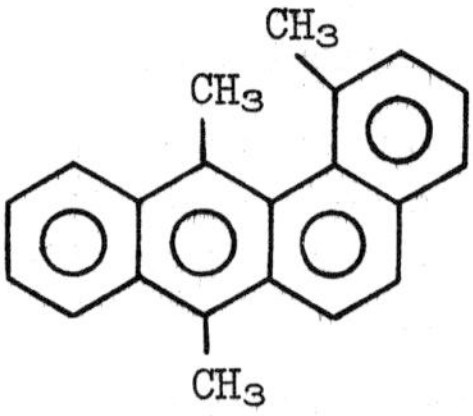

[7]

being tested

The applications of the concepts described in this paper may be extended to compounds in the dibenz(a, h)anthracene and benz(a)-pyrene series. Unfortunately, the requisite compounds have not yet been synthesized and tested.

In conclusion it is a pleasure to acknowledge the support of the National Cancer Institute of the Department of Health, Education, and Welfare for this work.

REFERENCES

1. M. S. Newman and R. Gaertner, J. Amer. Chem. Soc., 72, 264 (1950).
2. J. L. Hartwell, "Survey of Compounds Which Have Been Tested for Carcinogenic Activity," 2nd ed., U. S. Department of Health, Education, and Welfare, 1951; and P. Shubik, Supplement 1 to the above, 1957.

3. W. F. Dunning, M. R. Curtin, and M. Stevens, Proc. Soc. Exptl. Biol. Med., 128, 720 (1968).
4. J. L. Stevenson and E. von Haam, Amer. Ind. Hyg. Assoc. J., 26, 475 (1965).
5. C. B. Huggins, J. Pataki, and R. G. Harvey, Proc. Nat. Acad. Sci. U. S., 58, 2253 (1967).
6. Private communication from Dr. J. A. Miller and Dr. E. C. Miller.
7. L. F. Fieser and J. L. Hartwell, J. Amer. Chem. Soc., 60, 2555 (1938), and references therein.
8. M. S. Newman, D. MacPowell, and S. Swaminathan, J. Org. Chem., 24, 509 (1959).
9. M. S. Newman, S. Swaminathan, and R. Chatterji, J. Org. Chem., 24, 1961 (1959).
10. M. S. Newman and R. H. B. Galt, J. Org. Chem., 25, 214 (1960).
11. M. S. Newman, R. Chatterji, and S. Seshadri, J. Org. Chem., 26, 2667 (1961).
12. M. S. Newman and S. Seshadri, J. Org. Chem., 27, 76 (1962).
13. M. S. Newman and S. Blum, J. Org. Chem., 29, 1414 (1964).
14. E. C. Miller and J. A. Miller, Cancer Res., 20, 133 (1960).
15. J. A. Miller and E. C. Miller, Cancer Res., 23, 229 (1963).
16. M. S. Newman and S. Blum, J. Med. Chem., 7, 466 (1964).
17. M. S. Newman and R. F. Cunico, J. Med. Chem., 15, 323 (1972).
18. M. A. Frisch, C. Baker, J. L. Margrave, and M. S. Newman, J. Amer. Chem. Soc., 85, 2356 (1963).
19. Work in this area is underway.

Chapter 7

NEW TYPE OF CATALYZED REACTION BETWEEN POLYCYCLIC AROMATIC HYDROCARBONS AND PURINES OR PYRIMIDINES

Wolfgang Girke[*] and Manfred Wilk

Institut für organische Chemie
Johann Wolfgang Goethe Universität
Frankfurt/Main, Germany

Since 1966, when radical cations were first proposed as possible activated forms of carcinogenic polycyclic hydrocarbons, an increasing number of papers (1) have been published supporting this or similar aspects (2-8).

As organic chemists, we are particularly interested in the mode of activation of aromatic carcinogens and in their possible reactions with molecules of biological importance.

Our first model reaction, proposed in Jerusalem in 1968 (9), demonstrated that radical cations of benzo(a)pyrene, produced by iodine, react readily with different nucleobases to covalently bounded conjugates.

To test this proposition, Nagata (10) and associates injected mice with an iodine solution immediately after a single subcutaneous application of benzo(a)pyrene; the result was that no accelerating effect on the carcinogenicity of the hydrocarbon could be observed. However, in our opinion, this does not rule out radical cations as possible "ultimate carcinogens." Under the conditions of Nagata's experiment, i. e. , in the presence of hydroxyl ions, the very reactive radical cations have no chance of reaching a nucleophilic cell constituent of biological importance. These cations should be generated in the immediate neighborhood of the cell receptors. We cannot force this by experiment. We must try to elucidate if the cell itself, by enzymatic activation, produces radical cations as active intermediates.

---

[*]Present address: Institute for Organic Chemistry, The Hebrew University, Jerusalem, Israel.

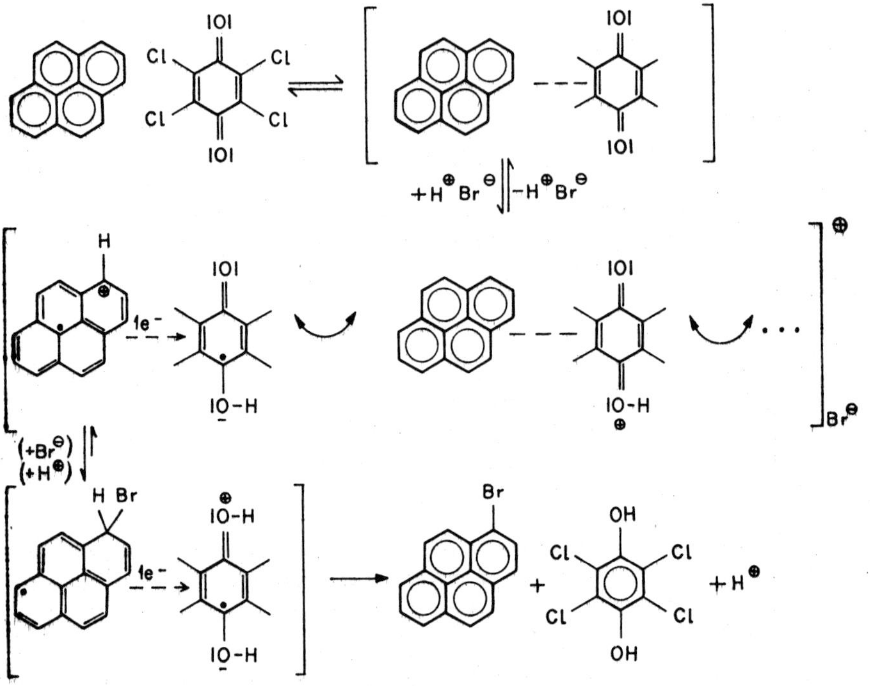

FIG. 1. Nucleophilic substitution of pyrene via an EDA complex in the presence of a nucleophilic anion (Br⁻).

After the "iodine experiments," we changed the electron acceptor and found that covalently bonded conjugates could be formed between a nucleophilic partner and polycyclic hydrocarbons by one-electron oxidation via electron-donor-acceptor (EDA) complexes.

By adding acids with nucleophilic anions to the benzene solution of an EDA complex composed of hydrocarbons with good donor-properties and tetrachlorobenzoquinone (both ortho and para), in some cases we obtained, at room temperature, in nearly quantitative yield, the substituted hydrocarbons (11). A possible mechanism for this reaction is proposed in Fig. 1.

We assume the first step to be the protonation of the quinone, leading to an increased electron affinity that enables the complete electron transfer from the donor to the acceptor molecule even in the ground state. The second step will be the electrophilic attack by the resulting radical cation on the nucleophilic anion of the present acid. A second one-electron uptake by the quinone leads to the substituted hydrocarbon.

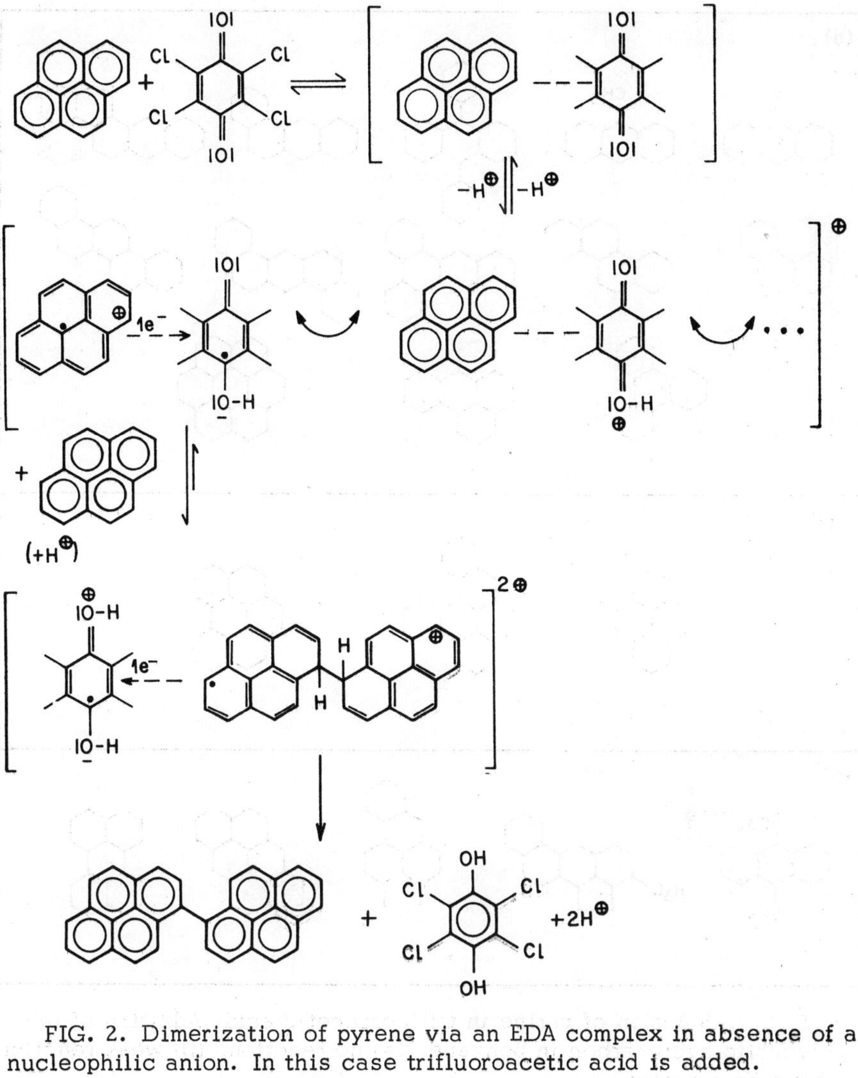

FIG. 2. Dimerization of pyrene via an EDA complex in absence of a nucleophilic anion. In this case trifluoroacetic acid is added.

If the anion of the added acid has no marked nucleophilic properties, then nearly quantitative dimerization is observed with some hydrocarbons (12). This mechanism is rationalized in Fig. 2.

In the presence of further nucleophilic partners, the reaction also yields products from the hydrocarbon and this compound. Furthermore, in such EDA complexes it is possible to transfer the electron, to

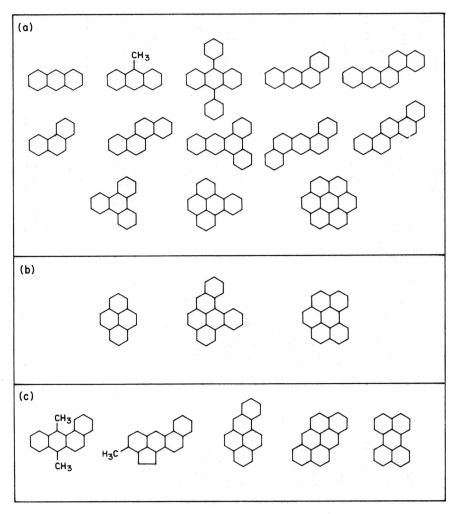

FIG. 3. Solution of purine in trifluoroacetic acid. Addition of the polycyclic hydrocarbon in benzene. (a) no reaction, (b) weak reaction, (c) strong reaction.

oxidize, by light. In the course of the so-called charge transfer absorption, a high concentration of radical ion pairs is available:

$$A^{\ominus} \ldots \ldots D^{\oplus}$$

In this case, too, the radical cations of a good donor also react with other nucleophilic partners added to the system (13). This may become a convenient way to substitute suitable hydrocarbons using nucleophilic compounds.

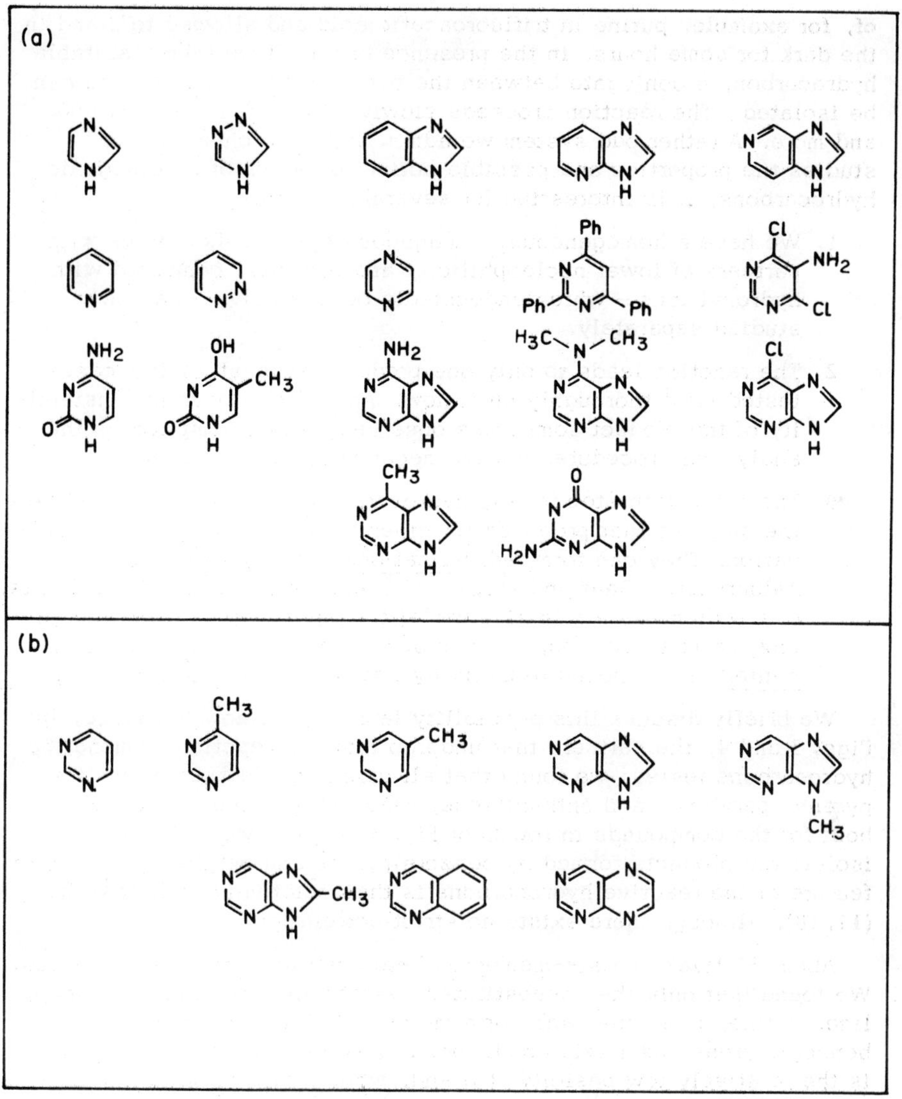

FIG. 4. Solution of perylene (or of benzo(a)pyrene) in benzene. Addition of the heterocyclic compound in trifluoroacetic acid. (a) no reaction, (b) reaction.

We now present more details of a very curious reaction that we have observed. This reaction is curious from the standpoint of the organic chemist. At present we are trying to clear up how it proceeds: A solution of a polycyclic aromatic hydrocarbon in benzene is mixed with a solution

of, for example, purine in trifluoroacetic acid and allowed to stand in
the dark for some hours, in the presence of air. If we take a suitable
hydrocarbon, a conjugate between the two partners is formed and can
be isolated. The reaction proceeds slowly with yields of about 60%
and more. A rather odd system we admit, but for a chemist who
studies the properties and possible activation steps of carcinogenic
hydrocarbons, it is interesting for several reasons:

1. We have a homogeneous, nonaqueous system. Reactions with
   partners of lower nucleophilicity and basicity, compared with
   hydroxyl ions — which undoubtedly occur in vivo — can be
   studied separately.

2. The reaction leads to only one product, at least in the cases
   tested most thoroughly until now. Another factor is the instability of the product sometimes observed, which complicates the
   analytical procedure, but not necessarily the reaction.

3. The activation step for the hydrocarbons in our system could be
   the same as that proposed for other models of biochemical activation: They can form radical cations, as demonstrated by
   Aalbersberg, Gaaf and Mockor (14) and by our own measurements,
   or a proton, as a primitive model for a positive oxygen atom in
   enzymatic activation, attacks and generates an electrophilic
   center, as proposed recently by Cavalieri and Calvin (15, 16).

We briefly discuss this possibility later; let us now introduce, in
Figs. 3 and 4, the partners that undergo that TFA reaction. Among the
hydrocarbons tested, we found that all carcinogenic ones as well as
pyrene, perylene, and anthanthrene, react with purine. The yield is
best for the compounds in row C of Fig. 3. At first we undertook to
isolate the products formed by benzo(a)pyrene and perylene. A common
feature of the reactive hydrocarbons is their relatively high basicity
(17, 18), although there exists no strict correlation.

About 30 five- and six-membered heterocyclic partners were tested.
We found that only the unsubstituted systems of pyrimidine, quinazo-
line, purine, pteridine, and some methyl derivatives, did react with
benzo(a)pyrene under this condition. A common feature in this case
is the relatively low basicity (19) and, what seems to be really significant, the presence of a pyrimidine structure in which the positions
N-1, C-2, N-3, and one neighboring C atom are unsubstituted.

The resulting products were found to be trifluoroacetates of
hydrocarbon-pyrimidine or -purine conjugates. Separation from the
educts and purification was achieved by repeated column chromatography on Sephadex LH20 with methanol. In the case of benzo(a)pyrene
and purine, the product is only sparingly soluble and forms pale yellow
needles that can be filtered off. The yield of this primary product before

further purification was found to be 86% in one case. Unfortunately, the purine products are far less stable than those with pyrimidine and methylpyrimidine. Mainly they decompose to one secondary product, which was found to be a neutral conjugate and no longer a trifluoro-acetate (TFA) salt.

The trifluoroacetates that formed in the largest amount can be trans-formed into perchlorates and picrates, too. Stability and purification can sometimes be increased that way. In each case, combustion analysis was in accordance with a 1:1:1-composition of hydrocarbon, heterocyclic compound, and acid.

UV-spectra of the reaction products in Figs. 5, 6, and 7 reveal the intact chromophore of the hydrocarbon moiety. The absorption bands are shifted to a longer wavelength in each case.

The primary products with pyrimidine and purine have nearly iden-tical UV-spectra. But the secondary products, easily obtained from the purine products, behave differently: The fine structure is lost; this should be due to a "loose-bolt" effect. Acidification does not return it, but results in a bathchromic effect. This process is reversible.

Analysis by mass spectroscopy afforded temperatures above 200°C, and brought the most intense signal at the mass number of the cationic part of the molecule. "Peak-matching" was in accordance with the precise masses calculated. The deviation was not more than 3 ppm.

If we compare the mass spectra of the stable secondary product of the TFA reaction between benzo(a)pyrene and purine with the spec-tra of one reaction product of the "iodine-reaction" between these two compounds (Fig. 8), they reveal a very similar fragmentation pattern. Loss of two molecules of hydrogen cyanide together with a hydrogen atom leads to the first two fragments observed. Fissure of the remaining substituent leaves the hydrocarbon moiety minus two hydrogen masses. We therefore hope to get more information about the iodine reaction, which is performed by radical cations, when we manage to determine the exact positions of the covalent linkage in the TFA products, which are much easier to prepare. The IR spectral data available until now indicate that the most reactive 6-position of the benzo(a)pyrene molecule is not substituted in the TFR product but that position 1 or 3 might be.

Although we are not yet able to rationalize the mechanism of the TFA reaction, let us demonstrate in Fig. 9 what possibilities we see and are trying to reduce to one by further experiments.

In our system, we expect an equilibrium between five different molecular species: the aromatic hydrocarbon, its protonated form,

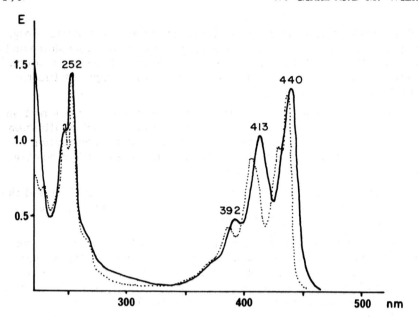

FIG. 5. Absorption spectra of perylene (. . . . . .) and the perylene-pyrimidine product, PE-PY.

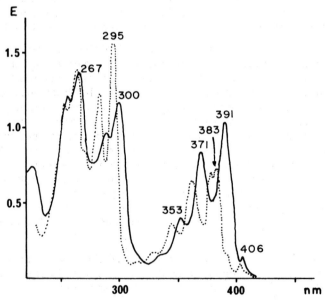

FIG. 6. Absorption spectra of benzo(a)pyrene (. . . . . .) and the benzo(a)pyrene-pyrimidine product, BP-PY.

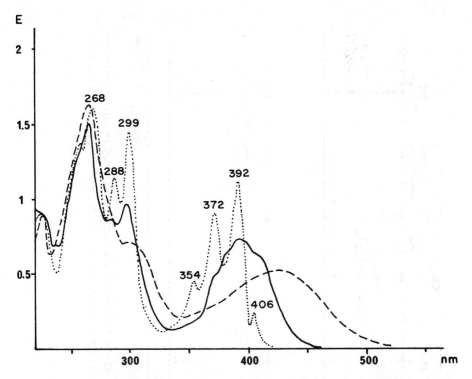

FIG. 7. Absorption spectra of the benzo(a)pyrene-purine products: Primary product BP-PU 1, ...; secondary product BP-PU 2, _____; acidified BP-PU 2 (x HCl), ------.

and its radical cation, which could form a dication by disproportionation (20, 21), and is formed by monovalent oxidation by oxygen of the air. The dication, on the other hand, could lose two protons and form a highly reactive aryne.

The heterocyclic compound, although of low basicity, is expected to be protonated to a certain extent, too. The realization of the first step is supported by the IR spectra of the two benzo(a)pyrene compounds that we isolated and in an experiment where oxygen was excluded by thorough flushing with nitrogen, the primary product was still formed.

We dared to present you our incomplete but fresh results in order to demonstrate that polycyclic aromatic hydrocarbons, especially the carcinogenic ones, react quite easily with suitable partners under relatively mild conditions if properly activated.

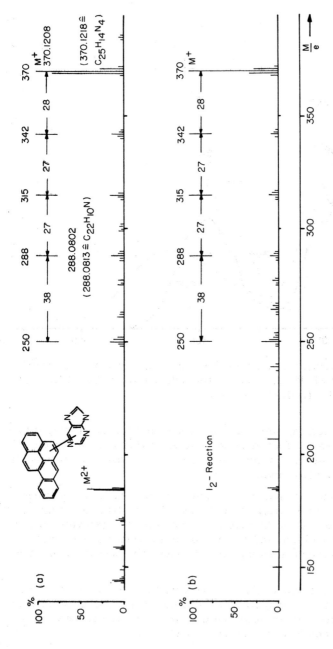

FIG. 8. Mass spectra. (a) Product BP-PU 2 of the trifluoroacetic acid-catalyzed reaction between benzo(a)pyrene and purine; (b) one main product of the iodine-oxidation of benzo(a)pyrene and purine, both adsorbed on silica.

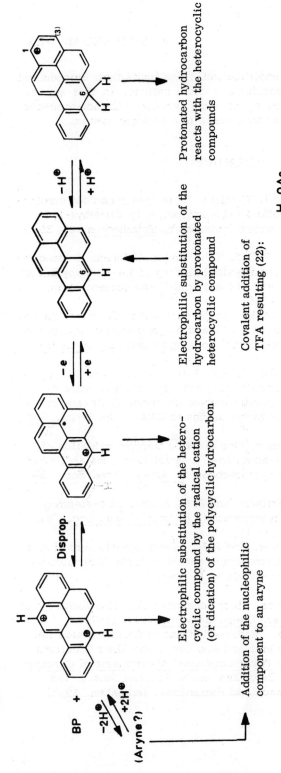

FIG. 9. Hypothetical activation steps in the TFA reaction.

193

It is perhaps an oversimplification if one limits their biochemical interactions to K-region epoxides or radical cations. In that sense, our system can perhaps demonstrate some aspects of the homogeneous catalysis, which is likely to take place in a biologic system.

REFERENCES

1. M. Wilk, W. Bez, and J. Rochlitz, Neue Reaktionen der carcinogenen kohlenwasserstoffe 3.4-benzpyren, 9,10-dimethyl-1,2-benzanthracen und 20-methylcholanthren, Tetrahedron, 22, 2599 (1966).

2. S.A. Lesko, A. Smith, P.O.P. Ts'o, and R.S. Umans, Interaction of nucleic acids. IV. The physical binding of 3.4-benzopyrene to nucleosides, nucleotides, nucleic acids, and nucleoprotein, Biochemistry, 7, 434 (1968).

3. H.D. Hoffmann, S.A. Lesko, and P.O.P. Ts'o, Chemical linkage of polycyclic hydrocarbons to DNA and polynucleotides in aqueous solution and in a buffer-ethanol solvent system, Biochemistry, 9, 2594 (1970).

4. V.M. Maher, S.A. Lesko, P.O.P. Ts'o, and P.A. Straat, Mutagenic action, loss of transforming activity, and inhibition of DNA template activity in vitro caused by chemical linkage of carcinogenic polycyclic hydrocarbons to DNA, J. Bacteriol., 108, 202 (1971).

5. J. Fried and D.E. Schumm, One electron transfer oxidation of 7,12-dimethylbenzo(a)anthracene, a model for the metabolic activation of carcinogenic hydrocarbons, J. Amer. Chem. Soc., 89, 5508 (1967).

6. L.S. Marcoux, J.M. Fritsch, and R.N. Adams, One-electron oxidation of aromatic hydrocarbons, J. Amer. Chem. Soc., 89, 5766 (1967).

7. G. Manning, V.D. Parker, and R.N. Adams, Anodic substitution reactions of aromatic hydrocarbon cation radicals. Unequivocal evidence for the ECE-mechanism, J. Amer. Chem. Soc., 91, 4584 (1969).

8. L. Jeftic and R.N. Adams, Electrochemical oxidation pathways of benzo(a)pyrene, J. Amer. Chem. Soc., 92, 1332 (1970).

9. M. Wilk and W. Girke, "Radical Cations of Carcinogenic Alternant Hydrocarbons, Amines and Azo Dyes, and Their Reactions with Nucleobases," in Physicochemical Mechanisms of Carcinogenesis, Vol. 1 (E.D. Bergmann and B. Pullman, eds.), The Israel Academy of Science and Humanities, Jerusalem, 1969, p. 91.

10. C. Nagata, Y. Tagashira, M. Inomata, and M. Kodama, Effect of iodine on the carcinogenicity of 3.4-benzpyrene, Gann, 62, 309 (1971).
11. M. Wilk and U. Hoppe, Nucleophile substitution carcinogener und nicht-carcinogener kohlenwasserstoffe über elektronen-donator-acceptor-komplexe, Liebigs Ann. Chem., 727, 81 (1969).
12. L. Schrott, Diplomarbeit, Frankfurt/Main, 1969.
13. L. Schrott, Dissertation Frankfurt/Main, in preparation.
14. W. I. Aalbersberg, J. Gaaf, and E. L. Mockor, Electron-transfer reactions between oxygen and aromatic hydrocarbons, J. Chem. Soc., 1961, 905.
15. E. Cavalieri and M. Calvin, Molecular characteristics of some carcinogenic hydrocarbons, Proc. Nat. Acad. Sci., 68, 1251 (1971).
16. E. Cavalieri, Charge-localization in the carbonium ion of the methyl benz(a)anthracenes. A clue to their mechanism of carcinogenesis, Proc. Cancer Res., 1972, Abstr. 499.
17. E. L. Mockor, A. Hofstra, and J. van der Waals, The basicity of aromatic hydrocarbons, Trans. Faraday Soc., 54, 66 (1958).
18. A. Streitwieser, Jr., A. Lewis, I. Schwager, R. Fish, and S. Labana, Rates of protodetritiation of polycyclic aromatic hydrocarbons in trifluoroacetic acid, J. Amer. Chem. Soc., 92, 6525 (1970).
19. A. Albert, Chemie der Heterocyclen, Verlag Chemie, Weinheim, Germany, 1962, p. 332.
20. C. V. Ristagno and H. J. Shine, Ion radicals. XXIII. Some reactions of the perylene cation radical, J. Org. Chem., 36, 4050 (1971).
21. V. D. Parker and L. Eberson, The active species in cation-radical reactions with nucleophiles: Cation radical or dication? J. Amer. Chem. Soc., 92, 7488 (1970).
22. A. Albert, Naturally occurring nitrogen heterocyclic compounds, Special Publication No. 3, Roy. Chem. Soc., London, 1955.

Chapter 8

ONE-ELECTRON OXIDATION OF POLYCYCLIC AROMATICS AS A MODEL FOR THE METABOLIC ACTIVATION OF CARCINOGENIC HYDROCARBONS

Josef Fried

Departments of Chemistry and Biochemistry and
The Ben May Laboratory for Cancer Research
The University of Chicago, Chicago, Illinois

There is now considerable agreement among investigators that one or more metabolic intermediates may be the proximate carcinogens responsible for the direct chemical interaction of an aromatic hydrocarbon with some vital macromolecule. Because of the complexity of investigating all the phases of the carcinogenic process, including metabolism of the carcinogen in the affected cell population, in mammalian systems we have chosen model systems in both the biologic and chemical spheres. The biologic model we have chosen for studying both metabolic and biologic activity is an E. coli-bacteriophage system. The chemical model involves an in vitro oxidizing system; there is a high degree of probability that it may be operative in bacterial and mammalian cells as well.

In selecting the biologic system, we were fortunate in having as a point a departure a most intriguing observation made by Weiss et al., who reported that carcinogenic hydrocarbons could inhibit the replication of the DNA bacteriophage ΦX174 and of the RNA bacteriophage MS 2, both single stranded, in E. coli (1, 2). They also observed that the infectivity of the DNA isolated from these bacteriophages toward E. coli spheroplasts was inhibited by these hydrocarbons. They demonstrated that the hydrocarbons did not affect entry of the DNA into the cell nor did they prevent the release of the phage from the host cell. In an important experiment they showed that when the phage DNA was first incubated with hydrocarbon and then permitted to enter the cell no inhibition could be observed, indicating that the host cell was required for the phenomenon to occur.

One of the remarkable aspects of this system was the discovery that there exists a clear correlation between viral inhibition and

carcinogenic activity in animals (1, 2). We have confirmed this by
comparing the inhibition of ΦX174 replication by all the 12 mono-
methylbenz(a)anthracenes with their carcinogenic properties in two
rat tumor systems. This is shown in Table 1. The correspondence is,
indeed, remarkable. It is particularly significant that the high activity of the 6-, 7-, 8-, and 12-monomethylbenz(a)anthracenes is accompanied by high inhibitory activity in the phage assay. The great
advantages of this system are that the assay is fast (24 hours), results are reproducible, and one can express the inhibitory activity of
a given compound in numerical form. Although we do not know the
precise relationship in molecular terms that phage inhibition bears to
carcinogenesis, these two types of biologic activity must be related
in a significant fashion, and we have used it forthwith in this work.

We now wish to introduce the second model system chosen to
simplify the problem of acquiring information regarding the possible

TABLE 1

Inhibition of ΦX174 Replication and Carcinogenicity of
Monomethyl Derivatives of Benz(a)anthracene (MBA)

Compound	ΦX-174 inhibition at 20 μg/ml, %	Carcinogenicity, rat	
		Sprague-Dawley[a]	Dunning[b]
1-MBA	0	0	+
2-MBA	0	0	0
3-MBA	0	0	0
4-MBA	19	0	+
5-MBA	16	0	+
6-MBA	99	+++++	++++
7-MBA	74	+++++	+++++
8-MBA	48	++++	++++
9-MBA	24	0	+
10-MBA	17	0	+
11-MBA	0	0	0
12-MBA	93	++++	++++

[a] Reference 9.
[b] Reference 10.

metabolic fate of these hydrocarbons. Our reasoning went as follows:
Polycyclic aromatics have low ionization potentials and are, therefore, expected to give up electrons readily to even the mildest
oxidizing agents. Thus, "one-electron oxidants" might be expected
to withdraw electrons from the π system in two discrete stages: first
producing a cation radical, which could further react with a nucleophilic constituent of the medium, to be followed by withdrawal of a
second electron to form a cation, which could again react with a
nucleophile. Examples of such oxidants are manganese dioxide,
ferricyanide, and ceric ion. The significance of this type of oxidative process for our purposes derives from the fact that it had been
shown, prior to this work, that oxidation of certain phenolic substances
by one-electron oxidants paralleled or even duplicated important
biogenetic processes operating in both bacterial and plant cells (3).
Thus, certain oxidative steps in the biogenesis of many families of
alkaloids, such as the morphine alkaloids, or antibiotics, e. g.,
griseofulvin, can be duplicated by the use of these oxidants. The
reactions involved in this process are exemplified by the conversion
of p-cresol to Pummerer's ketone [3]. The oxidant removes one
electron from the cresolate anion to form the radical, which can be
rewritten as [1] or [2], followed by dimerization, rephenolization,
and Michael addition of the phenolic hydroxyl to the α, β-unsaturated
ketone with the formation of Pummerer's ketone [3].

Having thus justified the use of this type of oxidation process in
biosynthetic terms, we have studied the oxidation of 7, 12-dimethyl-
benz(a)anthracene (DMBA) with three one-electron oxidants,
manganese dioxide, ferric ferricyanide, and ammonium ceric nitrate.
All three reagents gave the same products in somewhat differing
product ratios. A tracing of the gas chromatogram of the product
mixture obtained with ferric ferricyanide is shown in Fig. 1. It
reveals the complexity of the mixture obtained, showing at least
seven peaks.

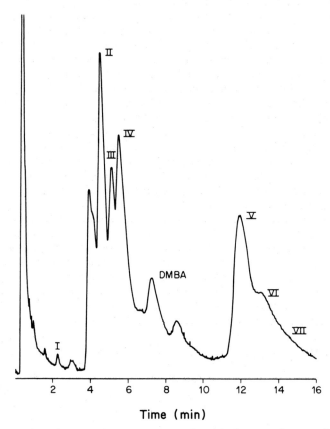

FIG. 1. Gas-liquid chromatogram of oxidation products of DMBA
with $Fe^{III}Fe^{III}(CN)_6$.

Before undertaking the oxidation experiments, we ventured some
predictions regarding the nature of the oxidation products: If the
reaction did indeed take the route via radical cations, knowledge of
the distribution of spin density around the molecule would provide
some information regarding the points of greatest reactivity. Such
information is essentially obtained from the EPR spectra of radical
cations. Model substances encompassing the structural features of
7-12-dimethylbenz(a)anthracene and whose EPR spectra in sulfuric
acid are known (4), are 9,10-dimethylanthracene [4] and phenanthrene [5]. The pertinent coupling constants derived from these
spectra are indicated at the appropriate positions in these structures.
According to the McConnell relationship, these coupling constants,
a_H, are proportional to the spin densities, ρ, at these sites. We

[4]

[5]

note that in 9,10-dimethylanthracene, highest spin density is associated with the two methyl groups and that in the phenanthrene molecule highest spin density is associated with the 9- and 10-positions, that is, the K-region. From the fact that the coupling constants are larger for the methyl substituents than for the K-region, we predicted that the points of greatest reactivity in DMBA would be the methyl groups and carbon atoms 7 and 12 to which they are attached.

We then proceeded to isolate and characterize the products obtained with the previously mentioned one-electron oxidants in an acetone-water medium (5). Careful thin-layer chromatography yielded all of them in pure and crystalline form. Some of them turned out to be known products, others did not. Their structures are shown in Fig. 2. Seven reaction products are depicted; an eighth, not shown, is 7-hydroxymethylbenz(a)anthracene (VIII). The roman numerals in this chart correspond to those designating the peaks in Fig. 1. It should be noted that all the products conform to our prediction in that they involve reactions at the meso-region, that is, at position 7 and 12 and at the methyl groups attached to these positions. Their structures can be readily rationalized on the basis of a radical cation intermediate [6], which in the aqueous acetone medium can react with water in the manner shown in Fig. 3. Loss of a proton would result in the methylene radical [7], which would be oxidized to the corresponding cation [8]. This cation can react further in three ways. With water it forms the hydroxymethyl methylene compound [9], which is then further oxidized to the isolated product III. Another reaction path involves its delocalized form [10], which on reaction with water would give the 7-hydroxy derivative, VIII, which is one of the isolated products. Oxidation of this benzylic alcohol leads in a well-known facile reaction to the isolated aldehyde V. A third reaction of the intermediate cation [8] is loss of a proton to form the dimethylene compound [11], which may be postulated to be oxidized to the isolated benz(a)anthraquinone II. Likewise one would, of course, expect to find among the isolated products those products derived from the symmetrical radical cation in which localization of the positive charge and the electron spin at the 7- and 12-positions are reversed.

There is one type of reaction postulated in this sequence for which there has been no precedent. This involves the removal of one or two

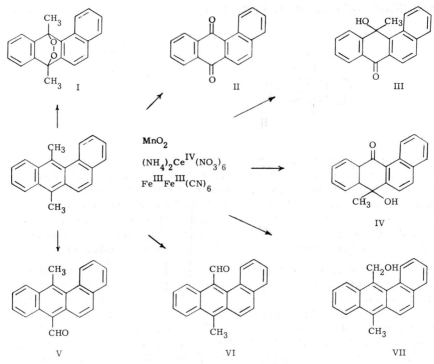

FIG. 2. Products isolated from one-electron oxidations of DMBA.

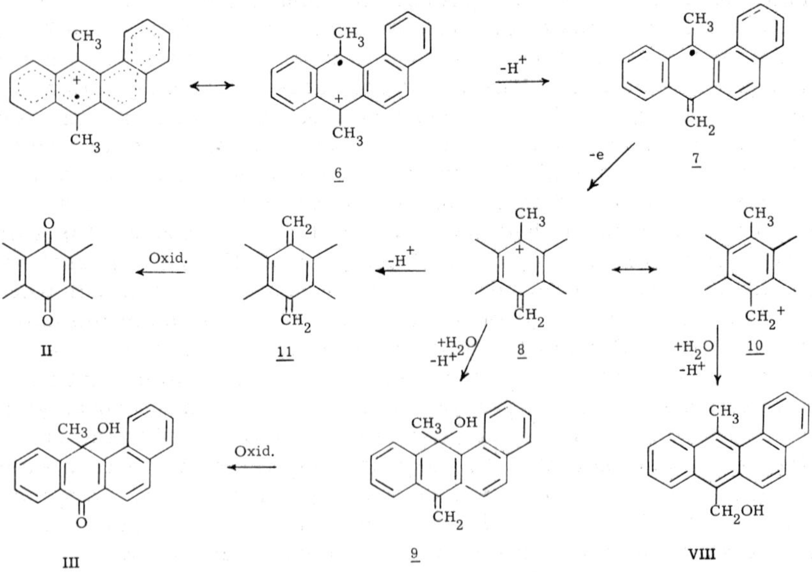

FIG. 3. Proposed mechanism for formation of oxidation products.

202

methylene carbons by these oxidants to form the methyl quinols III and IV and the quinone II. That these reactions do, indeed, take place was demonstrated by subjecting 10-methyleneanthrone [12] to oxidation by both manganese dioxide and ferric ferricyanide. In the former case the sole product was anthraquinone [13], the formation of

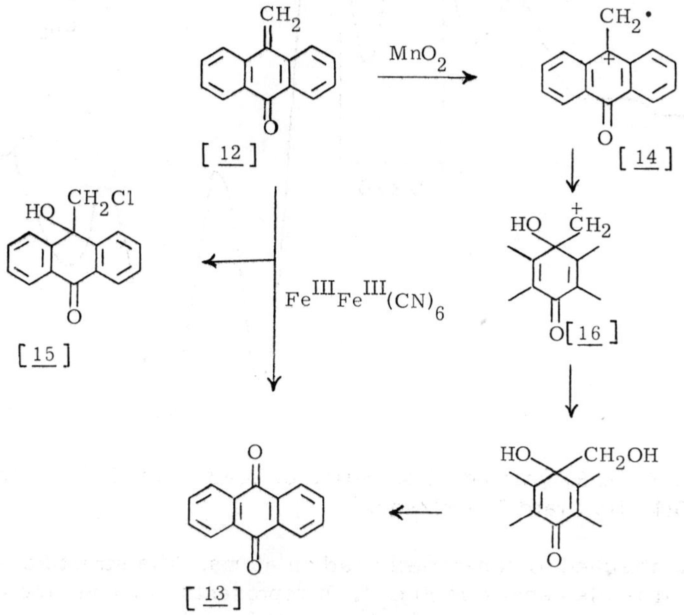

$$CH_2 \quad \xrightarrow{MnO_2} \quad CH_2^{\bullet}$$

[12]   [14]

$Fe^{III}Fe^{III}(CN)_6$

HO CH_2Cl

[15]

HO $\overset{+}{C}H_2$

O [16]

HO CH_2OH

O

[13]

which we formulate again via a radical cation [14]. That this is a reasonable assumption is documented by the presence of the chloro-methyl derivative [15] as a byproduct in the ferric ferricyanide oxida-tion. This product could readily arise by reaction of the cation [16], derived by oxidation of the corresponding radical, with chloride ion, the presence of which in the oxidation mixture results from the prepar-ation of ferric ferricyanide from ferric chloride and potassium ferri-cyanide. All of the isolated products are thus accounted for on the basis of the postulated radical cation intermediate.

It should be borne in mind that the alternative mechanism, i. e., loss of two electrons followed by proton loss, which would, of course, involve no radical but only cationic intermediates, would lead to the same products. We were therefore anxious to obtain evidence that radical cations were, indeed, intermediates in these oxidations. Through the courtesy of Dr. Landgraf of Varian Laboratories we were able to obtain the EPR spectrum of the mixture of DMBA with ammonium ceric nitrate in a spectrometer fitted with a flow cell. This spectrum is shown in Fig. 4. It shows a symmetric quintet with a coupling constant of 8.25 G, indicative of a radical possessing four equivalent

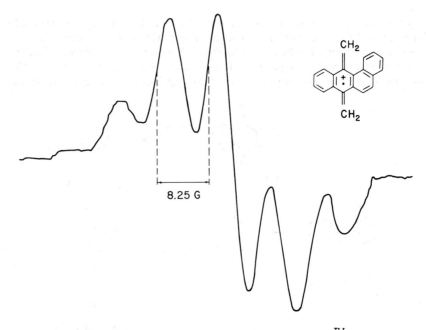

FIG. 4. EPR spectrum of oxidation of DMBA with Ce^{IV}. Acetone-water 3:1, flow rate 3. 5 ml/sec.

protons attached to nonaromatic carbon atoms. The structure of such a radical is also shown in Fig. 4. It represents, indeed, the radical of one of the intermediates ([11], Fig. 3) postulated in our scheme. Apparently, among several possible radical intermediates this is sufficiently long lived to be recognized in the spectrometer.

Having in hand now the isolated oxidation products derived from DMBA, they were subjected to assay in the E. coli-phage DNA system using, unless otherwise indicated, ΦX 174 DNA. The results obtained are shown in Table 2. Of all the products isolated, only two showed activity greater than the parent. These were the 7- and 12-formyl derivatives, V and VI (Fig. 2). Interestingly, the two corresponding alcohols VIII and VII were inactive in both the MS 2 RNA and the ΦX 174 DNA systems. This lack of activity misled us for some time, until it was discovered that the acetates derived from these alcohols were about equally as active as the corresponding aldehydes, leading to the presumption that the alcohols were not able to penetrate the spheroplasts, whereas the less polar acetates could do so. One would assume that abundant esterases present in E. coli would hydrolyze these acetates to the corresponding alcohols. The dose-response curves for the two highly active aldehydes are compared

TABLE 2

Inhibition of ΦX174 Replication and Carcinogenicity of
Oxidation Products of DMBA

Substance	ΦX174 bacteriophage inhibition	Carcinogenicity, Sprague-Dawley rat
	1	++++
	4	++++
	3	Inactive
	0.2	Inactive
	0	Inactive
	0[a]	++[b]
	0.1[a]	Inactive ++[b]
	3.5	
	2	
	0	

TABLE 2 (continued)

Substance	ΦX 174 bacteriophage inhibition	Carcinogenicity, Sprague–Dawley rat
	0	
	0.1	

[a] MS2, see Ref. 2.

[b] C57 mouse.

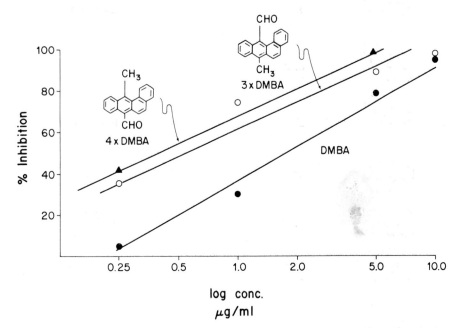

FIG. 5. Inhibition of ΦX174 replication by 7- and 12-formylmethyl-benz(a)anthracenes.

with that of DMBA in Fig. 5. It is seen that the important condition for proper assay evaluation, namely, straight line, parallel dose-response relationships, is obtained, and this has been true for the overwhelming majority of the compounds tested in this way (6).

To summarize at this point, we have demonstrated that substances derived by oxidation of one of the methyl groups of DMBA possess higher activity than their progenitor in a biologic assay, which has been shown to parallel classic carcinogenicity tests in animals. These substances were obtained by chemical oxidation reactions under conditions known to parallel enzymatic oxidation reactions occurring in both plants and microorganisms.

The next step, then, was to show whether E. coli spheroplasts were, indeed, capable of metabolizing DMBA to form these more active oxidation products. We now describe the experiments that showed that E. coli spheroplasts were, indeed, able to metabolize DMBA, not only to the highly active oxidation products, but to all the products elaborated by the chemical oxidizing system shown in Fig. 2 (6). For this purpose E. coli spheroplasts were incubated with tritiated DMBA of very high specific activity, which had been carefully purified by gas chromatography. The products resulting from this incubation were fractionated as shown in Figs. 6 and 7. After 3 hr at room temperature, the mixture was freeze-thawed to break up the cells, and the metabolites were extracted, first with benzene and then ethyl acetate. Both extracts contained essentially the same products. Chromatography on silica gel achieved separation into two major fractions, a slower-moving one containing the alcohol VII and its 7-isomer VIII and the quinols III and IV, and a faster-moving yellow fraction containing the aldehydes V and VI as well as benz(a)-anthraquinone (II, Fig. 2).

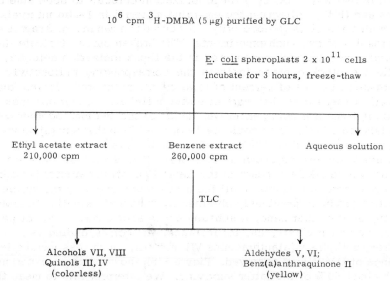

10^6 cpm ^{3}H-DMBA (5 μg) purified by GLC

E. coli spheroplasts 2 x 10^{11} cells
Incubate for 3 hours, freeze-thaw

Ethyl acetate extract
210,000 cpm

Benzene extract
260,000 cpm

Aqueous solution

TLC

Alcohols VII, VIII
Quinols III, IV
(colorless)

Aldehydes V, VI;
Benz(a)anthraquinone II
(yellow)

FIG. 6. Crude fractionation of metabolites from incubation of [^{3}H]DMBA with E. coli spheroplasts.

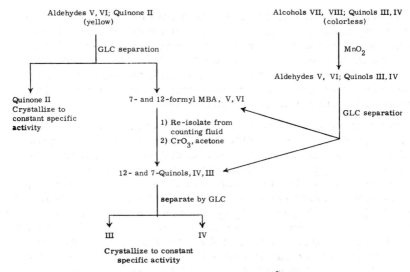

FIG. 7. Separation of TLC fractions from [^{3}H]DMBA incubation with E. coli spheroplasts.

The benzene extract was mixed with a small amount of the total reaction mixture of DMBA with ferric ferricyanide and injected into the column of a gas chromatograph. The effluent material was monitored in two ways: (a) by a flame ionization detector to determine total mass and (b) by collecting the emerging material in 1-min intervals for determination of its radioactivity. The curves shown in Fig. 8 represent the results of two such experiments. The broken curves indicate the emerging substances as measured in the flame ionization detector, while the blocked areas indicate the corresponding radioactivity expressed in terms of percent of total counts recovered. It was found in early experiments that more effective metabolic conversion took place if 1 mg of a cold carrier was added to the medium together with the labeled DMBA. This could be 7-formyl-12-methylbenz(a)anthracene (V), the corresponding 12-formyl-7-methylbenz(a)anthracene (VI), or a mixture of the two as shown in Fig. 8(a). It is seen that there are few counts where DMBA appears in the flame ionization detector (13 min), whereas there are counts in all the areas represented by the various reaction products previously obtained by chemical oxidation of DMBA. When, on the other hand, a substance was added that could not penetrate the spheroplasts, as, for instance, the corresponding 7- and 12-hydroxymethylbenz(a)anthracenes VII and VIII, much less metabolic change of DMBA was observed. Figure 8(b) shows such an experiment with about 50% of the latter surviving. We interpret this to mean that

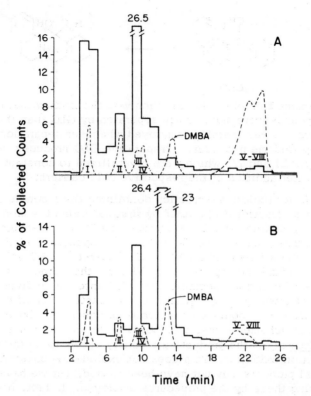

FIG. 8. (a) Radio gas-liquid chromatogram of the benzene extract of a spheroplast oxidation of [³H]DMBA in which the 7- and 12-aldehydes, compounds V and VI (Fig. 2) were added to the incubation mixture. (b) Same for a reaction in which the corresponding mono-alcohols VII and VIII were added to the incubation mixture. % of collected counts ———, detector response - - - -.

dilution of the very small amount (5 µg) of labeled DMBA with a large amount (1 mg) of carrier provides for better delivery into the spheroplasts.

The yellow and faster of the two TLC fractions containing the two aldehydes and benz(a)anthraquinone was further separated by preparative gas chromatography (GLC) as shown in Fig. 7. This furnished a mixture of the 7- and 12-aldehydes, V and VI, as well as pure benz(a)anthraquinone, which was crystallized to constant specific activity after addition of cold material. The aldehydes V and VI were reisolated from the scintillation fluid by thin layer chromatography and oxidized with chromium trioxide in acetone to form, in a clean reaction, the 12- and 7-methylquinols, III and IV. The rationale

for performing this oxidation reaction was the finding that the latter
two compounds were more easily separated by GLC than their aldehyde
precursors. It was therefore employed whenever separation of the
aldehydes became necessary. Preparative GLC produced the individual quinols III and IV, which were crystallized to constant specific
activity after addition of the respective cold carriers.

The slower (colorless) fraction containing the alcohols and quinols
(Fig. 6) was fractionated further by first oxidizing the mixture with
manganese dioxide, which transformed the 7- and 12-hydroxymethyl-
benz(a)anthracenes VII and VIII to the corresponding aldehydes leaving the quinols III and IV unchanged. Preparative GLC achieved
separation of the aldehydes V and VI from the quinols, which later
could then be further separated by GLC into the individual components followed by crystallization to constant specific activity
after dilution with nonlabeled material as described above. By following this scheme, it was thus possible to prove the presence as
metabolites of all the products previously shown to be the products of
one-electron oxidation. This does not exclude the possibility that
additional products may not have been formed, but we have no way of
discovering these by the procedures employed. In fact, had we not
had in hand the products obtained in the chemical oxidation, the
quantities available from the metabolic experiments would have been
too small to prove their presence with certainty.

Having shown that both 7- and 12-formylbenz(a)anthracene and
the corresponding alcohols VII and VIII are metabolites of DMBA in
E. coli — the organism in which phage replication is inhibited — and
having, moreover, demonstrated that both the aldehydes and the alcohols (the latter in the form of their acetates) were more active than
DMBA, the question arose as to which of these two groups of
compounds were the proximate "carcinogens." In considering this question
we tended toward the view that the alcohols were the more suitable
candidates for that designation in that they possessed functionality
that permitted their transformation into powerful alkylating agents,
for instance, by esterification with sulfuric acid or phosphoric acid.
E. coli is known to possess the enzymatic capacity to perform either
one of these reactions. The resulting powerful alkylating agents
might then be expected to react readily with ΦX 174 DNA, leading to
alkylated species, which would be subject to facile depurination,
resulting in inactive DNA. Such a hypothetical scheme is shown

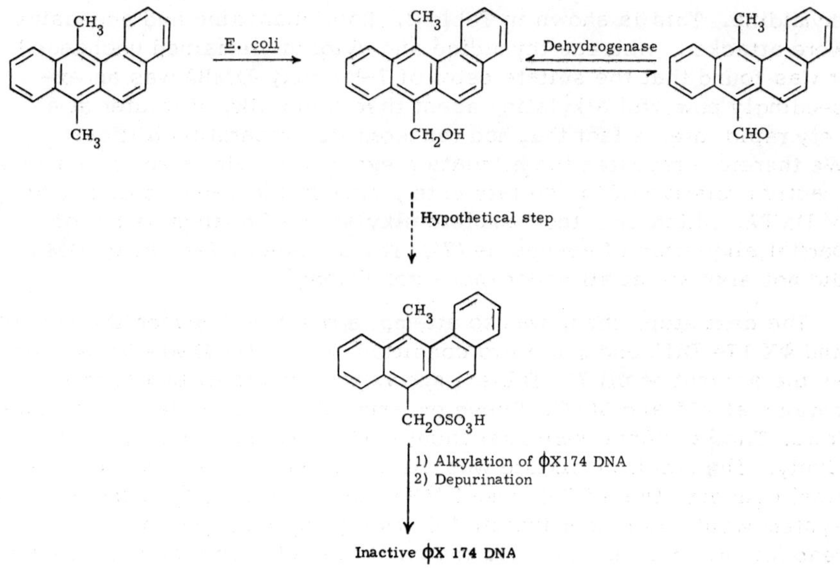

FIG. 9. Hypothetical scheme for metabolic activation of DMBA in E. coli and reaction with ΦX 174 DNA.

TABLE 3

Alkylation of Nucleosides with 7-Substituted 7,12-Dimethylbenz(a)anthracenes in DMF

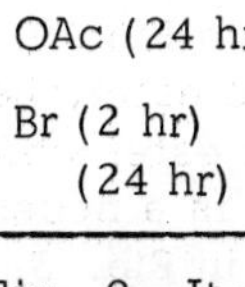	G	A	T	C
R = OSO₃H (18 hr)	100%	80%	0	0
R = OAc (24 hr)	0	0	0	0
R = Br (2 hr)	100%	+	0	0
(24 hr)	100%	++	0	0

in Fig. 9. It was, therefore, our next objective to ascertain whether the sulfate ester of 7-hydroxy-DMBA could, indeed, be prepared and found capable of inactivating ΦX 174 DNA in vitro without prior exposure to the E. coli spheroplasts. In advance of performing this experiment we examined the alkylating properties of this sulfate ester, prepared synthetically, toward the three ribonucleosides, guanosine, adenosine, and cytosine, and the deoxyribonucleoside

thymidine. This is shown in Table 3. Both guanosine and adenosine
were attacked, whereas thymidine and cytosine remained unchanged.
It was found that the sulfate ester of 7-hydroxy-DMBA was an ex-
ceedingly powerful alkylating agent that could alkylate water at a
very rapid rate, a fact that had rendered its preparation difficult.
We therefore repeated the alkylation experiment with a somewhat less
reactive relative of the sulfate ester, namely the 7-bromo derivative
of DMBA, which effected complete alkylation of guanosine but only
partial alkylation of adenosine (7). The acetate of 7-hydroxy-DMBA
did not alkylate at all under these conditions.

The next step, then, was to attempt a reaction between the bromide
and ΦX 174 DNA under in vitro conditions using 1:1 DMF-Tris buffer
as the solvent at pH 7. Table 4 shows the results of two such incubations at 25° and 30°C. These experiments were carried out as follows: The reactants were first incubated for 60 and 40 min, respectively. The reaction mixture was diluted to such an extent that the
final concentration of 7-bromo-DMBA when added to the complete test
system would no longer inhibit ΦX 174 replication, and the diluted
reaction mixture was added to the medium containing the spheroplasts.
Any inhibition of ΦX 174 replication that would now be observed must
thus have been the result of prior reaction between the alkylating
agent and the DNA in the absence of the cells. Table 4 shows that at
concentrations of 3×10^{-5} M the alkylating agent caused complete
inactivation of the ΦX 174 DNA, while at concentrations of 3×10^{-8} M
there was no inactivation. Fifty percent inactivation was achieved at
concentrations of between 3×10^{-6} and 3×10^{-7} M, that is, between
0.1 and 1 µg/ml. It should be mentioned here that a parallel series
of experiments carried out with DMBA showed no inactivation of ΦX
174 DNA. The time course of the reaction is shown in Table 5 at a
concentration of the alkylating agent of 1 µg/ml.

These experiments, indeed, demonstrate that an alkylating agent
of the type capable of being formed in E. coli from DMBA is able to
inactivate the ΦX 174 DNA at concentrations that could be generated
metabolically from DMBA. Only one reaction postulated in Fig. 9,
namely, the conversion of 7-hydroxy-DMBA to its sulfate ester, has
not been demonstrated experimentally. Although such an ester would
represent a possible intermediate, we do not feel that it is a necessary one. In fact, one of the cationic precursors shown in Fig. 3,
e.g., [11], could be the alkylating species that directly attacks one
or more nucleophilic centers of the nucleic acid.

In summary, we feel that metabolic conversion of DMBA to an
alkylating species in E. coli is compatible with all the experimental
data presented in this paper. The strict parallel of biologic responses
to hydrocarbons between the E. coli-ΦX 174 DNA test system, on the

TABLE 4

In Vitro Inactivation of ΦX 174 DNA by
7-Bromomethyl-12-methylbenz(a)anthracene

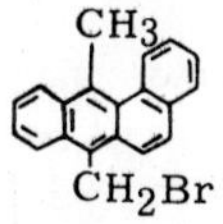

		% inactivation	
		3700 PFU[b]	3200 PFU
M[a]	μg/ml	25°, 60 min	30°, 40 min
3×10^{-5}	10	100	98
3×10^{-6}	1	75	52
3×10^{-7}	0.1	37	12
3×10^{-8}	0.01	0	0

[a] Solvent: 1:1 DMF/Tris buffer at pH 7.

[b] Plaque forming units (PFU).

TABLE 5

Time Course of in vitro Inactivation of ΦX 174 DNA by
7-Bromomethyl-12-methylbenz(a)anthracene

Time, min	% inactivation[a]	
	3400 PFU, 30°	4300 PFU, 37°
2	5	75
5	18	70
10	52	78
30	80	80

[a] Solvent: 1:1 DMF/Tris buffer at pH 7.5, 7-bromomethyl-12-methylbenz(a)anthracene, 1 μg/ml.

one hand, and conventional carcinogenesis assays, on the other, is suggestive that closely related chemical events are responsible for both biologic activities.

We have examined other polycyclic hydrocarbons as well, among them the related carcinogen 3-methylcholanthrene (8). When

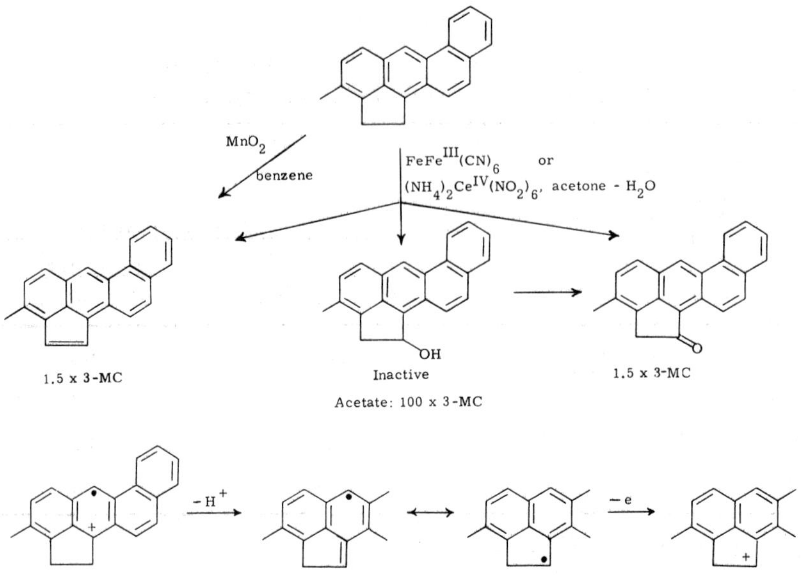

FIG. 10. One-electron oxidation of 3-methylcholanthrene.

subjected to one-electron oxidation under conditions identical to those described for DMBA, products analogous to those described for the latter were obtained. These are shown in Fig. 10. The most remarkable result of this study was the fact that the acetate of the hydroxylation product had 100 times the activity of its precursor, 3-methylcholanthrene, a finding that supports and extends our observations with DMBA.

REFERENCES

1. W. Hsu, J.W. Moohr, and S.B. Weiss, The influence of poly-cyclic aromatic hydrocarbons on bacteriophage development, Proc. Nat. Acad. Sci., 53, 517 (1965).
2. W. Hsu, J.W. Moohr, H.Y.M. Tsai, and J.B. Weiss, The influence of polycyclic aromatic hydrocarbons on bacteriophage development, II., Proc. Nat. Acad. Sci., 55, 1475 (1966).
3. A.J. Scott, Oxidative coupling of phenolic compounds, Quart. Rev. (London), 19, 1 (1965).

4. J. R. Bolton, H. Carrington, and A. D. McLachlan, Electron spin resonance studies of hyperconjugation in aromatic ions, Mol. Phys., 5, 31 (1962).
5. J. Fried and D. E. Schumm, One electron transfer oxidation of 7, 12-dimethylbenz[a]anthracene, a model for the metabolic activation of carcinogenic hydrocarbons, J. Amer. Chem. Soc., 89, 5508 (1967).
6. D.L. Schumm, In vitro and in vivo one-electron oxidation of 7, 12-dimethylbenz[a]anthracene, Dissertation, Univ. of Chicago, 1969.
7. F. Pochon and A. M. Michelson, Action of the carcinogen 7-bromomethylbenz[a]anthracene on synthetic polynucleotides, Europ. J. Biochem., 21, 144 (1971).
8. J. Fried and A. Shaffiee, unpublished work.
9. C.B. Huggins, J. Pataki, and R.G. Harvey, Proc. Nat. Acad. Sci., 58, 2253 (1967).
10. W. F. Dunning and M. R. Curtis, J. Nat. Cancer Institute, 25, 387 (1968).

Chapter 9

STRUCTURAL AND FUNCTIONAL CHANGES IN NUCLEIC ACIDS MODIFIED BY CHEMICAL CARCINOGENS

I. Bernard Weinstein and Dezider Grunberger

Institute of Cancer Research and
Departments of Medicine and Biochemistry
Columbia University College of Physicians and Surgeons
New York, New York

INTRODUCTION

It is now well established that several chemical carcinogens are covalently bound in vivo to cellular RNA, DNA, and protein (for a review of this subject see Refs. 1 and 2). It is not known which of these macromolecules, if any, is the critical target in the process by which the carcinogen converts a normal cell into a tumor cell. We favor the possibility that the nucleic acids, either RNA or DNA, rather than protein, constitute the critical target because of the widespread disturbance in gene expression that accompanies the transformation process (3, 4), as well as the usual stability of the transformed state once it has been established.

For these reasons we have addressed ourselves to the question: "When a carcinogen becomes covalently bound to a nucleic acid, what types of structural and functional changes occur in that nucleic acid?" We believe that the results of these studies at a molecular level allow us to make certain predictions about the cellular consequences of these events. In some of our studies we have employed transfer RNA, synthetic ribo-oligonucleotides, or polyribonucleotides as model compounds. This has been done for three reasons:

1. We are impressed with the fact that in vivo many carcinogens bind to cellular RNA to an extent that is equal to or greater than their binding to DNA (1-3, 5-7).
2. The possibility that cancer represents an aberration in differentiation rather than a somatic mutation suggests that the reaction with

RNA may be as (or more) critical than the reaction with DNA (3).
3. At the present time the analysis of base sequence and certain other
   aspects of nucleic acid chemistry are more readily performed with
   RNA than with DNA.

In view of certain gross structural similarities between all nucleic
acids, the data that we have obtained with carcinogen-modified RNA
allow us to make certain predictions about the structural changes that
would also occur in DNA and, therefore, have broad implications
should future studies reveal that DNA rather than RNA is the critical
target in carcinogenesis.

BASE DISPLACEMENT MODEL OF AAF-NUCLEIC ACID COMPLEX

All of the results described in the present study have employed the
N-acetoxy derivative of the liver carcinogen N-2-acetylaminofluorene
(AAF). This drug reacts primarily with the guanine residue of nucleic
acids to produce a derivative in which the acetylaminofluorene residue
is covalently bound to the 8-position of guanine (8, 9). This same
derivative has been isolated from liver nucleic acids following in vivo
administration of the carcinogen (8, 9). In our early studies, we found
that modification of certain tRNA's with N-acetoxy-AAF inhibited either
their amino acid acceptance capacities or their ability to function
during ribosomal binding and codon recognition (10). The presence of
AAF on guanosine residues in triplet codewords, such as G-U-U or
A-A-G, completely inhibited the ability of these synthetic codons to
stimulate ribosomal binding of their respective aminoacyl tRNA's (11,
12). These results, as well as several physical studies that are
reviewed below, have led us to propose a specific model for the conformation of nucleic acids modified by this carcinogen. These changes
are best illustrated in a computer-generated display of molecular
models; this allowed us to readily perform rotation around appropriate
bond angles while obtaining a three-dimensional display of the molecular structures on a video screen (13)(Fig. 1).

Figure 1(a) displays the conformation of a simple dinucleoside
monophosphate ApG (A-G) in which the ribose-phosphate-ribose backbone has a right-handed helical conformation analogous to a similar
segment in double helical DNA, with each of the bases in the anti
conformation (13). The covalent binding of AAF to the 8-position of
the G residue in A-G [see Fig. 1(b)] results in severe steric hindrance
between AAF and the guanosine ribose if the base is maintained in the
anti conformation. Therefore, the guanine base has been rotated around
the glycosidic bond to the syn conformation. In addition, the guanine
base has been displaced from its normal coplanar relation with the

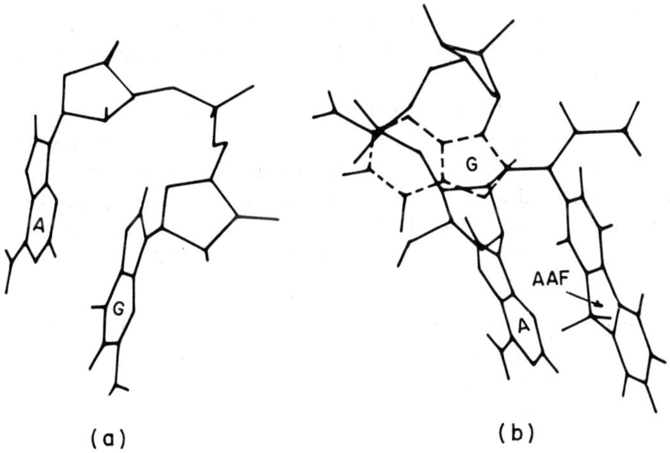

FIG. 1. Computer-generated three-dimensional structures of A-G and A-G$_{AAF}$. Only the base and acetyl hydrogen atoms are shown. (a) A probable conformation of A-G with the two bases coplanar to each other. (b) The base displacement model of A-G$_{AAF}$. The fluorene and adenine rings are closely stacked with optimum overlap in this structure. The dashed line represents the guanine ring structure, which has been displaced by the AAF. For additional details see Ref. 13.

adjacent adenine residue by the planar AAF molecule, and the latter is now stacked with the adjacent adenine residue. This model was developed in collaboration with Dr. Charles Cantor and Dr. James Nelson; additional features of this structure are described elsewhere (13).

We have designated this structure as the "base displacement model" to distinguish it from intercalation and other types of complexes between drugs and nucleic acids. This model makes certain specific predictions that can be tested by direct experimentation. These include the following.

1. The attachment of AAF to the 8-position of guanosine requires a rotation of the glycosidic bond from the anti to the syn conformation.
2. The guanine residue to which AAF is bound is displaced from its normal coplanar relation with adjacent bases in the polynucleotide strand and is therefore unavailable for base pairing.
3. There is a stacking interaction between the fluorene residue of the bound AAF and one of the next adjacent bases. This may also interrupt the normal base pairing capacity of the neighboring base.

4. Guanine residues in single-stranded regions of nucleic acid are more susceptible to AAF modification than are those in double-stranded regions.
5. AAF modification of double-stranded nucleic acids will produce localized denaturation because the displacement of the guanine residue must be associated with disruption of its base pairing with a cytosine residue in the complementary strand. This and the associated conformational changes in the backbone of the poly-nucleotide will cause a destabilization of that region of the double-stranded structure.

We now present specific evidence consistent with each of these predictions, and then relate our findings to certain biologic conse-quences predicted by the base displacement model.

EVIDENCE FOR A CONFORMATIONAL CHANGE FROM ANTI TO SYN

The first feature of this model is that the attachment of the AAF residue to the 8-position of guanosine is associated with a change in glycosidic [(N-9)-(C-1)] conformation from the anti conformation of nucleosides in nucleic acids with Watson-Crick geometry to the syn conformation. Evidence for this is restricted to a study of molecular models of AAF-guanosine that indicate severe steric hindrance be-tween AAF and the ribose, unless the guanosine base changes its orientation as described (7, 10, 11). This change to the syn conforma-tion is similar to the change that occurs with the substitution of bro-mine at the 8-position of GMP (14-16). Unfortunately, direct proof of the glycoside bond conformation by PMR studies (13) is not possible in the AAF-modified derivatives because of the loss of the C-8 proton.

EVIDENCE FOR STACKING INTERACTION BETWEEN FLUORENE AND AN ADJACENT BASE

The second major feature of our model is that there is a stacking interaction between AAF and a base adjacent to the substituted guano-sine residue. Direct evidence for this in oligonucleotides has been obtained from both circular dichroic (CD) and proton magnetic reso-nance (PMR) spectra (11, 13). The CD results are illustrated with A-G (ApG) in Fig. 2. At wavelengths greater than 290 nm, where most of the light absorption is due to AAF, the dichroism of AAF-modified A-G (A-G$_{AAF}$) is much greater than that of modified GMP (AAF-GMP). The optical activity in the 240 to 280 nm spectral region is also very

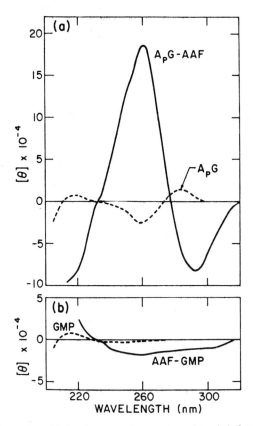

FIG. 2. Circular dichroic spectra comparing (a) ApG to ApG$_{AAF}$
and (b) GMP to AAF-GMP. For additional details see Ref. 11.

pronounced. The intense bands in the spectra of this and other modified oligomers that we have studied are probably the result of intramolecular interaction between the transition dipoles of fluorene and
the adjacent base residue. The possibility of intermolecular interactions is unlikely because the concentrations are relatively low (10^{-5}
M), there is no salt other than buffer in the solutions, and the spectra
are concentration independent over the 10^{-4} to 10^{-5} M range. A reversible temperature dependence of the circular dichroism of A-G$_{AAF}$ and
a loss of CD intensity of several other AAF-modified oligomers when
the solvent was changed from H_2O to MeOH (13) were observed.
These properties are also characteristic of stacking interactions.

We have observed a striking effect of the neighboring base on the
CD spectra of AAF-modified oligonucleotides, suggesting a stronger
base-fluorene interaction with A-G$_{AAF}$ than with U-G$_{AAF}$ (11, 13).

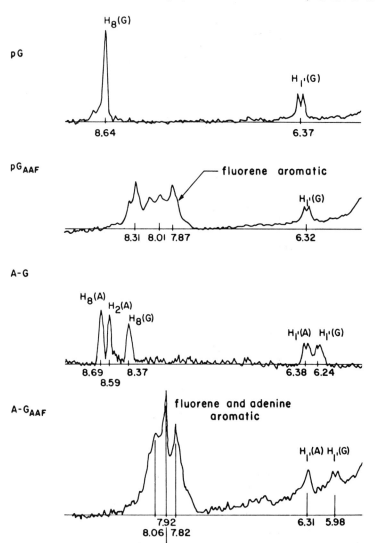

FIG. 3. Proton magnetic resonance spectra of the aromatic and
$H_{1'}$ protons of pG, pG$_{AAF}$, A-G, and A-G$_{AAF}$. Chemical shifts are
ppm downfield from external tetramethylsilane. Spectral assignments
are shown above the resonance signals with the appropriate nucleoside indicated in parentheses. The solvent is 0.005 M deuterated
phosphate buffer in D$_2$O at pD ~ 7. For further details see Ref. 13.

This is consistent with the fact that adenine base-stacked structures
are generally more stable than those of uracil. These findings suggest that base sequence in a nucleic acid may influence the type of

conformational changes that the carcinogen produces, and this may confer additional specificity to the drug in vivo. Studies described below indicate that this can be of functional significance, at least in the case of synthetic codons.

Additional evidence of a stacking interaction between AAF and the adjacent base was obtained from PMR measurements (13); this is illustrated in Fig. 3. Since both adenine and fluorene have significant aromaticity, we have been able to monitor the nature of possible fluorene-adenine interactions in A-G_{AAF} and G_{AAF}-A by comparing their PMR spectra with those of A-G, G-A, pG_{AAF}, and $_{AAF}Gp$. The H-2 and H-8 adenine signals of both A-G_{AAF} and G_{AAF}-A are shifted considerably upfield relative to the corresponding signals in the un-modified molecules. Analogous higher field shifts are observed for the fluorene ring protons of A-G_{AAF} and G_{AAF}-A when referenced to the corresponding protons of pG_{AAF} and $_{AAF}Gp$, respectively. These upfield shifts are characteristic of stacking (17, 18) and provide convincing evidence that the adenine and fluorene planes are intramolecularly stacked in the AAF-modified dinucleotides.

EFFECT OF AAF MODIFICATION OF GUANINE ON TRANSLATION OF THE NEIGHBORING BASE IN SYNTHETIC OLIGONUCLEOTIDES

We have previously demonstrated that AAF substitution of G residues present in synthetic codons inhibited the ability of these G residues to function normally in codon recognition (11, 12). The modification led to complete inactivation of function of the triplet containing the modified G residue rather than any miscoding. These results are also consistent with the base displacement model, since displacement of the modified G residue would prevent its proper alignment with a complementary base in the anticodon of the related tRNA.

It was also of interest to determine whether the strong stacking interaction between the fluorene residue and adjacent bases demonstrated in CD and PMR studies of oligonucleotides influenced the ability of these adjacent base(s) to function as components of synthetic codons when tested in a ribosomal binding assay. A series of oligonucleotides containing an AAF-modified G residue at either the 5' or the 3' end were prepared and tested (Tables 1 and 2). The control tetramers GAAA and AAAG coded efficiently for lysine since they contained the lysine codon AAA. Modification of the G residues of these tetramers with AAF led to about a 50% reduction in their coding capacities for lysine. This indicates that modification of the G residue interfered with the ability of the A residue(s) on the 3' or the

TABLE 1

Stimulation of Binding of [^{14}C]Lys-tRNA to
Ribosomes by Oligonucleotides[a]

Oligonucleotide,	[^{14}C]Lys-tRNA bound		
1.4 nmoles base res.	pmoles	Δpmoles	%
None	0.53	—	—
GAAA	5.63	5.10	100
G*AAA [b]	3.03	2.50	49
GAAAA	6.03	5.50	100
G*AAAA	5.23	4.70	85
AAAG	8.68	8.15	100
AAAG*	4.73	4.20	52
AAAAG	8.93	8.40	100
AAAAG*	8.03	7.50	90

[a] The incubation mixture (0.05 ml) for ribosomal binding and the processing of samples were as previously described (12). [^{14}C]Aminoacyl-tRNA and oligonucleotides were added as indicated.

[b] G* designates a guanosine residue modified by AAF.

TABLE 2

Stimulation of the Ribosomal Binding of
[^{14}C]aminoacyl-tRNAs by Oligonucleotides[a]

Oligonucleotide,	[^{14}C]Phe-tRNA bound			[^{14}C]Val-tRNA bound		
1.4 nmoles base res.	pmoles	Δpmoles	%	pmoles	Δpmoles	%
None	0.95	—	—	0.27	—	—
GUUU	5.37	4.42	100	1.98	1.71	100
G*UUU	5.40	4.40	100	0.29	0.02	0
UUUG	3.39	2.44	100	—	—	—
UUUG*	3.22	2.27	93	—	—	—

[a] Assays were performed as described in Table 1.

5' side of the modified G to function in base pairing with the anticodon of the lysine tRNA. This inhibition was less striking when
pentamers containing an additional A residue, GAAAA or AAAAG,
were modified with AAF, suggesting that the inhibitory effect was
limited mainly to the base immediately adjacent to the modified G
residue.

In contrast to these effects, the ability of a UUU triplet to function as a code word for phenylalanine was not influenced significantly
if an AAF-modified G residue was present on either the 5' or the 3'
side of the UUU triplet (Table 2). These results are entirely compatible with our CD data (as well as theoretical predictions), suggesting
that the stacking interaction between the fluorene moiety is much
stronger with a neighboring A residue than it is with a neighboring U
residue. As described previously (12), AAF modification of the G
residue completely inhibited the ability of the GUU sequence to code
for valine.

SINGLE-STRANDED GUANOSINE RESIDUES ARE MORE SUSCEPTIBLE
TO AAF MODIFICATION THAN DOUBLE-STRANDED ONES

The base displacement model predicts that guanosine residues
present in single-stranded regions of nucleic acid should be more
easily attacked by AAF than residues present in double-stranded
regions. Transfer RNA represents a convenient nucleic acid to test
this since it contains both double-stranded, or "stem regions," and
single-stranded, or "loop regions," as part of the cloverleaf structure. By reacting purified E. coli tRNA^{fMet} with [^{14}C]N-acetoxy-
AAF and degrading the modified tRNA with both T_1 and pancreatic
ribonuclease, we found (19) that the drug preferentially attacked a
guanosine residue at position 20, which is in the dihydrouridine
loop of the molecule (Fig. 4). This tRNA has 25 guanosine residues,
18 of which are thought to be in base-paired regions. None of the
latter reacted with the drug. There are seven non-base-paired
guanosine residues, and yet the drug preferentially attacked the G
residue present in the dihydrouridine loop. Studies in progress suggest that AAF also reacts preferentially with a guanosine residue in
the dihydrouridine loop of yeast tyrosine tRNA (Pulkrabek, Grunberger,
and Weinstein, unpublished studies).

Litt has found that kethoxal is bound preferentially to G in the
dihydrouridine loop of tRNA^{Phe} at position 20 (20). It is also of
interest to note that in Levitt's model of tRNA^{fMet} the G residue at
position 20 is in the syn conformation (21), since we would predict
that this would render this G residue particularly susceptible to AAF

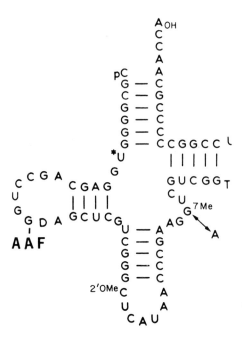

FIG. 4. Primary structure of tRNA^{fMet} indicating the presence of AAF on the G-20 residue. For details see Ref. 19.

modification. Several models have been proposed for the secondary and tertiary structure of tRNA (22). Most of these models place the dihydrouridine loop at the outer surface of the three-dimensional structure of the molecule. It becomes apparent from the results with AAF and tRNA that the attack of carcinogens on nucleic acids is a function of both the secondary and tertiary structure of the nucleic acid, and this may also have important biologic implications in terms of specificity.

Additional evidence that single-stranded regions are more suscep-tible to AAF modification than double-stranded regions was obtained by comparing the reactivity of native and denatured DNA with N-acetoxy AAF. We have found that denatured DNA is approximately twice as susceptible to AAF modification as native DNA. In addition, media of high ionic strengths are known to stabilize nucleic acid secondary structure, and we found that these led to a decrease in the reactivity of DNA with N-acetoxy AAF (23).

AAF MODIFICATION PRODUCES LOCALIZED
DENATURATION OF NUCLEIC ACIDS

The base displacement model predicts that AAF modification of double-stranded nucleic acids should produce a localized denaturation or loss of base pairing at the site of AAF modification. The distortion produced might result in a destabilization of double-stranded regions which could extend over a distance of several nucleotide residues adjacent to the modified G residue. We have demonstrated that this is the case in several different ways.

1. Heat denaturation studies indicate that a sample of calf thymus DNA in which 10% of the nucleotides had been modified with AAF had a 11° decrease in T_m when compared with a control sample of native DNA (23). A decrease in T_m with AAF-modified DNA has also been reported by Troll and Berkowitz (24).

   The decrease in T_m might be explained if we assume that AAF substitution of G residues simply displaces these G residues, thereby breaking single G-C base pairs and thus decreasing the effective G-C content of the DNA sample. A comparison of our data with the nomogram of Marmur and Doty (25) relating T_m to G+C content, however, indicates that the decrease in T_m, which we observed, is greater than that predicted by this assumption. It appears, therefore, that the destabilizing effect of AAF modification of double-stranded DNA extends beyond the immediate G residue that has been substituted.

   We have also found that AAF modification of tRNA also lowers its T_m during heat denaturation (19), but this is difficult to interpret directly in terms of the physical structure of the modified tRNA because of the complex nature of tRNA heat denaturation curves (26).

2. We have also studied the effects of AAF modification on the intrinsic viscosity of DNA. The viscosity of DNA is a function of both its flexibility and the length of the strands. Denaturation of native DNA is known to lead to a decrease in its intrinsic viscosity, whereas the noncovalent binding of acridines, Miracil D, or polycyclic hydrocarbons to DNA via intercalation results in an increase in intrinsic viscosity (27-30). This is explained by the fact that localized regions of denaturation provide flexible elbows in the DNA strand, whereas the sites of drug intercalation have a decreased flexibility, and intercalation is also associated with a lengthening of the DNA strand (28, 29).

   We modified 4% of the bases in a sample of native calf thymus DNA and compared its viscosity with control DNA across a range

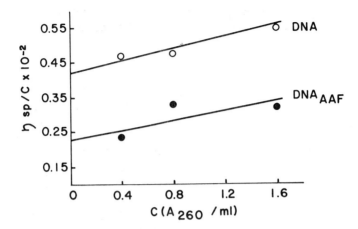

FIG. 5. Intrinsic viscosity of native calf thymus DNA compared with a sample of DNA in which 4% of the bases were modified with AAF. Viscosity was measured in a Zimm-Crothers viscometer as previously described (30) at three concentrations of DNA in 0.001 M phosphate (pH 7.0) - 0.1 M NaCl - 0.001 M EDTA at 25°C. C designates the concentration of DNA as A_{260}/ml $\eta_{sp} = \eta_{rel} - 1$, where $\eta_{rel} =$ (time for rotor to complete 10 revolutions in sample)/(time for rotor to complete 10 revolutions in solvent).

of DNA concentrations. Figure 5 indicates that AAF modification led to a marked decrease in the intrinsic viscosity of the DNA.

3. Other evidence for the denaturing effect of AAF was sought by examining whether AAF modification of double-stranded Rheo virus RNA (normally resistant to pancreatic ribonuclease in 0.3 M NaCl) renders regions of this RNA susceptible to pancreatic ribonuclease. Starting with Rheo virus RNA containing [³H]-uridine residues, we found that when approximately 3% of the bases of this RNA were modified with AAF, about 10% of the labeled uridine residues were rendered acid soluble after treatment with pancreatic ribonuclease (23). Under identical conditions, a sample of Rheo virus RNA that was not modified with AAF was completely resistant to pancreatic ribonuclease. Assuming that susceptibility to ribonuclease reflects the extent of denaturation and a random distribution of uridine and AAF-guanosine residues, these results indicate that the length of denaturation in the region of an AAF-modified guanosine extends over a distance of several nucleotides.

4. An alternate approach to determine the effect of AAF modification on the secondary structure of nucleic acids was to examine whether modification of a single-stranded nucleic acid with AAF would

impair hybridization with a complementary strand of nucleic acid. For this purpose, we modified purified ^{32}P-labeled 23S ribosomal RNA (rRNA) from E. coli with AAF and determined its ability to hybridize with E. coli DNA utilizing previously described methods (31). When control rRNA was hybridized to DNA with rRNA present in excess, 0.28% of the E. coli was complementary to the input RNA. This value is similar to that originally reported by Yankofsky and Spiegelman (31). Increasing modification of rRNA with AAF led to a progressive decrease in hybridizability to the DNA (23). With approximately 5% of the nucleotides modified, there was an approximately 50% reduction in hybridizability.

TABLE 3

Evidence that AAF Modification Produces Localized Denaturation

---

1. Decreased T_m of DNA

2. Decreased viscosity of DNA

3. Increased susceptibility of double-stranded RNA to RNAase

4. Decreased hybridization of rRNA to DNA

BIOLOGIC CONSEQUENCES OF THE BASE DISPLACEMENT MODEL

Our results clearly indicate that the conformational changes induced in nucleic acids by AAF modification interfere with the normal function of tRNA's in both amino acid acceptance and codon recognition in vivo. There is increasing evidence from bacterial systems that, in addition to its function as an adaptor in protein synthesis, tRNA may also play an important role as an intermediate in enzyme repression (see Ref. 32 for a review of this subject). If this proves to be the case in mammalian cells, then AAF-induced conformational changes in certain tRNA's might also lead to distortions in cell regulation and contribute to the transformation mechanism.

If subsequent studies indicate that AAF also modifies mRNA's in vivo, then our data with synthetic codons and mRNA's would predict that AAF could block mRNA translation in vivo. This may be of critical importance to transformation if the blocked mRNA's normally play a role in cell regulation, for example, in the synthesis of key repressor proteins.

Our results also bear on the mutagenic effects of AAF. Recent studies indicate that derivatives of AAF act as frame-shift mutagens in bacteria (33), and this has been interpreted by the authors as evidence for intercalation. It is important, however, to clearly distinguish the differences between the physical properties of intercalation and of base displacement, and these are compared in schematic form in Fig. 6. The data we have obtained with AAF are entirely consistent with our base displacement model; whereas certain findings, notably the decrease in T_m and decrease in intrinsic viscosity of AAF-modified DNA, are not consistent with the conventional model of intercalation. Recent studies by Fuchs and Daune (34) of AAF-modified DNA employing circular dichroism, thermal denaturation, and viscosity and light scattering measurements were also interpreted as indicating that the "modified bases are shifted out of the double helix, while the fixed carcinogen is inserted." Although the base displacement model differs appreciably from simple intercalation in terms of its physical structure, base displacement like intercalation could produce frame shift (as well as other types) of mutations during replication of the AAF-modified strand of DNA. This is indicated schematically in Fig. 7. If the replication mechanism randomly inserts a base when it encounters an AAF-modified G residue, then this would lead to a single base pair change. If the replication mechanism simply skips the modified G residue and then continues copying the modified

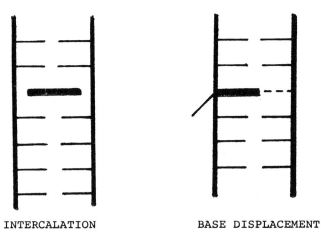

INTERCALATION   BASE DISPLACEMENT

FIG. 6. Schematic representation of a double-stranded nucleic acid with a planar drug, indicated by heavy line, inserted via intercalation or via base displacement. The vertical lines indicate the nucleic acid backbone and the horizontal lines complementary base pairs between the two strands.

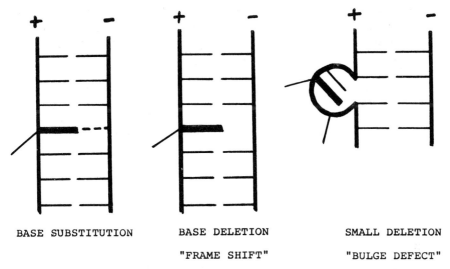

BASE SUBSTITUTION   BASE DELETION   SMALL DELETION

"FRAME SHIFT"   "BULGE DEFECT"

FIG. 7. Schematic representation of types of mutation that might occur as a consequence of the base displacement model. (+) designates a template strand during replication to which the drug (heavy line) is attached, and (-) designates the daughter strand.

strand in phase, then this would lead to a frame-shift mutation. If the AAF modification leads to an area of denaturation extending over a distance of several bases producing a small loop or bulge defect (35), then the replication mechanism may skip the entire defect, thereby resulting in a small deletion in the daughter strand.

Which one of the above processes prevails may depend on the local base sequence at the site of the AAF modification, the response of different polymerases when the replication mechanism encounters the site of AAF modification, and the efficiency and fidelity of DNA repair mechanisms.* As a matter of fact, single base pair errors and frame-shift mutations and deletions have all been described as muta-

---

*In terms of DNA repair mechanisms, it is of interest that cells from patients with xeroderma pigmentosum are defective in the repair of AAF-, ultraviolet light-, 4-nitroquinoline-1-oxide-, and polycyclic hydrocarbon-induced DNA lesions; yet these same cells normally repair lesions induced by point mutagens such as X ray and simple alkylating agents (36, 37). This suggests that the former group of agents all produce a bulky distortion in nucleic acid structure that is recognized by a repair mechanism that is distinct from that which repairs point mutations.

232   I. B. WEINSTEIN AND D. GRUNBERGER

genic effects of AAF or its derivatives in various test systems (33, 38-40). Although the mutagenic effects of AAF are often emphasized, our model predicts that AAF substitution could cause analogous defects in nucleic acid replication during the processes of DNA transcription into RNA or during reverse transcription of RNA into DNA.

Finally, we wonder whether the base displacement model we have formulated for AAF might also apply to other polycyclic carcinogens that bind covalently to nucleic acids, thereby providing a general mechanism by which this class of carcinogens distort nucleic acid structure and function.

ACKNOWLEDGMENTS

The authors wish to acknowledge the valuable contributions to the studies described in this paper made by Dr. Charles Cantor, Dr. Louis Fink, Dr. Shinji Fujimura, Dr. James Nelson, and Miss Augusta Flieg.

This research was supported by United States Public Health Service Grants CA-02332 and CA-05001 from the National Cancer Institute and the Alma Toorock Memorial for Cancer Research. Dr. Grunberger is a Scholar of the Leukemia Society of America.

REFERENCES

1. J. A. Miller, Carcinogenesis by chemicals: an overview —GHA Clowes Memorial Lecture, Cancer Res., 30, 559-576 (1970).
2. E. Farber, Biochemistry of carcinogenesis, Cancer Res., 28, 1859 (1968).
3. I. B. Weinstein, "Modifications in Transfer RNA during Chemical Carcinogenesis, " in Genetic Concepts and Neoplasia, Williams and Wilkins, Baltimore, Md., 1970, pp. 380-408.
4. S. Weinhouse, Glycolysis, respiration and anomalous gene expression in experimental hepatomas. GHA Clowes Memorial Lecture, Cancer Res., 32, 2007 (1972).
5. I. B. Weinstein and D. Grunberger, "RNA as the Target of Reactive

Forms of Chemical Carcinogens, " in Oncology, Vol. 1, Year Book
Medical Publishers, Inc. , Chicago, Ill. , 1971, pp. 47-57.

6. M. K. Agarwal and I. B. Weinstein, Modifications of ribonucleic
acid by chemical carcinogens. II. In vivo reaction of N-2-
acetylaminofluorene with rat liver ribonucleic acid, Biochemistry,
9, 503-508 (1970).

7. I. B. Weinstein, D. Grunberger, S. Fujimura, and L. M. Fink,
Chemical carcinogens and RNA, Cancer Res. , 31, 651 (1971).

8. E. C. Miller, U. Juhl, and J. A. Miller, Nucleic acid guanine:
reaction with the carcinogen N-acetoxy-2-acetylaminofluorene,
Science, 153, 1125 (1966).

9. E. Kriek, J. A. Miller, U. Juhl, and E. C. Miller, 8-(N-2-Fluorenyl-
acetamide)-guanosine, an arylamidation reaction product of
guanosine and the carcinogen N-acetoxy-N-2-fluorenyl-
acetamide in neutral solution, Biochemistry, 6, 177 (1967).

10. L. M. Fink, S. Nishimura, and I. B. Weinstein, Modifications of
ribonucleic acid by chemical carcinogens. I. In vitro modification
of transfer RNA by N-acetoxy-2-acetylaminofluorene, Biochemistry,
9, 496-502 (1970).

11. D. Grunberger, J. H. Nelson, C. R. Cantor, and I. B. Weinstein,
Coding and conformational properties of oligonucleotides modified
with the carcinogen N-2-acetylaminofluorene. Proc. Nat. Acad.
Sci. , 66, 488-494 (1970).

12. D. Grunberger and I. B. Weinstein, Modifications of ribonucleic
acid by chemical carcinogens. III. Template activity of polynucleotides modified by N-acetoxy-2-acetylaminofluorene,
J. Biol. Chem. , 246, 1123 (1971).

13. J. H. Nelson, D. Grunberger, C. R. Cantor, and I. B. Weinstein,
Modification of ribonucleic acid by chemical carcinogens. IV.
Circular dichroism and proton magnetic resonance studies of
oligonucleotides modified with N-2-acetylaminofluorene, J. Mol.
Biol. , 62, 331-346 (1971).

14. A. M. Kapuler and A. M. Michelson, The reaction of the carcinogen N-acetoxy-2-acetylaminofluorene with DNA and other polynucleotides and its stereochemical implications, Biochim.
Biophys. Acta, 232, 436 (1971).

15. C. E. Bugg and U. Thewalt, Effects of halogen substituents on
base stacking in nucleic acid components: The crystal structure
of 8-bromoguanosine, Biochem. Biophys. Res. Commun. , 37,
623 (1969).

16. S. S. Tavale and H. M. Sobell, Crystal and molecular structure of
8-bromoguanosine and 8-bromoadenosine, two purine nucleosides
in the syn configuration, J. Mol. Biol. , 48, 109 (1970).

17. S. I. Chan, M. P. Schweizer, P. O. P. Ts'o, and G. K. Helmkamp,
Interaction and association of bases and nucleosides in aqueous

solutions. III. A nuclear magnetic resonance study of the self-association of purine and 6-methyl-purine, J. Amer. Chem. Soc. 86, 4182 (1964).

18. S. I. Chan and J. H. Nelson, Proton magnetic resonance studies of ribose dinucleoside monophosphates in aqueous solution. I. The nature of the base-stacking interaction in adenylyl $(3' \rightarrow 5')$ adenosine, J. Amer. Chem. Soc., 91, 168 (1969).

19. S. Fujimura, D. Grunberger, G. Carvajal, and I. B. Weinstein, Modifications of ribonucleic acid by chemical carcinogens. Modification of Escherichia coli formylmethionine transfer ribonucleic acid with N-acetoxy-2-acetylaminofluorene, Biochemistry, 11, 3629 (1972).

20. M. Litt, Inactivation of yeast phenylalanine transfer ribonucleic acid by kethoxal, Biochemistry, 10, 2223 (1971).

21. M. Levitt, Detailed molecular model for transfer ribonucleic acid, Nature (London), 224, 759 (1969).

22. F. Cramer, Three dimensional structure of tRNA, Progr. Nucl. Acid Res. Mol. Biol., 11, 391 (1971).

23. L. M. Fink, A. Flieg, D. Grunberger, and I. B. Weinstein, Effect of N-2-acetylaminofluorene (AAF) modification of nucleic acids on their secondary structure, Proc. Amer. Assoc. Cancer Res., 12, 11 (1971).

24. W. Troll and E. M. Berkowitz, "Modification of DNA and poly rG by Carcinogenic Agents Assayed by Physical and Enzymatic Methods," Physico-Chemical Mechanisms of Carcinogenesis, Vol. 1 (E. D. Bergmann and B. Pullman, eds.), The Israel Academy of Sciences and Humanities, Jerusalem, 1969.

25. J. Marmur and P. Doty, Determination of the base composition of DNA from its thermal denaturation temperature, J. Mol. Biol., 5, 109-118 (1962).

26. P. E. Cole, S. K. Yang, and D. M. Crothers, Conformational changes in transfer ribonucleic acid. Equilibrium phase diagrams, Biochemistry, 11, 4358-4368 (1972).

27. L. S. Lerman, Structural considerations in the interaction of DNA and acridines, J. Mol. Biol., 3, 18 (1961).

28. S. Lerman, "The Combination of DNA with Polycyclic Aromatic Hydrocarbons," Proceedings of the Fifth National Cancer Conference, Lippincott, Philadelphia, 1964, pp. 36-48.

29. L. S. Lerman, Acridine mutagens and DNA structure, J. Cell. Comp. Physiol., 64 (Suppl. 1), 1-18 (1964).

30. R. A. Carchman, E. Hirschberg, and I. B. Weinstein, Miracil D: effect on the viscosity of DNA, Biochem. Biophys. Acta, 179, 158-164 (1969).

31. S. A. Yankofsky and S. Spiegelman, The identification of the ribosomal RNA cistron by sequence complementarity II, Proc. Nat. Acad. Sci., 48, 1466-1472 (1962).

32. M. Brenner, J. A. Lewis, D. S. Straus, F. De Lorenzo, and B. N. Ames, Histidine regulation in Salmonella typhimurium, J. Biol. Chem., 247, 4333 (1972).

33. B. N. Ames, E. G. Gurney, J. A. Miller, and H. Bartsch, Carcinogens as frameshift mutagens: metabolites and derivatives of 2-acetylaminofluorene and other aromatic amine carcinogens, Proc. Nat. Acad. Sci., 69, 3128 (1972).

34. R. Fuchs and M. Daune, Physical studies on deoxyribonucleic acid after covalent binding of a carcinogen, Biochim. Biophys. Acta, 14, 2659-2666 (1972).

35. T. R. Fink and D. M. Crothers, Free energy of imperfect nucleic acid helices. I. The bulge defect, J. Mol. Biol., 66, 1-2 (1972).

36. R. B. Setlow and J. D. Regan, Defective repair of N-acetoxy-2-acetylaminofluorene-induced lesions in the DNA of xeroderma pigmentosum cells, Biochem. Biophys. Res. Commun., 46, 1019 (1972).

37. H. F. Stich, R. H. C. San, J. A. Miller, and E. C. Miller, Various levels of DNA repair synthesis in xeroderma pigmentosum cells exposed to carcinogens N-hydroxy and N-acetoxy-2-acetylaminofluorene, Nature New Biol., 238, 9 (1972).

38. T. H. Corbett, C. Heidelberger, and W. F. Dove, Determination of the mutagenic activity to bacteriophage T4 of carcinogenic and noncarcinogenic compounds, Mol. Pharmacol., 6 (6), 667-679 (1970).

39. V. M. Maher, J. A. Miller, E. C. Miller, and W. C. Summers, Mutations and loss of transforming activity of Bacillus subtilis DNA after reaction with esters of carcinogenic N-hydroxy aromatic amides, Cancer Res., 30, 1473-1480 (1970).

40. O. G. Fahmy and M. J. Fahmy, Gene elimination in carcinogenesis: reinterpretation of the somatic mutation theory, Cancer Res., 30, 195-205 (1970).

Chapter 10

FORMATION AND REACTIONS OF EPOXY DERIVATIVES OF AROMATIC POLYCYCLIC HYDROCARBONS

P. Sims and P. L. Grover

Chester Beatty Research Institute
Institute of Cancer Research
Royal Cancer Hospital
Fulham Road, London

There have been a number of reports in recent years describing experiments in which metabolites of aromatic polycyclic hydrocarbons were biologically more active than their parent compounds (1-3). In the induction of tumors in whole animals, however, it is still not clear whether the hydrocarbons themselves are active or whether some metabolic activation within the cell precedes the initiation of carcinogenesis. When cells are treated with hydrocarbons, covalent binding of the hydrocarbon moieties to cellular constituents such as DNA, RNA, and proteins (4-7) occurs, and in these reactions some metabolic activating process is necessary since the hydrocarbons themselves do not possess reactive groups.

In experiments in which [^{3}H]-labeled hydrocarbons were incubated with a rat liver microsomal system in the presence of DNA, covalent binding of the hydrocarbon moieties to the nucleic acid was observed when cofactors for the NADPH-dependent mixed function oxidase were present (8), suggesting that the microsomal enzyme can convert aromatic hydrocarbons into reactive metabolites. In the metabolism of naphthalene in whole animals, the hydrocarbon is converted into trans-1, 2-dihydro-1, 2-dihydroxynaphthalene (9) and because of this, Boyland (10) suggested that naphthalene-1, 2-oxide was formed as a metabolic intermediate in the metabolism of naphthalene. Further support for this idea was provided by the isolation of the mercapturic acid, N-acetyl-S-(1, 2-dihydro-2-hydroxy-1-naphthyl)-L-cysteine from the urine of rabbits dosed with naphthalene (11). Thus, as shown in Fig. 1, naphthalene-1, 2-oxide could be an intermediate in the formation, from the hydrocarbon, of the dihydrodiol, of the mercapturic

237

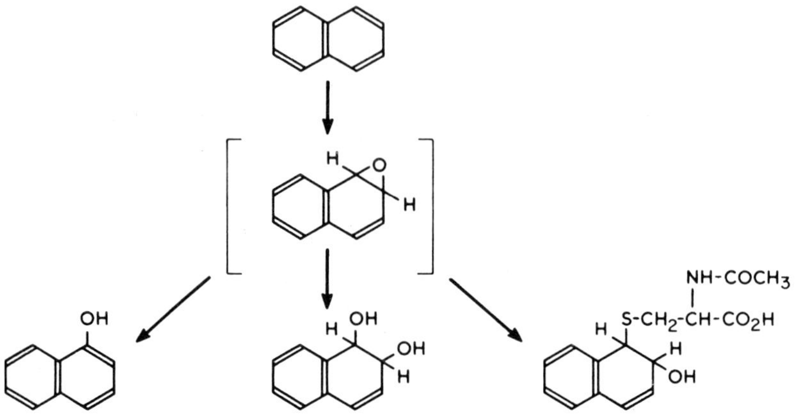

FIG. 1. Metabolism of naphthalene in whole animals.

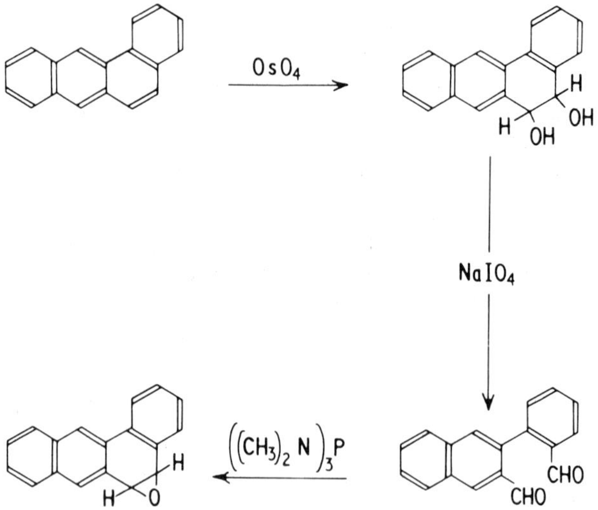

FIG. 2. Preparation of the K-region epoxide, benz(a)anthracene-
5, 6-oxide.

acid, and possibly of 1-naphthol. These findings made it likely that the reactive intermediates formed from polycyclic hydrocarbons by microsomal systems are arene oxides.

Using the method of Newman and Blum (12) outlined in Fig. 2, a number of these oxides have been synthesized. This method of synthesis yields "K-region" epoxides since the initial reaction in the synthetic route involves an oxidation of the parent hydrocarbon with osmium tetroxide: oxidations with this reagent take place at the "K-regions" of the hydrocarbons (13). Newman and Blum (12) first described the preparation of phenanthrene-9, 10-oxide, benz(a)-anthracene-5, 6-oxide, and 7-methylbenz(a)anthracene-5, 6-oxide. Other oxides synthesized by this method include chrysene-5, 6-oxide (14), 3-methylcholanthrene-10, 11-oxide (15), dibenz(a, h)anthracene-5, 6-oxide (16), and 7, 12-dimethylbenz(a)anthracene-5, 6-oxide (17). Two related compounds, 7-hydroxymethylbenz(a)anthracene-5, 6-oxide (18) and 7-hydroxymethyl-12-methylbenz(a)anthracene-5, 6-oxide (17) have also been synthesized because one of the routes by which the parent hydrocarbons, 7-methylbenz(a)anthracene and 7, 12-dimethylbenz(a)anthracene, are metabolized, by both rat liver preparations (19) and rodent embryo cells (20), involves hydroxylation of the methyl groups to give hydroxymethyl derivatives. A number of K-region epoxides have been prepared in the [³H]-labeled forms (21) since the parent hydrocarbons can readily be labeled with tritium by exchange reactions.

Although most of the aromatic polycyclic hydrocarbons that have been examined are metabolized by hepatic microsomal enzymes at the K-region, metabolism also occurs at other bonds in the molecules to yield dihydrodiols and phenols and, in many cases, these non-K-region products form the major components of the ethyl-acetate soluble metabolites (22). Since it appears likely that these metabolites also arise through the intermediate formation of arene oxides, a number of non-K-region epoxides have been synthesized, all of which are probably formed in the metabolism of their parent hydrocarbons. The non-K-region epoxides synthesized are benzo(a)pyrene-7, 8- and 9, 10-oxide (23), dibenz(a, c)anthracene-10, 11-oxide (24), and benz(a)-anthracene-8, 9-oxide (25). The synthetic route leading to the latter oxide is outlined in Fig. 3; the other non-K-region epoxides were synthesized by similar reactions. Dibenz(a, c)anthracene is of particular interest for while the parent hydrocarbon does not contain a K-region, binding of the hydrocarbon moiety to the nucleic acids of mouse skin and rodent embryo cells has been observed (4-7).

The arene oxides, both K-region and non-K-region, are all metabolized by similar routes in rat liver preparations (15-17, 23-26, 28): the metabolism of benz(a)anthracene-5, 6-oxide is shown in Fig. 4.

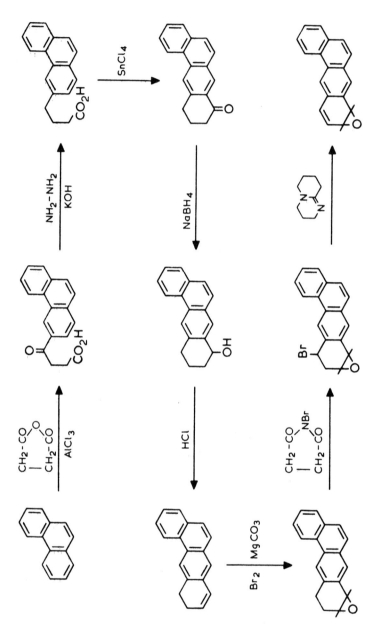

FIG. 3. Preparation of the non-K-region epoxide, benz(a)anthracene-8, 9-oxide.

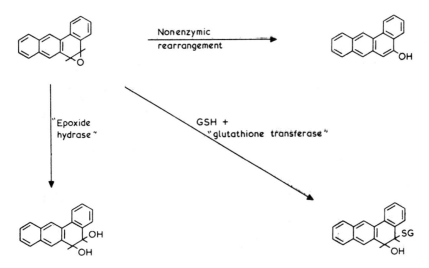

FIG. 4. Reactions of benz(a)anthracene-5, 6-oxide.

They are converted by epoxide hydrases, present in hepatic microsomal fractions (27), into the related trans-dihydrodiols and by a
glutathione transferase, present in hepatic soluble fractions (28),
into glutathione conjugates. These metabolites are identical with the
metabolites formed from the parent hydrocarbons by rat liver preparations. Although the oxides are rapidly rearranged into phenols by
mineral acid, they are only slowly converted into these phenols by
rat liver preparations, a reaction that is probably nonenzymic.

The enzymic conversion of a number of aromatic polycyclic hydrocarbons into their related K-region epoxides has been demonstrated
(29, 30) using a rat liver microsomal system containing the cofactors
necessary for the microsomal mixed function oxidase. The incubations,
using [^{3}H]-labeled hydrocarbons, were carried out in the presence of
1, 2-epoxy-1, 2, 3, 4-tetrahydronaphthalene, which, acting as an inhibitor of the epoxide hydrase, retards the enzymic conversion of the
oxides into dihydrodiols. The reaction products were chromatographed
on alumina using a system that separates the oxides from the unchanged
hydrocarbons and from hydroxylated metabolites such as dihydrodiols
and phenols. The identities of the epoxides were established by their
enzymic conversion into products with the chromatographic properties
of the related trans-dihydrodiols and by their chemical conversion
into products with the properties of the related phenols and glutathione
conjugates. Hydrocarbons that are now known to be converted into
K-region epoxides in the microsomal system include phenanthrene and
benz(a)anthracene (29), pyrene and benzo(a)pyrene (30), 7, 12-
dimethyl(a)anthracene (31), and 3-methylcholanthrene (32). An

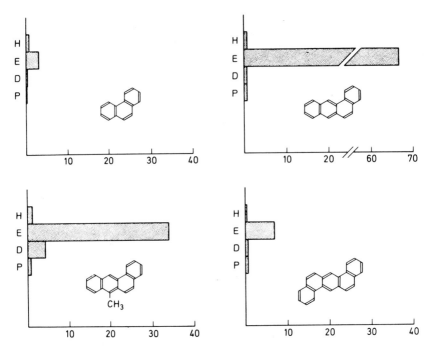

FIG. 5. Binding (μmoles/mole DNA P) of H, hydrocarbon; E, K-region epoxide; D, K-region cis-dihydrodiol; and P, K-region phenol to the DNA of polyoma virus-transformed BHK 21 cells in tissue culture.

unidentified oxide has also been detected in the microsomal oxidation of dibenz(a, h)anthracene (29, 33). The formation of non-K-region epoxides from hydrocarbons by the microsomal system could not be demonstrated, probably because epoxides of this type are less stable and rearrange to phenols on alumina columns.

As expected, all the arene oxides were alkylating agents and readily reacted with 4-(p-nitrobenzyl)pyridine, DNA, and protein (21). In experiments (34) using a polyoma-transformed line of BHK cells, in which the levels of the mixed function oxidase were low, the abilities of four [³H]-labeled polycyclic hydrocarbons and their K-region epoxides, cis-dihydrodiols, and phenols to react with DNA were compared. In each series of compounds, the highest levels of reaction with DNA were found with the oxides (Fig. 5).

The results shown in Table 1 indicate that K-region epoxides react chemically to varying extents with DNA and most of them with RNA.

TABLE 1

Reactions of [^{3}H]-Labeled K-Region Epoxides of
Polycyclic Hydrocarbons with DNA and RNA[a]

K-region epoxides	μmoles/mole-P	
	DNA	RNA
Phenanthrene-9, 10-oxide	15	7
Benz(a)anthracene-5, 6-oxide	680	505
7-Methylbenz(a)anthracene-5, 6-oxide	1630	960
Dibenz(a, h)anthracene-5, 6-oxide	327	417

[a]Nucleic acid (4.0 μmole-P) dissolved in distilled water (pH 7.4, 2.0 ml) was mixed with a solution of the epoxide (0.04 μmole) in ethanol (1 ml) and incubated at 37 °C for 2 hr. Extents of reaction were estimated following passage through a G25 Sephadex column.

The results of the reactions of K-region epoxides with polynucleotides are shown in Table 2 and suggest that guanine and adenine may be the principal sites of alkylation in the nucleic acids (35). The reactions of non-K-region epoxides with macromolecules, either chemically or in cells, have not been investigated because [^{3}H]-labeled oxides of this type have not yet been prepared.

It has so far been established that K-region epoxides are formed during the metabolism of aromatic polycyclic hydrocarbons by microsomal enzymes and that these epoxides will react with cellular constituents including DNA, RNA, and proteins. The metabolic formation of the non-K-region epoxides and their involvement in reactions with macromolecules has not been finally established. Although K-region epoxides are not as active as their parent hydrocarbons in the induction of cancer in mice (14, 36), they are more active than the parent hydrocarbons in some other biologic systems. Some are more active than their parent hydrocarbon in the induction of malignant transformations in rodent cells in culture (2, 3) and some will induce uncharacterized mutations in mammalian cells (37) and in bacteriophage (36). In Salmonella typhimurium, K-region epoxides have been found to revert to known frame-shift mutants (39).

Studies on a series of K-region epoxides have shown that there are wide variations in the rates at which the oxides will alkylate 4-(p-nitrobenzyl)pyridine, rearrange to phenols, and react enzymically

TABLE 2

Reactions of [³H]-Labeled K-Region Epoxides of Polycyclic Hydrocarbons with Polyribonucleotides[a]

K-Region Epoxide	μmoles/mole-P						
	Poly G	Poly A	Poly X	Poly I	Poly U	Poly C
Phenanthrene-9,10-oxide	280	22	31	42	9	9
Benz(a)anthracene-5,6-oxide	870	161	86	45	7	7
7-Methylbenz(a)anthracene-5,6-oxide	1310	566	265	80	27	8
Dibenz(a,h)anthracene-5,6-oxide	1860	35	90	51	5	5

[a]See footnote to Table 1 for experimental conditions.

with water (40, 41). Presumably, the relative rates at which the oxides are formed, react with cellular constituents, or are inactivated by further metabolism determines their effective concentration in the system and to some extent their biologic activities. There is as yet no direct evidence that arene oxides are involved in the carcinogenic activities of the polycyclic hydrocarbons, but there is sufficient indirect evidence to suggest that further studies on these compounds are worthwhile.

REFERENCES

1. E. Boyland, P. Sims, and C. Huggins, Induction of adrenal damage and cancer with metabolites of 7, 12-dimethylbenz[a]anthracene, Nature (London), 207, 816 (1965).
2. P. L. Grover, P. Sims, E. Huberman, H. Marquardt, T. Kuroki, and C. Heidelberger, In vitro transformation of rodent cells by K-region derivatives of polycyclic hydrocarbons, Proc. Nat. Acad. Sci., 68, 1098 (1971).
3. H. Marquardt, T. Kuroki, E. Huberman, J. K. Selkirk, C. Heidelberger, P. L. Grover, and P. Sims, Malignant transformation of cells derived from mouse prostate by epoxides and other derivatives of polycyclic hydrocarbons, Cancer Res., 32, 716 (1972).
4. P. Brookes and P. D. Lawley, Evidence for the binding of polynuclear aromatic hydrocarbons to the nucleic acids of mouse skin: Relation between carcinogenic power of hydrocarbons and their binding to deoxyribonucleic acid, Nature (London), 202, 781 (1964).
5. L. M. Goshman and C. Heidelberger, Binding of tritium-labeled polycyclic hydrocarbons to DNA of mouse skin, Cancer Res., 27, 1678 (1967).
6. M. E. Duncan and P. Brookes, Metabolism and macromolecular binding of dibenz[a, c]anthracene and dibenz[a, h]anthracene by mouse embryo cells in culture, Intern. J. Cancer, 9, 349 (1972).
7. T. Kuroki and C. Heidelberger, The binding of polycyclic aromatic hydrocarbons to the DNA, RNA and proteins of transformable cells in culture, Cancer Res., 31, 2168 (1971).
8. P. L. Grover and P. Sims, Enzyme-catalyzed reactions of polycyclic hydrocarbons with deoxyribonucleic acid and protein in vitro, Biochem. J., 110, 159 (1968).
9. J. Booth and E. Boyland, Metabolism of polycyclic compounds. 5. Formation of 1:2-dihydro-1:2-dihydroxynaphthalenes, Biochem. J., 44, 361 (1949).
10. E. Boyland, The biological significance of metabolism of polycyclic compounds, Symp. Biochem. Soc., 5, 40 (1950).

11. E. Boyland and P. Sims, Metabolism of polycyclic compounds.
    12. An acid-labile precursor of 1-naphthylmercapturic acid and
    naphthol: an N-acetyl-S-(1:2-dihydrohydroxynaphthyl)-L-cys-
    teine, Biochem. J., 68, 440 (1958).

12. M.S. Newman and S. Blum, A new cyclization reaction leading
    to epoxides of aromatic hydrocarbons, J. Amer. Chem. Soc., 86,
    5598 (1964).

13. J.W. Cook and R. Schoental, Oxidation of carcinogenic hydro-
    carbons by osmium tetroxide, J. Chem. Soc., 170 (1948).

14. E. Boyland and P. Sims, The carcinogenic activities in mice of
    compounds related to benz[a]anthracene, Intern. J. Cancer, 2,
    500 (1967).

15. P. Sims, The metabolism of 3-methylcholanthrene and some
    related compounds by rat liver homogenates, Biochem. J., 98,
    215 (1966).

16. E. Boyland and P. Sims, The metabolism of benz[a]anthracene
    and dibenz[a, h]anthracene and their 5, 6-epoxy-5, 6-dihydro
    derivatives by rat liver homogenates, Biochem. J., 97, 7 (1965).

17. P. Sims, Epoxy derivatives of aromatic polycyclic hydrocarbons.
    The preparation and metabolism of epoxides related to 7, 12-di-
    methylbenz[a]anthracene, Biochem. J., 131, 405 (1973).

18. P. Sims, The preparation of 7-hydroxymethylbenz[a]anthracene
    5, 6-oxide and its metabolism by rat liver preparations, Xeno-
    biotica, 2, 469 (1972).

19. E. Boyland and P. Sims, Metabolism of polycyclic compounds.
    The metabolism of 7, 12-dimethylbenz[a]anthracene by rat-liver
    homogenates, Biochem. J., 95, 780 (1965).

20. P. Sims, The metabolism of some aromatic hydrocarbons by mouse
    embryo cell cultures, Biochem. Pharmacol., 19, 285 (1970).

21. P.L. Grover and P. Sims, Interactions of the K-region epoxides
    of phenanthrene and dibenz[a, h]anthracene with nucleic acids
    and histones, Biochem. Pharmacol., 19, 2251 (1970).

22. P. Sims, Qualitative and quantitative studies on the metabolism
    of a series of aromatic polycyclic hydrocarbons by rat-liver prep-
    arations, Biochem. Pharmacol., 19, 795 (1970).

23. J.F. Waterfall and P. Sims, Epoxy derivatives of aromatic poly-
    cyclic hydrocarbons. The preparation and metabolism of epoxides
    related to benzo[a]pyrene and to 7, 8- and 9, 10-dihydrobenzo[a]-
    pyrene, Biochem. J., 128, 265 (1972).

24. P. Sims, Epoxy derivatives of aromatic polycyclic hydrocarbons.
    The synthesis of dibenz[a, c]anthracene 10, 11-oxide and its me-
    tabolism by rat-liver preparations, Biochem. J., 130, 27 (1972).

25. P. Sims, Epoxy derivatives of aromatic polycyclic hydrocarbons.
    The preparation of benz[a]anthracene 8, 9-oxide and 10, 11-di-
    hydrobenz[a]anthracene 8, 9-oxide and their metabolism by rat
    liver preparations, Biochem. J., 125, 159 (1971).

26. E. Boyland and P. Sims, Metabolism of polycyclic compounds. The metabolism of 9,10-epoxy-9,10-dihydrophenanthrene in rats, Biochem. J., 95, 788 (1965).

27. F. Oesch and J. Daly, Solubilization, purification, and properties of a hepatic epoxide hydrase, Biochim. Biophys. Acta, 227, 692 (1971).

28. E. Boyland and K. Williams, An enzyme catalyzing the conjugation of epoxides with glutathione, Biochem. J., 94, 190 (1965).

29. P. L. Grover, A. Hewer, and P. Sims, Epoxides as microsomal metabolites of polycyclic hydrocarbons, FEBS Letters, 18, 76 (1971).

30. P. L. Grover, A. Hewer, and P. Sims, Formation of K-region epoxides as microsomal metabolites of pyrene and benzo[a]pyrene, Biochem. Pharmacol., 21, 2713 (1972).

31. G. R. Keysell, J. Booth, P. Sims, P. L. Grover, and A. Hewer, The formation of an epoxide in the microsomal metabolism of 7,12-dimethylbenz[a]anthracene, Biochem. J., 129, 41P (1972).

32. P. L. Grover, A. Hewer, and P. Sims, unpublished work.

33. J. K. Selkirk, E. Huberman, and C. Heidelberger, An epoxide is an intermediate in the microsomal metabolism of the chemical carcinogen dibenz[a, h] anthracene, Biochem. Biophys. Res. Commun., 43, 1010 (1972).

34. P. L. Grover, J. A. Forrester, and P. Sims, Reactivity of the K-region epoxides of some polycyclic hydrocarbons towards the nucleic acids and proteins of BHK21 cells, Biochem. Pharmacol., 20, 1297 (1971).

35. P. L. Grover and P. Sims, Reactions of 'K'-region epoxides of polycyclic hydrocarbons with nucleic acids and polyribonucleotides, Biochem. J., 129, 41P (1972).

36. P. Sims, The carcinogenic activities in mice of compounds related to 3-methylcholanthrene, Intern. J. Cancer, 2, 505 (1967).

37. E. Huberman, L. Aspiras, C. Heidelberger, P. L. Grover, and P. Sims, Mutagenicity to mammalian cells of epoxides and other derivatives of polycyclic hydrocarbons, Proc. Nat. Acad. Sci., 68, 3195 (1971).

38. M. J. Cookson, P. Sims, and P. L. Grover, Mutagenicity of epoxides of polycyclic hydrocarbons correlates with carcinogenicity of parent hydrocarbons, Nat. New Biol., 234, 186 (1971).

39. B. N. Ames, P. Sims, and P. L. Grover, Epoxides of carcinogenic polycyclic hydrocarbons are frameshift mutagens, Science, 176, 47 (1972).

40. A. Swaisland, P. L. Grover, and P. Sims, Some properties of 'K-region' epoxides of polycyclic hydrocarbons, Biochem. Pharmacol.,

41. H. Pandov and P. Sims, The conversion of phenanthrene 9,10-oxide and dibenz[a, h]anthracene 5,6-oxide into dihydrodiols by a rat-liver microsomal enzyme, Biochem. Pharmacol., 19, 299 (1970).

Chapter 11

FLAVONES AND POLYCYCLIC HYDROCARBONS AS MODULATORS OF ARYL HYDROCARBON[BENZO(a)PYRENE] HYDROXYLASE

F. J. Wiebel and H. V. Gelboin

Chemistry Branch
National Cancer Institute
Bethesda, Maryland

N. P. Buu-Hoi
Institut du Radium
Paris, France

M. G. Stout and W. S. Burnham
ICN, Nucleic Acid Research Institute
Irvine, California

INTRODUCTION

Polycyclic hydrocarbons are metabolized by microsomal NADPH-requiring enzyme systems (1-5) that belong to the group of "mixed-function oxidases" (6). These "aryl hydrocarbon hydroxylases"[1] are present in most tissues of mammals (2-4, 7) and are inducible by a large number of aromatic compounds that can be divided into at least two major groups typified by phenobarbital (PB)[2] or methylcholanthrene (MC) (2, 3, 8).

It has become increasingly apparent that the enzymatic oxidation of polycyclic hydrocarbons can lead to both the detoxification and the activation to cytotoxic and carcinogenic derivatives (4, 9-15). Thus, the biologic effect of the hydrocarbon will partially depend on the qualitative and quantitative character of the enzyme system, e.g., its activity in the target tissues and the ratios of the various metabolites formed. These might be governed by factors such as constitutive levels, tissue specific forms, or the state and type of induction of the enzyme. We have searched for compounds that modulate the activity of the aryl hydrocarbon hydroxylases. These compounds may be used to distinguish between different forms of the enzyme, their distribution, and the nature of their development. Furthermore, they should be helpful in exploring the structure and function of the enzyme system. These compounds can also aid in defining the role of the enzyme in polycyclic hydrocarbon-induced toxicity and carcinogenicity. The present report describes a number of flavones and polycyclic hydrocarbons that are potent stimulators or inhibitors of the enzyme system and demonstrates their use in investigations on the occurrence of different forms of the enzyme and their mode of function.

METHODS

Sprague Dawley rats were used throughout the experiments. They were kept on a Wayne Blox diet ad libitum. Forty milligrams per kilogram body weight of MC in corn oil (0.3 ml/100 gm body weight) were injected intraperitoneally (i.p.). After 18 hr, animals were sacrificed by decapitation. Control animals received corn oil only. Eighty milligrams per kilogram of PB were injected i.p. in saline (0.2 ml/100 gm body weight) on three consecutive days and the animals were sacrificed 18 hr after the last injection. Microsomes of liver, lung, and kidney were isolated from 0.25 M sucrose-tris homogenates as described previously (16).

Aryl hydrocarbon hydroxylase (AHH) activity was determined by the measurement of the fluorescence of phenolic metabolites formed from benzo(a)pyrene (BP) by the method of Wattenberg et al. (17) with modifications described previously (18, 19). AHH activity is expressed as nanomoles of phenolic products formed per milligram protein per 30 min. None of the flavonoid compounds or other polycyclic hydrocarbons used nor their metabolites caused significant fluorescence at the wavelengths that were employed for the determination of the BP metabolites (395 nm excitation/520 nm emission). Protein concentrations were determined by the method of Lowry et al. (20) using ribonuclease as standard.

RESULTS AND DISCUSSION

7,8-Benzoflavone as Probe for Different Forms of
Benzo(a)pyrene Hydroxylase

Preliminary studies suggested that the synthetic flavone, 7,8-benzoflavone (7,8-BF, see structure in Table 3), could be used as an agent to differentiate hepatic forms of the enzyme system (21). The

TABLE 1

Effect of 7, 8-Benzoflavone on Aryl Hydrocarbon Hydroxylase
Activity in Hepatic Microsomes from Normal and Phenobarbital-
or Methylcholanthrene-Treated Rats[a]

Addition	nmoles of product formed/mg protein/20 min		
	Normal	PB	MC
None	3.00	8.25	37.50
7, 8-BF (10^{-5})	4.26 (+42)	9.15 (+11)	19.87 (-53)
(10^{-4})	4.35 (+45)	9.16 (+12)	8.82 (-78)

[a] Values in parentheses give the percentage of inhibition (-) or
stimulation (+) of AHH activity in the presence of 7, 8-BF. Substrate
concentration was 10^{-4} M BP. 7, 8-BF was added in 0.010 ml of
methanol. Other conditions and treatment of rats with phenobarbital
(PB) or methylcholanthrene (MC) as described in Methods.

following discussion demonstrates the usefulness of 7, 8-benzoflavone
in distinguishing the enzyme systems of rats of different ages and
sexes and after different modes of induction.

The activity of aryl hydrocarbon [benzo(a)pyrene] hydroxylase (AHH)
is induced three- or ten-fold by pretreatment of rats with PB or MC,
respectively (Table 1). In vitro addition of 7, 8-BF to hepatic microsomes from either normal, PB-, or MC-treated male rats influences
AHH activity in various ways.

Enzyme activity of microsomes from untreated rats is increased in
the presence of 7, 8-BF. Similarly, enzyme activity in microsomes
from PB-treated animals is somewhat stimulated by 7, 8-BF. In contrast, AHH activity in microsomes from MC-treated rats is strongly
inhibited by 7, 8-BF. At a concentration of 10^{-5} M, which is one-
tenth of the substrate BP concentration, 7, 8-BF reduces the hydroxylating activity by 50%.

This effect, differentiating the constitutive and the MC-induced
enzyme, is not observed in extrahepatic tissues. As described
earlier (22), microsomes of lung and kidney from normal rats exhibit
low AHH activity that is markedly increased by pretreatment with an
inducer of the polycyclic hydrocarbon type (see legend Fig. 1). As
shown in Fig. 1, 7, 8-benzoflavone inhibits the microsomal enzyme
of lung and kidney from both normal and MC-treated animals, similar
to the inhibition of MC-induced enzyme in liver. This has also been

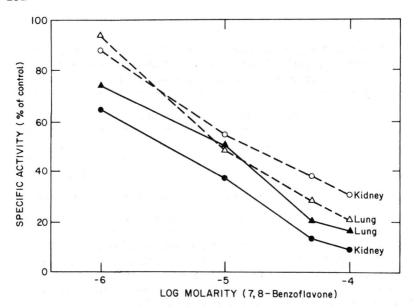

FIG. 1. Effect of 7, 8-benzoflavone on aryl hydrocarbon hydroxylase activity in lung and kidney microsomes from MC-treated and normal rats. Open symbols, microsomes from normal rats; closed symbols, microsomes from MC-treated rats. Ordinate: 100% refers to the specific AHH activity (nmoles of product formed/mg protein/30 min) in microsomal preparations from MC-treated and normal rats in the absence of 7, 8-BF: Amounts of microsomal protein used (mg/ml incubation mixture): lung, normal microsomes = 0.70, MC microsomes = 0.80; kidney, normal microsomes = 1.03, MC microsomes = 0.90. Specific AHH activities were as follows: Normal microsomes of lung and kidney, 0.025 and 0.007, MC microsomes of lung and kidney, 0.620 and 0.770. Other conditions as described in Methods (19).

found with the constitutive and induced enzyme activities from skin of untreated mice and mice pretreated topically or intraperitoneally with a polycyclic hydrocarbon inducer (19, 23). In these extrahepatic tissues, however, we always observed that the inhibition of the constitutive enzyme is somewhat less than that of the induced enzyme (Fig. 1). This indicates that extrahepatic tissues also contain two forms of hydroxylases, one form of which, the flavone-resistant form, comprises only a small fraction. In addition to the different sensitivity of the hydroxylases to the 7, 8-BF probe, hepatic and extrahepatic tissues appear to differ in the genetic regulation of the enzyme system (30).

Benzoflavones induce AHH activity in vitro by prior application in vivo, similar to MC and BP (24-26), and inhibit the metabolism of

TABLE 2

Effect of 7, 8-Benzoflavone on Hepatic Aryl Hydrocarbon
Hydroxylase: Age and Sex Dependency[a]

	AHH specific activity			
	Normal microsomes		MC microsomes	
Age and sex	In vitro addition			
of rats	None	7, 8-BF	None	7, 8-BF
Newborn (6 days)				
Female	0.17	0.64 (+273)	5.45	0.93 (-83)
Male	0.17	0.61 (+265)	6.06	1.07 (-82)
Adult (30 days)				
Female	0.56	0.14 (-75)	9.19	1.26 (-86)
Male	2.09	1.69 (-19)	9.39	2.15 (-77)

[a] Enzyme activities were determined in the supernatants of liver
homogenates from three to four rats after centrifugation at 8000 × g
for 15 min. Amounts of protein were 0.85 to 1.20 mg/ml of incubation
mixture. Incubation period was 10 min. AHH specific activity is expressed as nanomoles of phenolic products formed/mg of protein/30
min. Other conditions as in Materials and Methods.

polycyclic hydrocarbons in cells in culture (21, 26) and presumably
in vivo (23). These activities have previously been related to their
effect on the cytotoxicity and the tumorigenicity of polycyclic hydrocarbons (23, 25-29).

Hepatic AHH during the Development of Rats

Table 2 shows the effect of 7, 8-BF on hepatic AHH activity from
rats of different sex and age. Hepatic enzyme activity from newborn
animals (six days postpartum) is greatly increased in the presence of
7, 8-BF. In contrast, 7, 8-BF inhibits the enzyme from young adult
females by 75% and to a small degree also reduces the enzyme activity of the young adult male. These data clearly indicate that the
differential effect of the flavone is due to factors other than the
amount of enzyme present in the liver. Treatment with MC induces
hydroxylase activity of newborn and adult male and female animals
to high levels relatively independent of the widely differing constitutive levels. Unlike the constitutive enzyme, the induced enzyme of

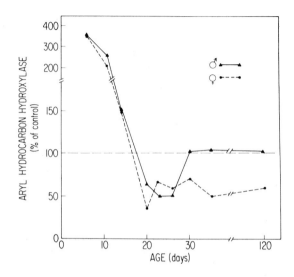

FIG. 2. Effect of 7, 8-benzoflavone on hepatic aryl hydrocarbon hydroxylase: postnatal development in male and female rats. One hundred percent of control refers to the specific activities (phenolic products formed/mg of protein/30 min) in tissue preparations from rats of different ages and sexes in the absence of 7, 8-BF (see Table 2). Experimental conditions as described in Table 2 and in Methods. Note the change in the scale of the ordinate.

rats of either sex or either age is inhibited 70 to 80% by the benzo-flavone.

The development of the different constitutive forms of AHH was examined using the benzoflavone as probe (Fig. 2): The stimulation of AHH activity by 7, 8-BF in newborn rats decreases as the animal approaches weaning. At that time, about 18 days after birth, the 7, 8-BF exerts some inhibitory effect on the enzyme. Somewhat later the difference between the enzymes in male and female rats becomes apparent. Whereas in mature male rats enzyme activity in the presence of the flavone approaches or exceeds (Table 1) the control levels, the enzyme from the female rat is inhibited about 50%. This sex difference in response to 7, 8-BF is also found in older animals weighing 300 g. Thus the enzyme systems in mature male and female rats not only differ quantitatively as observed by others (31) and shown in this study (Table 2), but they are also qualitatively different.

Our data indicate the existence of at least two forms of aryl hydro-carbon hydroxylase in rats and these vary in their relative amounts in different tissues: One type (form I), which is stimulated by 7, 8-BF in vitro, is typified by the hepatic enzyme in immature animals. This type predominates in the liver of the normal adult male rat and is inducible by phenobarbital. The other type (form II), which is inhibited by the flavone, predominates in extrahepatic tissues. It comprises a sizable fraction of the AHH activities in the liver of the normal adult female rat and is highly inducible by polycyclic hydrocarbons in both hepatic and extrahepatic tissues. Further evidence for the existence of two types of BP hydroxylases in liver comes from the kinetic analysis of the normal and polycyclic hydrocarbon-induced enzymes that show considerable differences in their maximum velocities and Michaelis constants (32, 33). Differences in the kinetic constants of the enzyme from male and female rats are consistent with the view that the liver of untreated animals contains both forms of hydroxylases (49).

Age- and sex-dependent differences are common in the metabolism of drugs and steroids by microsomal oxidases (3, 34, 35) and have also been observed for the metabolism of polycyclic hydrocarbons such as 7, 12-dimethylbenz(a)anthracene (36). The change from the stimulation of AHH by 7, 8-BF to inhibition during the period of weaning may be primarily due to the intake of exogenous inducers contained in the diet that cause induction of the enzyme (36, 37), most likely of the type sensitive to 7, 8-BF inhibition. This is supported by the finding that the decrease in total AHH activity in female rat liver observed after 18 hr of starvation is accompanied by a lower degree of inhibition by 7, 8-BF (49). The findings of others (37, 38) furthermore suggest that what we observe as "constitutive" enzyme activity in extrahepatic tissues of adult animals might be largely the result of a continuous low level induction by exogenous compounds taken up through lung, skin, or the intestinal tract.

POLYCYCLIC HYDROCARBONS AS MODULATORS OF BENZO(a)PYRENE HYDROXYLASE

A large number of polycyclic hydrocarbons were tested for their potency as modulators of AHH activity, i. e. , as either inducers or inhibitors of the enzyme system in hamster embryo cells in culture. These compounds included acridines, carbazoles, dibenzofuranes, and phenothiazines (unpublished results). Among the many compounds tested, two polycyclic hydrocarbons were found to be particularly potent inhibitors of the enzyme. These are 9-chloro-7H-dibenzo-(a, g) carbazole (9-Cl-7H-DBC) and 6-aminochrysene.

The effect of 9-Cl-7H-DBC on AHH in hepatic microsomes from male adult rats is shown in Fig. 3. Concentrations of 5×10^{-7}, i. e. , a hundredth of the substrate concentration, are sufficient to inhibit MC-induced enzyme activity by 50%. In contrast, enzyme activity

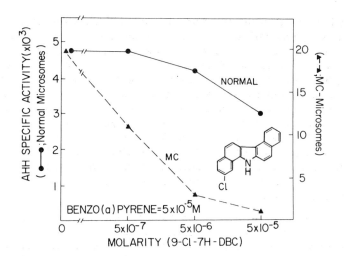

FIG. 3. Inhibition of aryl hydrocarbon hydroxylase from normal
and MC-treated rats by 9-chloro-7H-dibenzo(a, g)carbazole. Microsomal preparations from livers of male, adult rates that were treated
with methylcholanthrene (=MC microsomes) or corn oil (=normal
microsomes) as described in Methods, were incubated with various
amounts of 9-chloro-7H-dibenzo(a, g)carbazole (=9-Cl-7H-DBC),
added in 0.010 ml DMSO, in the presence of 5×10^{-5} M BP. Control
samples contained 0.010 ml of DMSO. Note the different AHH specific activities (nmoles of phenolic products/mg protein/30 min) of
normal microsomes (● —— ●) and MC microsomes (▲ —— ▲) indicated
by different scales of the ordinates.

in normal microsomes is far less sensitive to the inhibitor: The concentrations of the inhibitor that cause a 50% reduction of BP-
hydroxylation in normal and MC microsomes differ by a factor of 100.
Thus the marked differential effect on the hepatic hydroxylases is
not unique to the 7, 8-BF.

The effect of 6-aminochrysene on the two forms of hepatic
hydroxylases is shown in Fig. 4. Concentrations of the compound as
low as 5×10^{-6} M inhibit BP hydroxylation by 50%; but in contrast to
7, 8-BF and 9-Cl-7H-DBC, the normal and induced enzyme type of
liver are both affected similarly by the inhibitor.

9-Cl-7H-DBC and 6-aminochrysene are far more potent inhibitors
of BP hydroxylation than the other polycyclic hydrocarbons that were
previously tested in this system, such as 7, 12-dimethylbenz(a)-
anthracene, dibenz(a, c)anthracene (39), 3-methylcholanthrene, benz-
(a)anthracene (39, 40), pyrene, or benzo(e)pyrene (40).

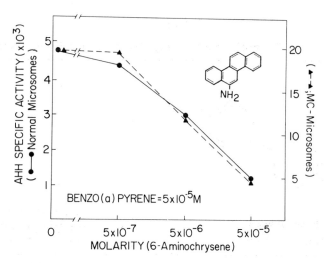

FIG. 4. Inhibition of aryl hydrocarbon hydroxylase from normal and MC-treated rats by 6-aminochrysene. 6-Aminochrysene was added in 0.010 ml of DMSO. Other conditions as described under Fig. 3 and in Methods. Note the different AHH specific activities (nmoles of phenolic products formed/mg protein/30 min) of normal microsomes (●——●) and MC microsomes (▲——▲) indicated by different scales of the ordinates.

Neither 9-Cl-7H-DBC nor 6-aminochrysene appeared to be inducers of the enzyme system in hamster embryo cell cultures. However, the apparent lack of induction may well be due to the presence of residual amounts of these compounds in the cell homogenates and hence in the reaction mixture interfering with the in vitro assay of enzyme activity. Indeed, in a different system, where the compound is applied topically to the skin (25), 9-Cl-7H-DBC and 6-amino-chrysene cause a several-fold induction of the enzyme during a few hours (51).

The structural similarity of 6-aminochrysene to the substrate, BP, is apparent and may account for the lack of a discriminatory effect on the normal and the induced enzyme form, i.e., it may share with BP most characteristics of interaction with the enzyme. The data suggest the possibility of exploring the nature of the enzyme sites responsible for carcinogen metabolism by the selectively modified inhibitory compounds. An approach has been made with a series of structurally related flavones and benzoflavones subsequently described.

TABLE 3

Effect of 7, 8-Benzoflavones on Aryl Hydrocarbon Hydroxylase[a]

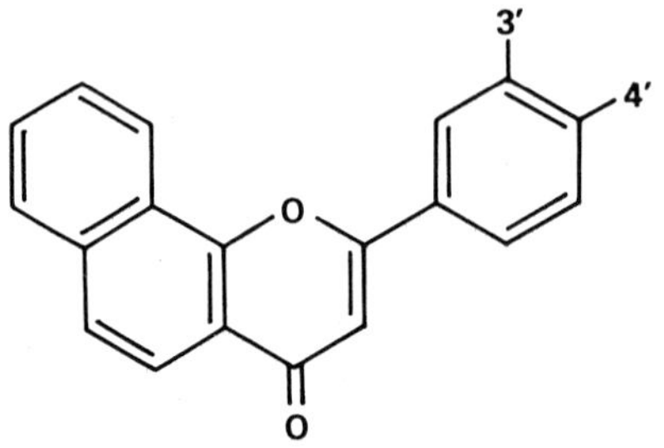

7,8-benzoflavone

Addition (10^{-5} M)	7,8-benzoflavone	Enzyme activity (fraction of control)	
		Normal	MC induced
	7, 8-Benzoflavone	1.32	0.46
4'-fluoro-	7, 8-Benzoflavone	1.12	0.43
4'-Bromo-	7, 8-Benzoflavone	1.18	0.57
4'-Benzyloxy-	7, 8-Benzoflavone	1.42	1.03
4'-Benzyloxy-3'-methoxy-	7, 8-Benzoflavone	1.88	1.03
4'-Hydroxy-	7, 8-Benzoflavone	0.70	0.50
4'-Hydroxy-3'-methoxy-	7, 8-Benzoflavone	0.57	0.42

[a] 7, 8-BF and the derivatives were added in 0.010 ml dimethyl-sulfoxide (DMSO). The flavone effect is expressed as fraction of "controls, " i.e., of samples that received the appropriate solvent only. The specific AHH activity of the controls in the experiments shown in Tables 3 to 6 were: 1.30 to 1.60 in microsomes from normal adult, male rats (= normal) and 7.20 to 8.50 in microsomes from MC-treated rats (= MC-induced). Incubation period was 10 min. Other conditions as described in Methods. 7, 8- and 5, 6-BF were obtained from Aldrich Chemical Co. The various flavone derivatives were synthesized by two of us (M.G.S. and W.S.B.) in the laboratory of the ICN, Nucleic Acid Research Institute (manuscript in preparation) unless stated otherwise.

Flavones as Modulators of Benzo(a)pyrene Hydroxylase

Two aspects of the effects of flavonoids on hepatic AHH of male rats were investigated: (a) their stimulatory or inhibitory effect and (b) their effectiveness in differentiating between the constitutive ("normal") and the polycyclic hydrocarbon induced ("MC-induced")

TABLE 4

Effect of 5, 6-Benzoflavones on Aryl Hydrocarbon Hydroxylase[a]

| 5,6-benzoflavone | Enzyme activity (fraction of control) | |
Addition (10^{-4} M)	Normal	MC-induced
5, 6-Benzoflavone	1. 11	0. 59
4'-Fluoro- 5, 6-Benzoflavone	0. 98	0. 70
4'-Bromo- 5, 6-Benzoflavone	1. 01	0. 51
4'-Benzyloxy-5, 6-Benzoflavone	0. 96	0. 92
4'-Hydroxy- 5, 6-Benzoflavone	0. 29	0. 22

[a] 5, 6-Benzoflavone and its derivatives were added in 0. 010 ml DMSO. Other conditions as under Table 3.

enzyme. Table 3 shows a series of 3'- and 4'-substituted derivatives of 7, 8-BF and their effect on the enzyme system. The 4'-halogenated derivative exhibits a differential effect on the control and induced enzyme that is similar to that of the parent compound. The introduction of a benzyloxy group increases somewhat the stimulating activity on the normal enzyme and diminishes the inhibitory effect on the induced form of the enzyme. Addition of a methoxy group in the adjacent 3'-position inhibits both the induced enzyme and to a lesser degree the normal enzyme. The 4'-derivatives of 5, 6-benzoflavone behave similarly to their 7, 8-BF isomers (Table 4). The parent compound stimulates the normal enzyme and inhibits the induced form. Addition of a hydroxyl group converts the compound into a strong inhibitor for the normal and the induced enzyme type. Substitution of the benzyloxy group eliminates the inhibitory effect on the induced enzyme but does not enhance the stimulation of the control enzyme as is seen with the 7, 8-BF derivative (Table 3).

The 3'- and 4'-methoxy- or halogenated derivatives of 5, 6, 7, 8-tetramethoxyflavone have qualitatively similar effects to the benzoflavones except for the 4'-methoxy-3'-bromo-derivative (Table 5).

TABLE 5

Effect of Tetramethoxyflavones on Aryl Hydrocarbon Hydroxylase[a]

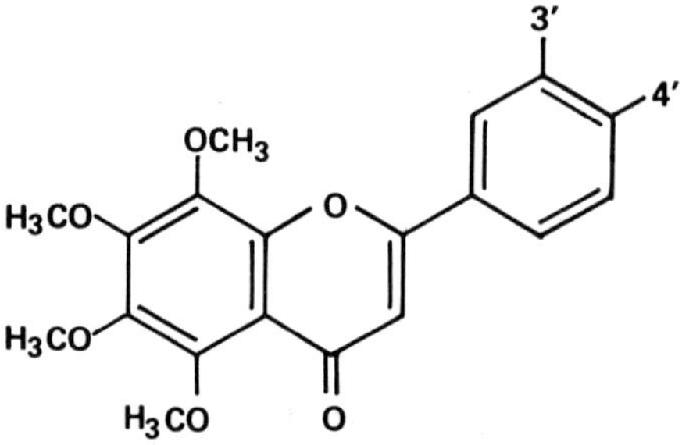

5,6,7,8-tetramethoxyflavone

Addition (10^{-4} M)		Enzyme activity (fraction of control)	
		Normal	MC-induced
4'-Methoxy- (= Tangeretin)	5, 6, 7, 8-Tetramethoxyflavone	1.54	0.72
3', 4'-dimethoxy- (= Nobiletin)	5, 6, 7, 8-Tetramethoxyflavone	1.12	0.74
4'-Bromo-	5, 6, 7, 8-Tetramethoxyflavone	1.39	0.89
4'-Chloro-	5, 6, 7, 8-Tetramethoxyflavone	1.32	0.86
4'-Fluoro-	5, 6, 7, 8-Tetramethoxyflavone	1.43	0.81
4'-Methoxy-3'-bromo-	5, 6, 7, 8-Tetramethoxyflavone	0.81	1.03
4'-Hydroxy-	5, 6, 7, 8-Tetramethoxyflavone	0.59	0.83

[a] The tetramethoxyflavones were added in 0.010 ml acetone. Tangeretin and Nobiletin were obtained from the U.S. Fruit and Vegetable Product Laboratory (Winter Haven, Florida). Other conditions as in Table 3.

The 4'-hydroxylated derivative evokes a different type of response: Not only does it inhibit both the normal and the induced enzyme form, but it also appears to be a more potent inhibitor of the normal than of the induced enzyme. This is even more apparent with two other hydroxylated flavones, Apigenin and Quercetin, shown in Table 6: These two naturally occurring flavones strongly inhibit the normal constitutive form and to a lesser degree the induced form, i.e., their effects are opposite to those of the benzoflavones.

Thus the modification of flavones, particularly in the 4'-position, provides a series of compounds that allow the alteration of AHH in different ways: the stimulation or inhibition of the enzyme and the differential modulation of the two hepatic forms of hydroxylases.

TABLE 6

Effect of 5, 7-Dihydroxyflavones on Aryl Hydrocarbon Hydroxylase[a]

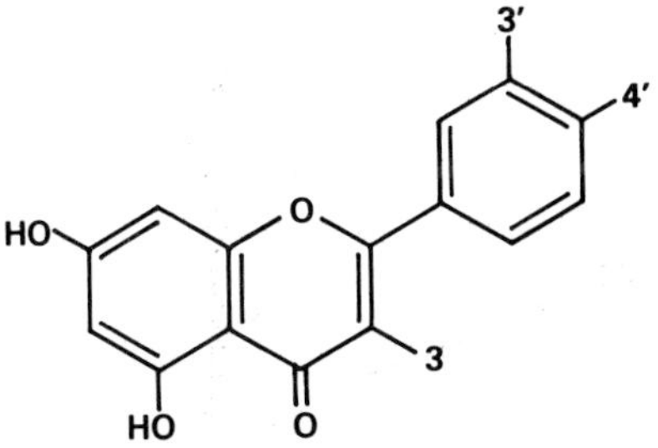

5,7-dihydroxyflavone

Addition		Concen-tration, M	Enzyme activity (fraction of control)	
			Normal	MC-induced
4'-Hydroxy- (= Apigenin)	5, 7-Dihydroxyflavone	10^{-4} 10^{-5}	0.17 0.38	0.18 0.63
3, 3', 4'-Trihydroxy-5, 7-Dihydroxyflavone (= Quercetin)		10^{-4} 10^{-5}	0.08 0.30	0.21 0.82

[a] Apigenin (Aldrich Chemical Co.) and Quercetin (Calbiochem) were added in 0.010 ml DMSO. Other conditions as in Table 3.

The different effects of substituted flavones do not appear to be primarily related to steric factors since considerable structural varia-tion, e.g., the shift of the benzyl group (Tables 3 and 4, 7, 8-BF and 5, 6-BF) or substitution by several methoxy groups (Table 5, Tangeretin), does not change the particular pattern of inhibition and stimulation of the two enzyme forms. The change in inhibition characteristics observed after substitution of the methoxy group by a hydroxyl group in the 4' position (Table 5) indicates that other factors such as the polarity of the compounds may determine their specific action on the enzyme system. We have found earlier that aliphatic alcohols, simi-lar to the phenolic flavones, strongly inhibit the control enzyme and have less effect on the MC-induced form (19). The different effects of the hydroxy- or methoxy-substituted flavonoids appear to be re-flected also in their properties as inducers of the enzyme system in vivo (24).

Stimulation of Benzo(a)pyrene Hydroxylase by 4'-Benzyloxy-
3'-methoxy-7, 8-BF

In order to study the nature of the enzyme system, we have ex-amined in detail the stimulatory effect of the flavones and have used

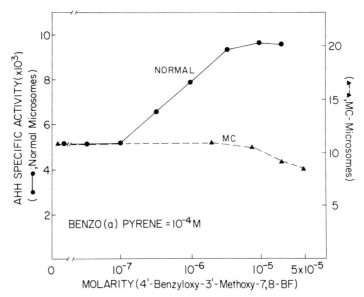

FIG. 5. Stimulation of aryl hydrocarbon hydroxylase from normal and MC-treated rats by 4'-benzyloxy-3'-methoxy-7, 8-BF. BP concentration was 10^{-4} M. Other conditions as described under Fig. 3, and in Methods. Note the different AHH specific activities (nmoles of phenolic product formed/mg protein/30 min) in normal microsomes (●——●) and MC microsomes (▲——▲) indicated by different scales of the ordinates.

the most potent derivative, 4'-benzyloxy-3'-methoxy-7, 8-BF (Table 3), as a model compound. The effect of various concentrations of this compound on BP hydroxylation in hepatic microsomes from normal and MC-treated male rats is shown in Fig. 5: Concentrations below 5 × 10^{-7} M are sufficient to produce some stimulation of the hydroxylation of 10^{-4} M BP in normal microsomes and maximum stimulation is reached at flavone concentrations of 10^{-6} to 10^{-5} M. In contrast there is very little effect of this compound on the induced enzyme: Concentrations one to two orders of magnitude higher are needed to cause a slight inhibition of 10 to 20% (Fig. 5).

Our assay measures the production of phenolic metabolites from BP and does not determine the appearance of other known metabolites such as dihydrodiols, various water soluble conjugates, and possibly quinones (1, 5, 41). A stimulation of the hydroxylation rate by the flavone could be due to the inhibition of a nonphenolic pathway leading to a corresponding increase in phenol formation. In this case the overall metabolism of the substrate might remain the same or even be

TABLE 7

Effect of 4'-Benzyloxy-3'-methoxy-7, 8-BF on [^{3}H]Benzo(a)pyrene
Metabolism in Microsomes of Rat Liver[a]

Products of BP	Control	picomoles of products formed/minute 4'-Benzyloxy- 3'-methoxy- 7, 8-BF	Ratio: BF/control
Organic soluble			
Phenolic	14	38	2. 7
Nonphenolic	29	68	2. 3
Aqueous soluble	12	32	2. 7
Total	55	1 38	2. 5

[a] The incubation mixture contained in 1 ml: 50 μmoles Tris-HCl
buffer, pH 7. 6; 0. 50 μmoles NADPH, 3 μmoles $MgCl_2$, 0. 150 mg
microsomal protein, and 0. 325 mg protein of the 100, 000 × g supernatant fraction, both from livers of untreated male rats. Five nanomoles of the substrate [^{3}H]benzo(a)pyrene (25 Ci/mmole) were added
in 0. 020 ml of methanol. One nanomole of 4'-benzyloxy-3'-methoxy-
7, 8-BF was added in 0. 010 ml of DMSO prior to the substrate. The
profile of BP metabolites was determined essentially as described by
Kinoshita et al. (41). After a 3-min incubation at 37°, samples were
extracted with acetone: ethylacetate (1:2). Metabolites in the extract
separated by thin-layer chromatography [silica gel, CAMAC, Inc.,
developed with methanol: benzene (5:95) for 90 min] and quantitated
by liquid scintillation counting. Radioactivity in aliquots of the
aqueous phase was determined using Aquasol solution (New England
Nuclear).

decreased. In order to examine this, we used tritium-labeled substrate
and studied the effect of the stimulating flavone on the major metabolic
pathways in normal hepatic microsomes (Table 7): The amounts of nonphenolic organic soluble derivatives, comprising mainly dihydrodiols
and quinones, and of the aqueous soluble metabolites increased
roughly in parallel to the amount of phenolic metabolites formed in the
presence of the flavone. The increase in total metabolites was further
reflected by a faster rate of disappearance of the substrate from the
reaction mixture. These results indicate that the stimulating agent
does not act only on the phenol formation but rather on a step leading
to all of the major oxidation products. This step could be the initial

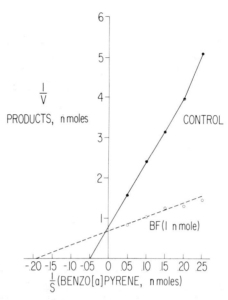

FIG. 6. Stimulation of aryl hydrocarbon hydroxylase by 4'-benzyloxy-3'-methoxy-7, 8-BF: dependency on the substrate concentration (Lineweaver-Burk plot). Reciprocal plots of the substrate, benzo(a)pyrene, concentration versus product formation (nmoles of phenolic products) in the presence of 10^{-6} M 4'-benzyloxy-3'-methoxy-7, 8-BF ($=$ BF) or of 0.010 ml of the solvent, DMSO ($=$ control). Amounts of protein/ml of incubation mixture were: microsomal protein $=$ 0.15 mg; 100,000 $\times$ g̲ supernatant $=$ 0.75 mg. The reaction mixtures were incubated for 3 min. Other conditions as described in Methods.

oxidation of the substrate, which may occur through the formation of an epoxide (14, 42, 43) or a preceding event.

The dependency of the stimulatory effect on substrate concentration is shown in Fig. 6: The reciprocal plots of substrate concentration versus product formation (Lineweaver-Burk) indicate a decrease of the apparent K_m from 2×10^{-5} M to 5×10^{-6} M BP in the presence of the flavone and show only a slight increase in the V_{max}. These changes in kinetics clearly differ from those observed for the stimulation of another function of the microsomal oxidase, aniline hydroxylation, where the V_{max} as well as the K_m are increased in the presence of the stimulating agent (44). Although the complexity of this multicomponent enzyme system makes difficult the derivation of a specific mode of activation from the kinetic data, several mechanisms can be envisioned. For example, the stimulating flavone could facilitate the reduction of the cytochrome P-450, the terminal oxidase of the enzyme system. This step is believed to be rate limiting for the oxidative metabolism of various compounds (45-47). It can be stimulated by a group of substrates that cause a particular difference spectrum (Type I) in liver microsomes (45). Both benzoflavones (50) and BP produce the Type I spectrum and enhance the rate of cytochrome P-450 reduction in microsomes from normal and MC-treated rats (48). Thus, the benzoflavone might increase the rate of P-450 reduction by binding to a site different from the catalytic center and with differing affinities for BP and the flavone. However, by binding to the enzyme, the flavone could conceivably alter other steps involving the interaction of enzyme and substrate. It is also possible that the compound does not bind to the cytochrome itself but interferes with other metabolic processes competing with BP-hydroxylase for a common intermediate and channels the flow of electrons into the oxidation of the polycyclic hydrocarbon. Finally, competition for unspecific binding sites might increase the availability of the substrate, BP, and contribute to the apparent stimulation of its metabolism.

In further studies the inhibitors and stimulators described above should be helpful for exploring the oxidation mechanism of polycyclic hydrocarbons and for establishing its relationship to the oxidative metabolism of other exogeneous and endogeneous compounds.

SUMMARY

The microsomal aryl hydrocarbon [benzo(a)pyrene] hydroxylase is important in the detoxification of polycyclic hydrocarbons as well as their activation to cytotoxic or carcinogenic derivatives. We have searched for compounds that can modify the activity of this enzyme system.

Three major groups of flavone derivatives are distinguished with respect to their in vitro effect on hepatic enzyme activity from untreated rats and enzyme activity induced by prior treatment with a polycyclic hydrocarbon: (a) the 5, 6- and 7, 8-benzoflavones and their more hydrophobic derivatives inhibit the induced enzyme and increase or do not affect the activity of the constitutive enzyme; (b) derivatives typified by the 4'-hydroxylated benzoflavones decrease to a similar degree the induced and constitutive enzyme activities. (c) Poly-hydroxyflavones inhibit the constitutive enzyme more than the induced enzyme. Two polycyclic hydrocarbons, 9-chloro-7H-dibenzo(a, g)-carbazole and 6-aminochrysene, both potent inhibitors of the enzyme system, affect the constitutive and induced enzyme similarly to compounds in group (a) and (b), respectively.

7, 8-Benzoflavone was used to probe the distribution and development of two forms of aryl hydrocarbon hydroxylases in rats: (a) Form I,
which is stimulated in the presence of the flavone, occurs in the liver
of newborn rats, predominates in the liver of the normal adult male
animal, and is inducible by phenobarbital; (b) Form II, which is
inhibited by the 7, 8-benzoflavone, comprises a major fraction of the
enzyme activity in extrahepatic tissues and in the liver of the normal
adult female rat. This form is inducible by polycyclic hydrocarbons
in hepatic and extrahepatic tissues.

NOTES

1. In the present studies we have chosen benzo(a)pyrene as a model
   substrate for the enzyme system, and the terms "aryl hydrocarbon
   hydroxylase" (AHH) and "benzo(a)pyrene hydroxylase" are used
   interchangably. It should be kept in mind that the findings made
   with this substrate might not extend to the hydroxylation of every
   other aryl hydrocarbon by this enzyme system.

2. Abbreviations: 5, 6-benzoflavone (β-naphthoflavone) = 5, 6-BF;
   7, 8-benzoflavone (α-naphthoflavone) = 7, 8-BF; benzo(a)pyrene =
   BP; 9-chloro-7H-dibenzo(a, g)carbazole = 9-Cl-7H-DBC; 7, 12-
   dimethyl-benz(a)anthracene = DMBA; 3-methylcholanthrene = MC;
   dimethylsulfoxide = DMSO; phenobarbital = PB; aryl hydrocarbon
   hydroxylase = AHH .

REFERENCES

1. A. H. Conney, E. C. Miller, and J. A. Miller, Substrate-induced
   synthesis and other properties of benzpyrene hydroxylase in rat
   liver, J. Biol. Chem., 228, 753 (1957).
2. J. R. Gillette, Factors that affect the stimulation of the microsomal drug enzyme induced by foreign compounds, Advan.
   Enzyme Regulation, 1, 215 (1963).
3. A. H. Conney, Pharmacological implications of microsomal
   enzyme induction, Pharm. Rev., 19, 317 (1967).
4. H. V. Gelboin, Carcinogens, enzyme induction, and gene action,
   Advan. Cancer Res., 10, 81 (1967).
5. P. Sims, Qualitative and quantitative studies on the metabolism
   of a series of aromatic hydrocarbons by rat-liver preparations,
   Biochem. Pharmacol., 19, 795 (1969).

6. H. S. Mason, Mechanism of oxygen metabolism, Advan. Enzyme, 19, 79 (1957).
7. D. W. Nebert and H. V. Gelboin, The in vivo and in vitro induction of aryl hydrocarbon hydroxylase in mammalian cells of different species, tissues, strains, and developmental and hormonal states, Arch. Biochem. Biophys., 134, 76 (1969).
8. H. Remmer, Drugs as activators of drug enzymes, Proc. 1st Intern. Pharmacol. Meeting, Stockholm, Vol. 6, 1962, pp. 235-249.
9. D. N. Wheatley, Enhancement and inhibition of the induction by 7,12-dimethylbenz(a)anthracene of mammary tumours in female Sprague-Dawley rats, Brit. J. Cancer, 22, 787 (1968).
10. L. W. Wattenberg, Chemoprophylaxis of carcinogenesis: A review, Cancer Res., 26, 1520 (1966).
11. J. A. Miller, Carcinogenesis by chemicals: An overview. G. H. A. Clowes Memorial Lecture, Cancer Res., 30, 559 (1970).
12. H. V. Gelboin and F. J. Wiebel, Studies on the mechanism of aryl hydrocarbon hydroxylase induction and its role in cytotoxicity and tumorigenicity, Ann. N. Y. Acad. Sci., 179, 529 (1971).
13. B. B. Brodie, W. D. Reid, A. K. Cho, G. Sipes, G. Krishna, and J. R. Gillette, Possible mechanism of liver necrosis caused by aromatic organic compounds, Proc. Nat. Acad. Sci., 68, 160 (1971).
14. J. K. Selkirk, E. Huberman, and C. Heidelberger, An epoxide is an intermediate in the microsomal metabolism of the chemical carcinogen dibenz(a, h)anthracene, Biochem. Biophys. Res. Commun., 43, 1010 (1971).
15. H. V. Gelboin, N. Kinoshita, and F. J. Wiebel, Microsomal hydroxylases: induction and role in polycyclic hydrocarbon carcinogenesis and toxicity, Fed. Proc. Fed. Soc. Exptl. Biol., 31, 1298 (1972).
16. H. V. Gelboin, Studies on the mechanism of methylcholanthrene induction of enzyme activities. II. Stimulation of microsomal and ribosomal amino acid incorporation: The effects of polyuridylic acid and actinomycin-D, Biochim. Biophys. Acta, 91, 130 (1964).
17. L. W. Wattenberg, J. L. Leong, and P. J. Strand, Benzpyrene hydroxylase activity in the gastrointestinal tract, Cancer Res., 22, 1120 (1962).
18. D. W. Nebert and H. V. Gelboin, Substrate-inducible microsomal aryl hydroxylase in mammalian cell culture, J. Biol. Chem., 243, 6242 (1968).
19. F. J. Wiebel, J. C. Leutz, L. Diamond, and H. V. Gelboin, Aryl hydrocarbon (benzo[a]pyrene) hydroxylase in microsomes from rat tissues: Differential inhibition and stimulation by benzoflavones and organic solvents, Arch. Biochem. Biophys., 144, 78 (1971).

268   WIEBEL ET AL.

20. O. H. Lowry, N. J. Rosebrough, A. L. Farr, and R. J. Randall, Protein measurement with the Folin phenol reagent, J. Biol. Chem., 193, 265 (1951).
21. L. Diamond and H. V. Gelboin, Alpha-naphthoflavone: An inhibitor of hydrocarbon cytotoxicity and microsomal hydroxylase, Science, 166, 1023 (1969).
22. H. V. Gelboin and N. R. Blackburn, The stimulatory effect of 3-methylcholanthrene on benzpyrene hydroxylase activity in several rat tissues: Inhibition by actinomycin D and puromycin, Cancer Res., 24, 356 (1964).
23. N. Kinoshita and H. V. Gelboin, The role of aryl hydrocarbon hydroxylase in 7, 12-dimethylbenz(a)anthracene skin tumorigenesis: On the mechanism of 7, 8-benzoflavone inhibition of tumorigenesis, Cancer Res., 32, 1329 (1972).
24. L. W. Wattenberg, M. P. Page, and J. L. Leong, Induction of increased benzpyrene hydroxylase activity by flavones and related compounds, Cancer Res., 28, 934 (1968).
25. H. V. Gelboin, F. J. Wiebel, and L. Diamond, Dimethylbenzanthracene tumorigenesis and aryl hydrocarbon hydroxylase in mouse skin: Inhibition by 7, 8-benzoflavone, Science, 170, 169 (1970).
26. L. Diamond, R. McFall, J. Miller, and H. V. Gelboin, The effects of two isomeric benzoflavones on aryl hydrocarbon hydroxylase and the toxicity and carcinogenicity of polycyclic hydrocarbons, Cancer Res., 32, 731 (1972).
27. L. W. Wattenberg and J. L. Leong, Inhibition of the carcinogenic action of benzo(a)pyrene by flavones, Cancer Res., 30, 1922 (1970).
28. N. Kinoshita and H. V. Gelboin, Aryl hydrocarbon hydroxylase and polycyclic hydrocarbon tumorigenesis: Effect of the enzyme inhibitor 7, 8-benzoflavone on tumorigenesis and macromolecule binding, Proc. Nat. Acad. Sci., 69, 824 (1972).
29. H. Marquardt and C. Heidelberger, Influence of "feeder cells" and induction and inhibition of microsomal mixed-function oxidases on hydrocarbon-induced malignant transformation of cells derived from C3H mouse prostate, Cancer Res., 32, 721 (1972).
30. F. J. Wiebel, J. C. Leutz, and H. V. Gelboin, Aryl hydrocarbon (benzo[a]pyrene) hydroxylase: Inducible in extrahepatic tissues of mouse strains not inducible in liver, Arch. Biochem. Biophys., 154, 292 (1973).
31. R. Kuntzman, L. C. Mark, L. Brand, M. Jacobson, W. Levin, and A. H. Conney, Metabolism of drugs and carcinogens by human liver enzymes, J. Pharmacol. Exptl. Therap., 152, 151 (1966).

32. A. P. Alvares, G. R. Schilling, and R. Kuntzman, Differences in the kinetics of benzpyrene hydroxylation by hepatic drug-metabolizing enzymes from phenobarbital and 3-methylcholanthrene-treated rats, Biochem. Biophys. Res. Commun., 30, 588 (1968).
33. H. L. Gurtoo and T. C. Campbell, A kinetic approach to a study of the induction of rat liver microsomal hydroxylase after pretreatment with 3, 4-benzpyrene and aflatoxin B_1, Biochem. Pharmacol., 19, 1729 (1969).
34. R. Kato and J. R. Gillette, Sex differences in the effects of abnormal physiological states on the metabolism of drugs by rat liver microsomes, J. Pharmacol. Exptl. Therap., 150, 285 (1965).
35. J. B. Schenkman, I. Frey, H. Remmer, and R. W. Estabrook, Sex differences in drug metabolism by rat liver microsomes, Mol. Pharmacol., 3, 516 (1967).
36. P. Sims and L. Grover, Quantitative aspects of the metabolism of 7, 12-dimethylbenz(a)anthracene by liver homogenates from animals of different age, sex and species, Biochem. Pharmacol., 17, 1751 (1968).
37. L. W. Wattenberg, Studies of polycyclic hydrocarbon hydroxylases of the intestine possibly related to cancer, Cancer, 28, 99 (1971).
38. P. Sims and P. L. Grover, Variations dependent on age and diet in the metabolism of 7, 12-dimethylbenz(a)anthracene by rat liver homogenates, Nature, 216, 77 (1967).
39. R. Tomingas, W. Dehnen, and S. Jackson, Untersuchung zur Kinetik der Hemmung des Benzo(a)pyrene Abbaus, Z. Krebforsch., 74, 279 (1970).
40. D. Williams, F. J. Wiebel, J. C. Leutz, and H. V. Gelboin, Effect of polycyclic hydrocarbons in vitro on aryl hydrocarbon (benzo-[a]pyrene) hydroxylase, Biochem. Pharmacol,, 20, 2130 (1971).
41. N. Kinoshita, B. Shears, and H. V. Gelboin, K-region and non-K region metabolism of benzo(a)pyrene by rat liver microsomes, Cancer Res., 33, 1937 (1973).
42. D. M. Jerina, J. W. Daly, B. Witkop, P. Zaltzman-Nirenberg, and S. Udenfriend, 1, 2-Naphthalene oxide as an intermediate in the microsomal hydroxylation of naphthalene, Biochemistry, 9, 147 (1970).
43. D. M. Jerina, N. Kaubisch, and J. W. Daly, Arene oxides as intermediates in the metabolism of aromatic substrates: Alkyl and oxygen migrations during isomerization of alkylated arene oxides, Proc. Nat. Acad. Sci., 68, 2545 (1971).
44. M. W. Anders, Acetone enhancement of microsomal aniline para-hydroxylase activity, Arch. Biochem. Biophys., 126, 269 (1968).
45. P. L. Gigon, T. E. Gram, and J. R. Gillette, Studies on the rate of reduction of hepatic microsomal cytochrome P-450 by reduced nicotinamide adenine dinucleotide phosphate: Effect of drug substrates, Mol. Pharmacol., 5, 109 (1969).

46. D. S. Davies, P. L. Gigon, and J. R. Gillette, Species and sex differences in electron transport systems in liver microsomes and their relationship to ethylmorphine demethylation, Life Sci., 8, 85 (1969).

47. J. B. Schenkman and D. L. Cinti, The rate-limiting step in aminopyrine demethylase of rat liver microsomes, Biochem. Pharmacol., 19, 2396 (1970).

48. Y. Gnosspelius, H. Thor, and S. Orrenius, A comparative study on the effects of phenobarbital and 3, 4-benzpyrene on the hydroxylating enzyme system of rat-liver microsomes, Chem. - Biol. Interactions, 1, 125 (1969-70).

49. F. J. Wiebel and H. V. Gelboin, manuscript in preparation.

50. F. J. Wiebel, B. Stripp, and H. V. Gelboin, unpublished observations.

51. N. Kinoshita and H. V. Gelboin, unpublished observations.

Chapter 12

AROMATIC HYDROCARBON-PRODUCED TUMORIGENESIS AND THE GENETIC DIFFERENCES IN ARYL HYDROCARBON HYDROXYLASE

Daniel W. Nebert and William F. Benedict[*]

Section on Development Pharmacology
Laboratory of Biomedical Sciences
National Institute of Child Health and Human Development
National Institutes of Health
Bethesda, Maryland

Richard E. Kouri

Department of Viral-Chemical Oncology
Microbiological Associates, Inc.
Bethesda, Maryland

As documented by numerous other reports, it has become increasingly evident that the metabolism of lipophilic foreign substances by the liver microsomal mixed-function (1, 2) oxygenase system does not necessarily result in detoxification (3). Rather, the parent compound — whether it be a chemical carcinogen, halogenated hydrocarbon, or drug — may be mono-oxygenated to a chemically active epoxide intermediate (arene oxide) (Fig. 1), which can (a) rearrange spontaneously to phenols (4), (b) be converted to trans-dihydrodiols by microsomal epoxide hydrases (5), (c) conjugate with glutathione (4, 6, 7), or (d) combine covalently with cellular macromolecules (8-10). In cell culture, K-region epoxides are generally many times more reactive than the parent polycyclic hydrocarbons, the corresponding phenols, or the cis- and trans-dihydrodiols, in producing malignant transformation (11-13). Further, the magnitude

---

[*]Present address: Division of Hematology, Children's Hospital of Los Angeles, Los Angeles, California.

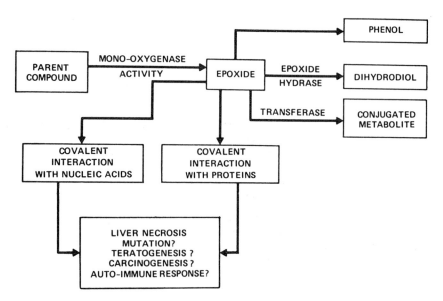

FIG. 1. Possible in vivo subcellular pathways for reactive
epoxide intermediates of carcinogenic polycyclic hydrocarbons.

of mutagenicity produced by K-region epoxides (14, 15) correlates well
with the known carcinogenicity of the parent aromatic hydrocarbons in
vivo. Therefore, if these metabolic pathways for polycyclic hydrocarbons are etiologically important in the initiation of chemical carcinogenesis, any marked changes in the rates of formation of
epoxides[1], phenols, dihydrodiols, glutathione conjugates, or covalently bound metabolites should affect the host's susceptibility to
cancer. In order to test this hypothesis, at least three possible types
of experimental manipulation could be performed in vivo: (a) alteration
of appropriate enzyme cofactors or glutathione content in the tissue,
(b) selective inhibition of each of the three enzymes shown in Fig. 1,
and (c) examination of animals possessing genetically mediated differences in the activities of each of the three enzymes. The first
possibility is currently under investigation in several laboratories.
The second possibility is also being tested (17), although nonspecific
effects of the inhibitors may cloud interpretation of the data (cf. Ref.
18 for discussion). In the chapter, we offer a model based on the third
possibility: i. e., testing the correlation between genetically controlled
differences in mono-oxygenase activity and susceptibility to tumorigenesis.

Induction[2], or increase, in aryl hydrocarbon hydroxylase activity
segregates as a single autosomal dominant gene in crosses involving
the inbred mouse strains C57BL/6 and DBA/2 (19, 26-32). We propose

$$Ah^b Ah^b \times Ah^d Ah^d \qquad\qquad Ah^b Ah^d \times Ah^b Ah^b$$
$$\downarrow \qquad\qquad\qquad\qquad\qquad \downarrow$$
$$Ah^b Ah^d \qquad\qquad\qquad Ah^b Ah^b : Ah^b Ah^d$$

$$Ah^b Ah^d \times Ah^b Ah^d \qquad\qquad Ah^b Ah^d \times Ah^d Ah^d$$
$$\downarrow \qquad\qquad\qquad\qquad\qquad \downarrow$$
$$Ah^b Ah^b : Ah^b Ah^d : Ah^d Ah^d \qquad\qquad Ah^b Ah^d : Ah^d Ah^d$$

FIG. 2. Diagram of the four possible genetic crosses between inbred strains ($\underline{Ah}^b/\underline{Ah}^b$) having the aromatic hydrocarbon-inducible hydroxylase activity and strains ($\underline{Ah}^d/\underline{Ah}^d$) not having the aromatic hydrocarbon-inducible hepatic enzyme. With the use of C57BL/6 mice as the prototype inbred strain homozygous for the $\underline{Ah}^b$ allele and DBA/2 mice as the prototype inbred strain homozygous for the $\underline{Ah}^d$ allele, genetic expression of aromatic hydrocarbon-inducible aryl hydrocarbon hydroxylase activity has been shown (19, 26-32) to segregate as a single autosomal dominant gene. Hence, all F_1 hybrids (upper left box) and all progeny from the F_1 heterozygote backcrossed with the B6 parent (upper right box) possess in the liver, kidney, bowel, lung, and skin the mono-oxygenase activity that is as inducible as the inbred B6 parent; the magnitude of induction ranges from three- to sixfold in liver and from two- to more than 80-fold in the nonhepatic tissues (19, 26-32). Hydroxylase induction among the F_2 generation (lower left box) and among the offspring from the F_1 hybrid backcrossed with the inbred $\underline{Ah}^d/\underline{Ah}^d$ parent (lower right box) occurs with an approximate frequency of three-fourths and one-half, respectively, whereas the enzyme activity in liver, kidney, and bowel from the remaining aromatic hydrocarbon-treated mice is not significantly different from control values. The hydroxylase activity in lung and skin from certain aromatic hydrocarbon-treated $\underline{Ah}^d/\underline{Ah}^d$ mice is not inducible, or only slightly inducible, compared with that found in lung or skin from aromatic hydrocarbon-treated $\underline{Ah}^b/\underline{Ah}^b$ or Ah^b/Ah^d mice (32). We presently have evidence for a possible third allele at the $\underline{Ah}$ locus (unpublished data).

this locus be designated $\underline{Ah}$ (Fig. 2); the allele carried by the C57BL/6 mouse is Ah^b and the allele carried by the DBA/2 mouse is $\underline{Ah}^d$. Following aromatic hydrocarbon treatment in vivo, the differences between the hydroxylase in various tissues of $\underline{Ah}^b/\underline{Ah}^b$ or $\underline{Ah}^b/\underline{Ah}^d$ mice are twofold to more than 80-fold greater than that of $\underline{Ah}^d/\underline{Ah}^d$ animals (26-32). Taking advantage of these findings, we show in this report that we can evaluate tumor susceptibility among littermates in which the presence or absence of aryl hydrocarbon hydroxylase induction is expressed in their tissues. With the use of such a model, other nonspecific phenomena — such as characteristic

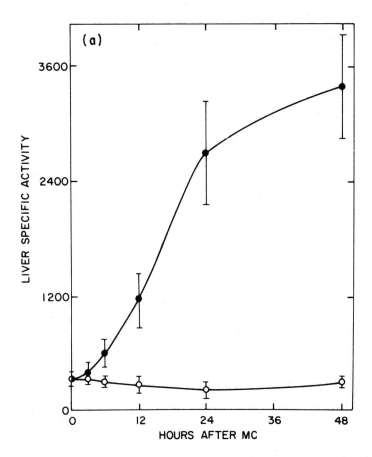

FIG. 3. Kinetics of aryl hydrocarbon hydroxylase induction by
MC in (a) liver and (b) skin from Ah^b/Ah^b, Ah^b/Ah^d, or Ah^d/Ah^d
weanling mice (32). The closed circles represent means of Ah^b/Ah^b
or Ah^b/Ah^d animals; the open circles depict means of Ah^d/Ah^d mice;
brackets depict the standard deviation for each mean. For each time
point, each mean $\pm$ standard deviation represents 12 to 23 individual
determinations from single mice; about an equal number of the inbred
mice and the offspring from the backcross or intercross were tested.
Each mouse received simultaneously 80 mg of MC per kg body weight
intraperitoneally and 300 μg of MC to the nape of the neck, and
enzyme activities from liver (19, 26) and skin (19, 33) of each mouse
were determined. One unit of aryl hydrocarbon hydroxylase activity
is defined (19) as that amount of enzyme catalyzing per minute at 37°
the formation of hydroxylated product causing fluorescence equivalent

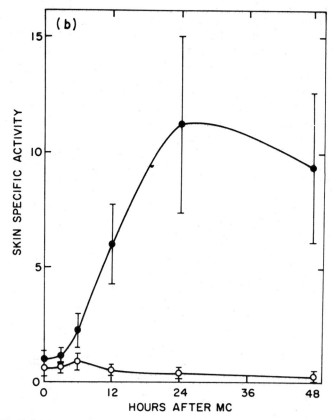

FIG. 3.b.

to that of 1 pmole of 3-hydroxylbenzo(a)pyrene. Throughout this paper
the specific activity of the hepatic enzyme is expressed as units per
milligram of microsomal protein, and the specific activities of the
nonhepatic hydroxylase are shown as units per milligram of tissue
homogenate protein.

mouse strain differences involving immunology, latent viral infections,
nutrition, hormones, stress, or levels of other enzymes — will theoretically be cancelled. With the use of this experimental model, we
show in this report that the genetically mediated presence of this
inducible hydroxylase is correlated with tumor susceptibility produced
by one carcinogen and is not correlated with tumor susceptibility
caused by two other carcinogens at the dosages tested.

In many tissues of the B6[3] inbred mouse, the hydroxylase is inducible by MC, whereas in D2 inbred mice the enzyme is relatively

nonresponsive to MC (26). Figure 3 shows the rate at which the
enzyme activity accumulates in liver and skin of MC-treated B6 and
D2 inbred animals and their progeny. In those inbred mice or their
offspring having at least one Ah^b allele, the hepatic specific oxygenase activity increased about threefold in 12 hr, about sixfold in
24 hr, and about eightfold in 48 hr, following MC administration. The
magnitude of the enzyme induction in skin from these same weanlings
was markedly similar, except for considerably larger standard devia-
tions and except for some decrease in the value at the 48-hr time
point. In mice presumed to be homozygous for the Ah^d allele, both
the hepatic and skin hydroxylase specific activities became slightly
depressed during the 48-hr experiment. Similar results were obtained
with the use of BP or β-naphthoflavone as the inducer (32). Similar
kinetics, but with a smaller magnitude of hydroxylase induction, was
also found with DMBA as the inducer (32).

Figure 4 shows that there is a high correlation between the
presence of the inducible enzyme in skin, peritoneal lining, lung,
and bowel. As noted previously (26, 30, 32), the differences in specific hydroxylase activities between MC-treated Ah^b/Ah^d and Ah^d/Ah^d
mice were more striking in bowel (15- to 80-fold) than in skin (two-
to 10-fold). The differences were much less pronounced in lung and
peritoneal lining. However, the enzyme activity in lung, peritoneal
lining, and lymph nodes (32) was generally higher in MC-treated
Ah^b/Ah^d mice than in MC-treated Ah^d/Ah^d animals. Actually, the
term "twofold" or "20-fold" to denote magnitude of induction should
be used with reservation if one is dealing with amounts of enzyme
that are barely detectable. The limit of sensitivity of the hydroxylase
assay is about 0.10 unit of enzyme per milligram of protein (19). If
one finds a specific enzyme activity of 0.40 in an MC-treated animal,
for example, the magnitude of induction may be "twofold" or "20-fold,"
depending on whether the control specific activity for that assay is
0.20 or 0.02. Therefore, in the bowel, the specific hydroxylase
activity in MC-treated Ah^b/Ah^d mice was greater than 10 and in
MC-treated Ah^d/Ah^d mice was less than 0.60; in the peritoneal
lining, on the other hand, the specific enzyme activity in MC-treated
Ah^b/Ah^d mice was greater than 0.45 and in MC-treated Ah^d/Ah^d
animals was less than 0.55. In any event, we conclude that aryl
hydrocarbon hydroxylase induction in lung and peritoneal lining by
MC among progeny of the B6 and D2 inbred strains probably segregates as a single autosomal dominant trait — as is the case in liver,
bowel, kidney, and skin (19, 26-32). However, other factors apparently influence the extent of hydroxylase induction in lung, peritoneal
lining, and perhaps even skin; these factors may include hormonal
levels, stress, nutrition, environmental exposure to pharmacologically
or toxicologically active substances (34), or differences in the subcellular mechanisms of transcription or translation (19, 22).

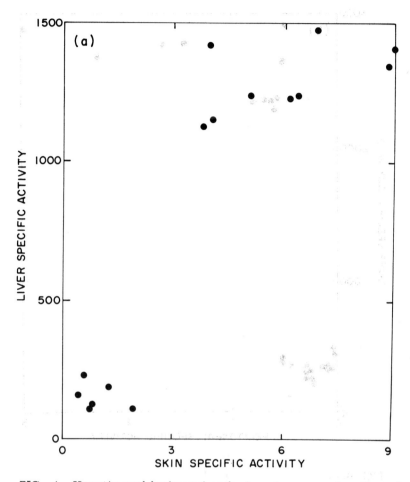

FIG. 4. Hepatic aryl hydrocarbon hydroxylase as a function of the hydroxylase activities in (a) skin, (b) peritoneal lining, (c) lung, and (d) bowel from MC-treated $\underline{Ah}^b/\underline{Ah}^d$ or $\underline{Ah}^d/\underline{Ah}^d$ weanling mice (32). Each point in Fig. 2(a) depicts a single mouse 12 hr after receiving simultaneously 80 mg of MC intraperitoneally per kilogram of body weight and 300 μg of MC in 0.20 μl acetone to the nape of the neck. Each point in Figs. 2(b), 2(c), and 2(d) represents an individual weanling 24 hr after intraperitoneal treatment with MC; the enzyme activities were derived from the peritoneal lining, lung, and bowel from the same 27 mice. Offspring from the B6D2 F_1 × D2 backcross were used. Correlation coefficients r for Figs. 2(a), 2(b), 2(c), and 2(d) were 0.89, 0.71, 0.78, and 0.78, respectively (P < 0.001 for each of the four relationships). In each tissue the specific hydroxylase activity from control animals was not significantly (P > 0.05) different from that found in MC-treated $\underline{Ah}^d/\underline{Ah}^d$ mice.

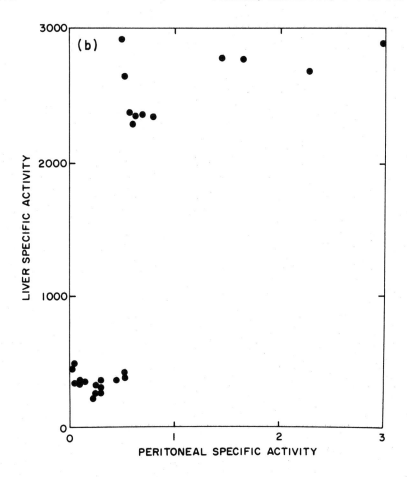

FIG. 4. b.

It was recently reported (17) that α-naphthoflavone inhibits
DMBA-produced skin tumorigenesis only if the inhibitor is applied
less than 12 hr after application of DMBA to mouse skin. In view of
this finding, it must be kept in mind that if polycyclic hydrocarbon-
evoked carcinogenesis requires metabolic activation by the aryl
hydrocarbon hydroxylase system, those changes in the skin specific
enzyme activity during the first 12 hr would be far more important than
those changes occurring after 12 hr. It was because of this finding,
therefore, that the changes in liver and skin hydroxylase after only
12 hr of MC treatment are shown in Fig. 4(a).

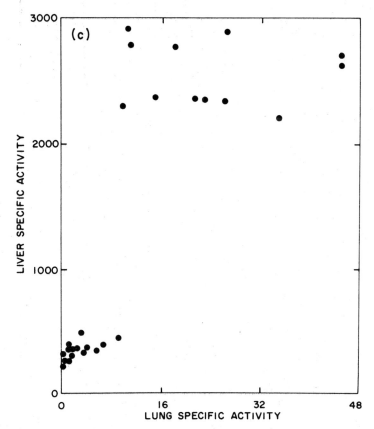

FIG. 4.c.

We have summarized in Table 1 the results carried out in both laboratories (28, 32, 35, 39) with respect to tumor incidence among the B6 and D2 inbred strains and their progeny treated with various carcinogens in various ways. The topical application of DMBA or BP, combined with promotion by phorbol ester, produced tumors without any apparent correlation with the presence or absence of inducible hydroxylase activity. It is noteworthy that inbred D2 mice were more susceptible to DMBA- or BP-evoked tumorigenesis than inbred B6 mice when they received the promotor phorbol ester. The intraperitoneal administration of a 3-mg dose of BP to weanlings resulted in significantly (0.02 < P < 0.05) more tumors in progeny having the noninducible hydroxylase than in offspring having the inducible enzyme.

On the contrary, tumor susceptibility to a 150-μg subcutaneous dose of MC was highly correlated with the gentically regulated

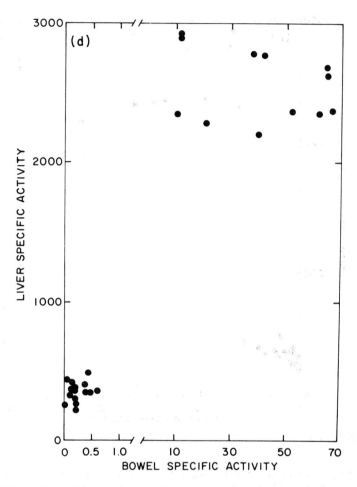

FIG. 4.d.

presence of hydroxylase induction among both the inbred B6 and D2
strains and their progeny. Upon careful examination, however, a
gene-dose relationship may exist: i. e. , the heterozygotes displayed
a susceptibility to MC-evoked tumors that was intermediate between
that found in the two inbred strains. Thus, we suspect that at least
one other gene plays a role in this phenomenon. The presence of
group-specific (or gs) antigens characteristic of type C RNA viro-
gene expression has been examined (40) and does not contribute to
this codominant effect.

Figure 5 shows the carcinogenic index[4] as a function of hepatic
aryl hydrocarbon hydroxylase induction for 14 inbred strains of mice
treated with MC. Whereas the correlation coefficient r was 0.90

TABLE 1

Tumor Incidence among Parents and Progeny of C57BL/6 and DBA/2 Mice after Initiation with 7,12-Dimethylbenz(a)anthracene, Benzo(a)pyrene, or 3-Methylcholanthrene[a]

Compound, route of administration	Promotion with phorbol ester	Mice with tumors/total in group				Ref.
		Parents		Progeny[b]		
		$\underline{Ah}^b/\underline{Ah}^b$	$\underline{Ah}^d/\underline{Ah}^d$	$\underline{Ah}^b/\underline{Ah}^b$ or $\underline{Ah}^b/\underline{Ah}^d$[c]	$\underline{Ah}^d/\underline{Ah}^d$	
DMBA, topical	yes	0/13	19/21	20/34	16/25	28
BP, topical	yes	0/40	2/33	12/62	8/34	32
BP, intraperitoneal	no			3/36	5/19	32
MC, subcutaneous	no	25/30	2/29	10/26	2/21	39

[a] The experimental details can be found in the references noted in the right-hand column.

[b] Includes both B6D2 F_1 × D2 backcross and B6D2 F_1 × B6D2 F_1 intercross.

[c] Among these offspring, we cannot distinguish whether they are homozygous or heterozygous for the dominant $\underline{Ah}^b$ allele.

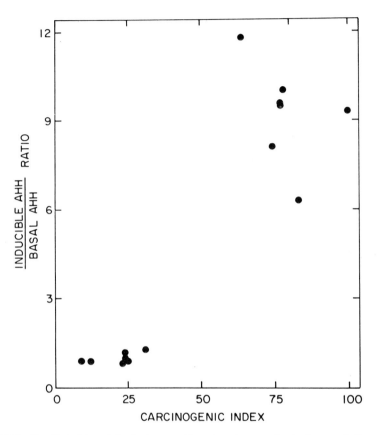

FIG. 5. Relationship between the carcinogenic index and the genetically mediated induction of aryl hydrocarbon hydroxylase activity by MC for each of 14 inbred mouse strains; the correlation coefficient r is 0.90 (P < 0.001). Each closed circle represents a particular inbred mouse strain. The carcinogenic index was evaluated after a subcutaneous dose of 150 μg of MC had been given to a minimum of 30 weanling mice of each strain (35). The "inducible AHH/basal AHH ratio" reflects the mean of hepatic hydroxylase activity in MC-treated mice divided by the mean hepatic enzyme activity in control mice (N ≥ 5 for each of the two groups). Whether the MC-inducible hydroxylase activity in the nonhepatic tissues segregates as a single gene with the inducible hepatic enzyme activity has not been examined for many of these strains.

(P < 0.001) for tumors produced by a 150-μg subcutaneous dose of MC, r was 0.28 and 0.22 for tumors produced by the same subcutaneous dose of DMBA and BP, respectively (P > 0.20 for both). These data for DMBA and BP (35), therefore, are in accord with the data in Table 1 for DMBA and BP and indicate that important differences exist in the metabolic activation of the three carcinogens, DMBA, BP, and MC. These differences might reflect dissimilarities in the position of epoxidation[1] by the basal hydroxylase, as compared with that by the aromatic hydrocarbon-induced enzyme, or might be a manifestation of any other changes in the metabolic pathways outlined in Fig. 1. Recently, the same sort of conclusion has been reached for differences in DMBA- and BP-produced tumorigenesis in mouse skin with the use of α-naphthoflavone as an inhibitor of aryl hydrocarbon hydroxylase activity (17, 37). Such differences may help to explain the seemingly contradictory results (cf. Ref. 32 for discussion) from various laboratories as to whether activation or detoxification of the parent polycyclic hydrocarbon molecule is important in the etiology of chemically initiated carcinogenesis.

The susceptibility or resistance to chemically evoked pulmonary tumors is linked to specific genes on six different linkage groups (38). However, the molecular basis has not been delineated for any of these loci. We suggest that the Ah locus is one of these specific loci. Genes regulating the other steps in the metabolic pathways for chemical carcinogens, as shown in Fig. 1, may coincide with other of these specific loci. This genetically mediated difference in the activity of aryl hydrocarbon hydroxylase is therefore offered as an experimental model for understanding chemical carcinogenesis. We hope that variations of this model can be developed. For example, the levels of epoxide hydrase or glutathione transferase may also be under monogenic regulation.

SUMMARY

The susceptibility to tumorigenesis produced by the subcutaneous administration of 3-methylcholanthrene is highly correlated with the genetically mediated presence of aryl hydrocarbon hydroxylase induction in 14 strains of mice. There is no such relationship among inducible hydroxylase activity and (a) subcutaneous treatment with 7,12-dimethylbenz(a)anthrene or benzo(a)pyrene, (b) intraperitoneal administration of benzo(a)pyrene, or (c) topical application of 7,12-dimethylbenz(a)anthracene or benzo(a)pyrene and promotion by phorbol ester.

ACKNOWLEDGMENT

We thank Dr. Paul O. P. Ts'o and Dr. Joseph A. DiPaolo for thoughtfully inviting us to participate in this work. Work was supported in part by Contract NIH 70-2068 within the Special Virus-Cancer Program of the National Cancer Institute and the Council for Tobacco Research.

NOTES

1. In addition to changes in the formation rate of polycyclic hydrocarbon epoxides, a change in the position of epoxidation may drastically affect a molecule's reactivity to bind covalently to cellular macromolecules and therefore may be etiologically important in carcinogenic initiation. For example, phenobarbital-induced mono-oxygenase activities preferentially produce 3, 4-epoxidation of bromobenzene (16) and ω and ω-1 hydroxylations of n-hexane (V. Ullrich, unpublished data), whereas the polycyclic hydrocarbon-induced enzyme systems cause predominantly 2, 3-epoxidation of bromobenzene (16) and ω-2 hydroxylation of n-hexane (V. Ullrich, unpublished data).

2. The process of induction denotes a relative increase in the rate of de novo synthesis or in the rate of activation of enzyme activity from pre-existing moieties, or in the rate of both, compared with the rate of breakdown. Since this enzyme may be a multicomponent membrane-bound system, there are technical difficulties in attempting to distinguish between enzyme de novo synthesis and activation. Thus, the rate of enzyme induction is used here only to express the rate of whatever induced hydroxylase activity accumulates. It has been established (19) that the synthesis of an induction-specific RNA takes place in the first 20 min after exposure of cells to the polycyclic hydrocarbon inducer (20), that the rise in hydroxylase activity and the appearance of a new spectrally distinct cobinding cytochrome are concomitantly dependent on translation involving this RNA species (21), that this RNA species in all likelihood is not rRNA (22), and that the inducer is actively metabolized by both the control and induced enzymes (23). Moreover, fusion of cultured cells possessing the inducible enzyme with cells having no detectable hydroxylase activity produces somatic-cell hybrids in which the enzyme is as inducible (24) or more inducible (25) than the inducible hydroxylase in the parent cell line.

3. Abbreviations used are: MC, 3-methylcholanthrene; BP, benzo-
   (a)pyrene; DMBA, 7,12-dimethylbenz(a)anthracene; B6, the
   C57BL/6 inbred mouse strain; D2, the DBA/2 inbred mouse strain;
   phorbol ester, 12-O-tetradecanoyl-phorbol-13-acetate.

4. The carcinogenic index (CI) provides a means for relating the
   latency period to tumor incidence (36) by the equation
   $$CI = (P/T) \times 100$$
   where
         P is the percent of mice developing tumors within eight
         months
         T is the average latency period (in days) for a tumor of
         1.5- to 2.0-cm dimensions to develop.

REFERENCES

1. H. S. Mason, Mechanisms of oxygen metabolism, Advan. Enzymol.,
   19, 79 (1957).
2. O. Hayaishi, Enzymic hydroxylation, Ann. Rev. Biochem., 38,
   21 (1969).
3. J. W. Daly, D. M. Jerina, and B. Witkop, Arene oxides and the
   NIH shift: the metabolism, toxicity and carcinogenicity of aromatic compounds, Experientia, 28, 1129 (1972).
4. D. Jerina, J. Daly, B. Witkop, P. Zaltzman-Nirenberg, and S.
   Udenfriend, Role of the arene oxide-oxepin system in the metabolism of aromatic substrates. I. In vitro conversion of benzene
   oxide to a premercapturic acid and a dihydrodiol. Arch. Biochem.
   Biophys., 128, 176, 1968.
5. F. Oesch, D. M. Jerina, and J. Daly, A radiometric assay for
   hepatic epoxide hydrase activity with [7-^{3}H]styrene oxide, Biochem.
   Biophys. Acta, 227, 685 (1971).
6. D. Jerina, J. Daly, B. Witkop, P. Zaltzman-Nirenberg, and S.
   Udenfriend, 1,2-Naphthalene oxide as an intermediate in the
   microsomal hydroxylation of naphthalene, Biochemistry, 9, 147
   (1970).
7. P. L. Grover, A. Hewer, and P. Sims, Epoxides as microsomal
   metabolites of polycyclic hydrocarbons, FEBS Letters, 18, 76
   (1971).
8. P. L. Grover and P. Sims, Enzyme-catalysed reactions of polycyclic hydrocarbons with deoxyribonucleic acid and protein in
   vitro, Biochem. J., 110, 159 (1968).

9. P. L. Grover and P. Sims, Interactions of the K-region epoxides of phenanthrene and dibenz(a, h)anthracene with nucleic acids and histone, Biochem. Pharmacol., 19, 2251 (1970).

10. G. Krishna, M. Eichelbaum, and W. D. Reid, Isolation and characterization of liver proteins containing covalently bound ^{14}C-bromobenzene metabolites, Pharmacologist, 13, 196, 1971 [abstract].

11. P. L. Grover, P. Sims, E. Huberman, H. Marquardt, T. Kuroki, and C. Heidelberger, In vitro transformation of rodent cells by K-region derivatives of polycyclic hydrocarbons. Proc. Nat. Acad. Sci., 68, 1098 (1971).

12. E. Huberman, L. Aspiras, C. Heidelberger, P. L. Grover, and P. Sims, Mutagenicity to mammalian cells of epoxides and other derivatives of polycyclic hydrocarbons, Proc. Nat. Acad. Sci., 68, 3195, 1971.

13. E. Huberman, T. Kuroki, H. Marquardt, J. K. Selkirk, C. Heidelberger, P. L. Grover, and P. Sims, Transformation of hamster embryo cells by epoxides and other derivatives of polycyclic hydrocarbons, Cancer Res., 32, 1391 (1972).

14. M. J. Cookson, P. Sims, and P. L. Grover, Mutagenicity of epoxides of polycyclic hydrocarbons correlates with carcinogenicity of parent hydrocarbons, Nature New Biol., 234, 186 (1971).

15. B. N. Ames, P. Sims, and P. L. Grover, Epoxides of carcinogenic polycyclic hydrocarbons are frameshift mutagens, Science, 176, 47 (1972).

16. J. R. Mitchell, D. J. Jollow, J. R. Gillette, and B. B. Brodie, Drug metabolism as a cause of drug toxicity, Drug Metab. Dispos., 1, 418 (1973).

17. N. Kinoshita and H. V. Gelboin, The role of aryl hydrocarbon hydroxylase in 7, 12-dimethylbenz(a)anthracene skin tumorigenesis: on the mechanism of 7, 8-benzoflavone inhibition of tumorigenesis, Cancer Res., 32, 1329 (1972).

18. W. F. Benedict, J. E. Gielen, and D. W. Nebert, Polycyclic hydrocarbon-produced toxicity, transformation, and chromosomal aberrations as a function of aryl hydrocarbon hydroxylase activity in cell cultures, Intern. J. Cancer, 9, 435 (1972).

19. D. W. Nebert and J. E. Gielen, Genetic regulation of aryl hydrocarbon hydroxylase induction in the mouse, Fed. Proc. Fed. Amer. Soc. Exptl. Biol., 31, 1315 (1972).

20. D. W. Nebert and L. L. Bausserman, Fate of inducer during induction of aryl hydrocarbon hydroxylase activity in mammalian cell culture. II. Levels of intracellular polycyclic hydrocarbon during enzyme induction and decay, Mol. Pharmacol., 6, 304 (1970).

21. D. W. Nebert, Microsomal cytochromes b_5 and P_{450} during induction of aryl hydrocarbon hydroxylase activity in mammalian cell culture, J. Biol. Chem., 245, 519 (1970).

22. D. W. Nebert and J. E. Gielen, Aryl hydrocarbon hydroxylase induction in mammalian liver cell culture. II. Effects of actinomycin D and cycloheximide on induction processes by phenobarbital or polycyclic hydrocarbons, J. Biol. Chem., 246, 5199 (1971).

23. D. W. Nebert and L. L. Bausserman, Fate of inducer during induction of aryl hydrocarbon hydroxylase activity in mammalian cell culture. I. Intracellular entry, binding, distribution, and metabolism, Mol. Pharmacol., 6, 293 (1970).

24. W. F. Benedict, B. Paul, and D. W. Nebert, Expression of benz(a)-anthracene-inducible aryl hydrocarbon hydroxylase activity in mouse-hamster and mouse-human somatic-cell hybrids, Biochem. Biophys. Res. Commun., 48, 293 (1972).

25. W. F. Benedict, D. W. Nebert, and E. B. Thompson, Expression of aryl hydrocarbon hydroxylase induction and suppression of tyrosine aminotransferase induction in somatic-cell hybrids, Proc. Nat. Acad. Sci., 69, 2179 (1972).

26. J. E. Gielen, F. M. Goujon, and D. W. Nebert, Genetic regulation of aryl hydrocarbon hydroxylase induction. II. Simple Mendelian expression in mouse tissue in vivo, J. Biol. Chem., 247, 1125 (1972).

27. D. W. Nebert, F. M. Goujon, and J. E. Gielen, Aryl hydrocarbon hydroxylase induction by polycyclic hydrocarbons: simple autosomal dominant trait in the mouse, Nature New Biol., 236, 107 (1972).

28. D. W. Nebert, W. F. Benedict, J. E. Gielen, F. Oesch, and J. W. Daly, Aryl hydrocarbon hydroxylase, epoxide hydrase, and 7, 12-dimethylbenz(a)anthracene-produced skin tumorigenesis in the mouse, Mol. Pharmacol., 8, 374 (1972).

29. P. E. Thomas, R. E. Kouri, and J. J. Hutton, The genetics of aryl hydrocarbon hydroxylase induction in mice: a single gene difference between C57BL/6J and DBA/2J, Biochem. Genet., 6, 157 (1972).

30. D. W. Nebert, J. E. Gielen, and F. M. Goujon, Genetic expression of aryl hydrocarbon hydroxylase induction. III. Changes in the binding of n-octylamine to cytochrome P-450, Mol. Pharmacol., 8, 651 (1972).

31. F. M. Goujon, D. W. Nebert, and J. E. Gielen, Genetic expression of aryl hydrocarbon hydroxylase induction. IV. Interaction of various compounds with different forms of P-450 and the effect of benzo(a)-pyrene metabolism in vitro, Mol. Pharmacol., in press, 8, 667 (1972).

32. W. F. Benedict, N. Considine, and D. W. Nebert, Genetic differences in aryl hydrocarbon hydroxylase induction and benzo(a)-pyrene-produced tumorigenesis in the mouse, Mol. Pharmacol., 9, 266 (1973).\

288 NEBERT, BENEDICT, AND KOURI

33. D. W. Nebert, L. L. Bausserman, and R. R. Bates, Effect of 17-β-estradiol and testosterone on aryl hydrocarbon hydroxylase activity in mouse tissues in vivo and in cell culture, Intern. J. Cancer, 6, 470 (1970).
34. A. H. Conney, Pharmacological implications of microsomal enzyme induction, Pharmacol. Rev., 19, 317 (1967).
35. R. E. Kouri, R. A. Salerno, and C. E. Whitmire, Relationships between aryl hydrocarbon hydroxylase inducibility and sensitivity to chemical-induced subcutaneous sarcomas in various strains of mice, J. Nat. Cancer Inst., 50, 363 (1973).
36. J. Iball, The relative potency of carcinogenic compounds, Amer. J. Cancer, 35, 188 (1939).
37. N. Kinoshita and H. V. Gelboin, Aryl hydrocarbon hydroxylase and polycyclic hydrocarbon tumorigenesis: effect of the enzyme inhibitor 7, 8-benzoflavone on tumorigenesis and molecular binding, Proc. Nat. Acad. Sci., 69, 824 (1972).
38. W. E. Heston, "Genetics of Neoplasia," Methodology in Mammalian Genetics (W. J. Burdett, ed.), Holden-Day, Inc., San Francisco, 1963, p. 247.
39. R. E. Kouri, H. Ratrie, and C. E. Whitmire, J. Nat. Cancer Inst., 51, 197 (1973).
40. R. E. Kouri, H. Ratrie, W. F. Benedict, and D. W. Nebert, unpublished data.

Chapter 13

CHEMICAL AND BIOCHEMICAL FACTORS THAT CONTROL THE TOXICITY AND CARCINOGENICITY OF ARENE OXIDES

Donald M. Jerina

Laboratory of Chemistry
National Institute of Arthritis, Metabolism
and Digestive Diseases
National Institutes of Health
Bethesda, Maryland

INTRODUCTION

Several years ago, efforts at the National Institutes of Health to develop convenient radiometric assays for the measurement of aryl hydroxylase activity catalyzed by monoxygenase enzymes were thwarted by the occurrence of a unique and unexpected phenomenon, which was subsequently termed the "NIH shift" (1). The principle of these enzyme assays was based on the stoichiometric release of tritium from a ring position into the medium during hydroxylation [Eq. (1)]. Since electrophilic and radical substitution reactions of the

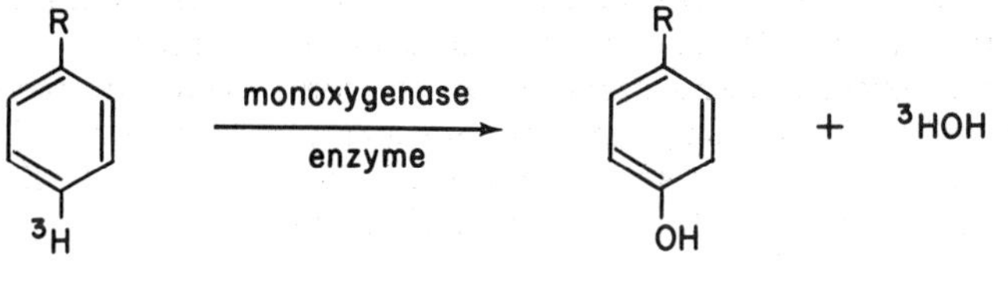

$$\text{(substrate with } {}^3\text{H)} \xrightarrow[\text{enzyme}]{\text{monoxygenase}} \text{(phenol with OH)} + {}^3\text{HOH} \qquad (1)$$

aromatic ring were known to release the hydrogen from the ring position attached (2), there was no reason to suspect that monoxygenases would behave otherwise. Release of tritium from the substrate, however, was not stoichiometric, and the phenolic product was found highly radioactive. Several lines of evidence conclusively established that the tritium migrated from its initial position to either adjacent ring carbon and was thus retained in the phenolic product [Eq. (2)]. Examination of several monoxygenase enzymes that catalyze the

$$\text{>90\% }^3\text{H retained}$$

formation of phenols soon demonstrated the phenomenon to be general;
such intramolecular migrations and retentions of substituents during
the course of aryl hydroxylation became known as the "NIH shift" in
honor of the institution at which these studies were conducted (1).
The numerous examples of migrations of hydrogen isotopes, halogens,
and alkyl groups, catalyzed by enzymes (3) from animals, plants, and
microorganisms and by chemical model systems (4) for these enzymes,
have been reviewed.

Undoubtedly, the most important aspect of the discovery and subsequent studies on the NIH shift has been the use of this phenomenon
as a probe to elucidate the mechanism(s) by which oxidative enzymes
convert aromatic substrates to phenols, a process intimately associated with the detoxification of xenobiotic substances (e. g., drugs,
pesticides, herbicides, carcinogens, etc.), the biosynthesis of regulatory molecules, and (in the case of certain microorganisms) the
catabolic production of energy. An understanding of the unique mechanism which produces the NIH shift would then lead the way to understanding the overall process of phenol formation. Subsequently, arene
oxides (an aromatic compound in which one of the formal double bonds
has been converted to an epoxide) were demonstrated as obligatory
intermediates in the formation of phenols and recently have been implicated as plausible causative agents in carcinogenesis, mutagenesis,
and necrosis. In the discussion that follows, the factors that control
the enzymatic formation and disposition of arene oxides as well as
the propensity of these compounds to isomerize to phenols and react
with nucleophiles are discussed since the relative rates of all these
steps will determine the biologic activity of arene oxides.

ARENE OXIDES AS MEDIATORS OF METABOLISM

Formation of a cationoid intermediate [Eq. (3)] seemed a highly
probable mechanism for the NIH shift since rearrangements (and migrations) involving carbonium ions are well known throughout organic
chemistry. The cationoid species, generated as a result of enzymatic
oxidation, could then undergo rearrangement to the keto form of the

$$\text{(3)}$$

product phenol. This mechanism seemed particularly attractive since it supplied a driving force for the NIH shift; stabilization of this ion by an additional resonance contributor with positive charge on oxygen is shown in Eq. 3. Support for this mechanism was found in the acid-catalyzed dehydration (5) of [1-^{2}H]-trans-1,2-dihydroxy-1,2-dihydro-4-chlorobenzene to 4-chlorophenol [Eq. (4)]. Indeed, the 4-chloro-phenol produced was found to contain a substantial portion (25%) of

$$\text{(4)}$$

25% ^{2}H migrated
and retained

the initial deuterium that had now migrated and was retained at the 3-position. Dihydrodiols such as that shown in Eq. (4) have been known for many years as metabolites in mammalian systems (6). However, despite the realization that acid-catalyzed dehydration of such diols is compatible with the NIH shift, such diols cannot be the intermediates leading to phenols in biologic systems because of their relatively high stabilities. Some other intermediate had to be found. An attractive possibility for such an intermediate was an arene oxide. Several arene oxides had been synthesized (7, 8) and were known to undergo facile rearrangement to the corresponding isomeric phenols.

If arene oxides function as the obligatory intermediates in the metabolism of aromatic hydrocarbons by mammals, they necessarily must be converted to several classes of metabolites (9), including phenols, mercapturic acids (S-substituted-N-acetylcysteines), dihydrodiols, and catechols [Eq. (5)]. It should, therefore, be possible to demonstrate enzymes in the livers of mammals that catalyze the addition of glutathione (GSH) and of water to arene oxides to form mercapturic acids and dihydrodiols, respectively. In addition, the rearrangement of arene oxides to phenols must be accompanied by the NIH shift. The enzymatic dehydrogenation of dihydrodiols to catechols was already known (10). Incubation of benzene oxide with liver microsomes (11) resulted in formation of a trans-dihydrodiol, while the soluble supernatant from liver catalyzed the addition of glutathione to benzene oxide [Eq. (6)]. Furthermore, rearrangement of

$$(5)$$

[1-^{2}H]4-methylbenzene oxide (12) to p-cresol and of [1 - ^{2}H]naph-
thalene-1,2-oxide (13) to 1-naphthol were both accompanied [see
Eq. (7)] by a NIH shift of deuterium with retentions as high as 80%
in each case.

A particularly attractive feature of arene oxides as intermediates
is that they explain the ratios of isomeric phenols obtained during
metabolism. For example, incubation of toluene with liver microsomes
produces only o- and p-cresol [Eq. (8)]; significant amounts of m-cre-
sol are not formed.

(6)

(7)

(8)

Synthesis of the three possible arene oxides of toluene and study of their phenolic rearrangement products has shown that only o- and p-cresols are formed (14) in agreement with the metabolic results. The correlation was extended by comparison of the phenolic metabolites from the three xylenes with the rearrangement products of the nine possible arene oxides. Electronic stabilization of the intermediate ions formed during isomerization was postulated (14) as the cause for the directed openings [Eq. (8)] observed for these arene oxides. Studies of the rearrangement products from arene oxides with substituents other than methyl are in progress. The mechanisms by which these facile rearrangements of arene oxides occur are discussed later.

Despite the indirect evidence for the intermediacy of arene oxides, the key experiment remained — the direct demonstration of the formation of an arene oxide in a metabolic system. This was achieved by incubating [^{14}C] naphthalene with the liver microsomal system in the presence of added naphthalene oxide (15). Isolation of the carrier naphthalene oxide and purification to remove the radioactive naphthalene, naphthol, and dihydrodiol showed that radioactivity was incorporated into the carrier as naphthalene oxide. Thus, the 20-year-old theory that arene oxides are intermediates in metabolism (16) was finally proven (15) for the case of naphthalene. Subsequent experiments have indicated that K-region arene oxides are formed from several polycyclic aromatic hydrocarbons (17).

CHEMICAL AND BIOLOGIC REACTIONS OF ARENE OXIDES

The demonstration that naphthalene oxide was actually formed in a biologic system (15) stimulated considerable interest in arene oxides. To date, arene oxides have been implicated as potent carcinogens in cell culture systems (18), as frame-shift mutagens (19), and as causative agents in tissue necrosis (20). Since the pharmacologic and toxicologic effects of arene oxides must be related to the chemical and biochemical reactions of these compounds, a comprehensive understanding of the properties of arene oxides has become essential. Factors such as lifetime in biologic fluids, chemical stability toward rearrangement to phenols, reactivity with cellular nucleophiles, and enzymatic disposition must be understood.

The kinetics and mechanism of isomerization of a number of arene oxides have now been studied in detail. The mechanisms that have been discovered are, in effect, the mechanisms that cause the NIH shift. Plots of log k (where k is the rate of disappearance of the arene oxide) versus pH have shown (21) that the isomerizations both of benzene and naphthalene oxides occur by two different pathways,

the choice of pathway being governed by pH [Eq. (9)]. In the neutral
to basic region, a pH independent or <u>spontaneous</u> (k_n) rearrangement

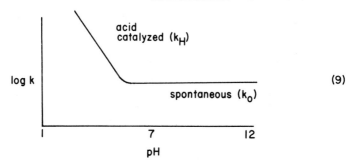

(9)

occurs, which is thought to proceed via the stepwise formation of the
zwitterion [Eq. (10)]; opening of the arene oxide to the zwitterion is

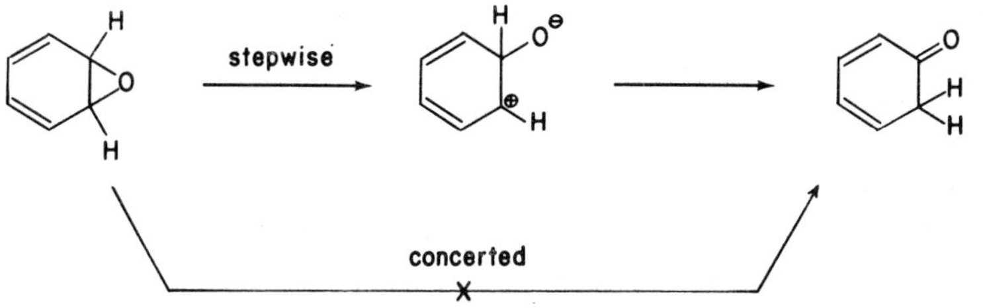

(10)

considered the rate-determining step (22). Below neutrality, the rate
is directly proportional to the acid concentration. The <u>acid</u> catalyzed
(k_H) rearrangement is thought to proceed via rate-determining collapse
of the protonated arene oxide to a carbonium ion [Eq. (11)]. The
occurrence of both pH-dependent and pH-independent pathways for

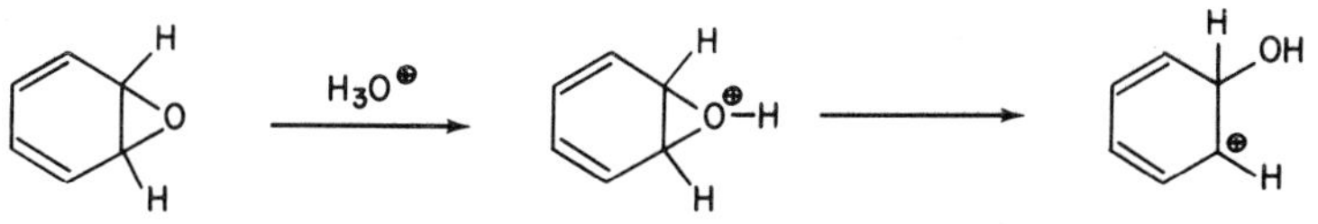

(11)

isomerization has been observed for naphthalene oxide and a wide
number of substituted benzene oxides (21-24). Of particular interest
to this discussion is the fact that spontaneous (uncatalyzed) isomerization does occur in the physiologic pH range. Enzyme catalysis is
not required in this step, and as yet no such enzyme activity has
been detected. Initial studies suggested that the rate of isomerization
of benzene oxide to phenol was greater in the presence of microsomes
than in buffer alone (11). The effect was thought due to catalysis by
the amide group. However, a subsequent careful kinetic analysis (21)
has indicated that protein has no significant effect on the rate of
spontaneous isomerization.

Stability of an arene oxide toward rearrangement to the corresponding phenol(s) is a critical factor in determining its biologic
activity. For substituted benzene oxides, enough examples have now
been studied to permit predictions. Hammett plots of log k_H or k_0
versus σ^+ show good correlations, with rho values near -7 (Fig. 1).
Such large negative rho values for both the spontaneous and acid-
catalyzed rearrangements are indicative that electron-donating groups
stabilize the carbonium ion formed during the reaction. Thus, electron-
donating groups facilitate the isomerization and decrease the lifetime
of an arene oxide, while electron-withdrawing groups increase its
lifetime. The biologic consequence of this fact is discussed later in
relationship to the necrosis caused by aromatic compounds.

Comparison of the rates of isomerization of arene oxides with
deuterium versus hydrogen on the oxirane ring (22) have indicated
that stepwise formation of the carbonium ion in the acid region or of
the zwitterion in the spontaneous region are the rate-determining
steps for these reactions. In addition to the direct reaction of a
nucleophile with an arene oxide (S_N2 mechanism), the carbonium ions
produced during isomerization could capture nucleophiles by an S_N1
mechanism.

To date, only one K-region arene oxide, phenanthrene 9,10-oxide,
has been examined kinetically. The isomerization does not occur

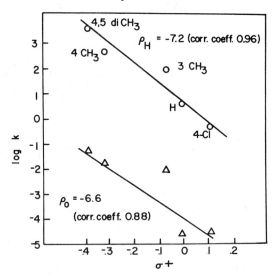

FIG. 1. Plots of the acid-catalyzed isomerization, k_H + (0), and
the spontaneous isomerization, k_0 ($\triangle$), rate constants versus $\sigma+$ for
4,5-dimethylbenzene oxide (4,5-diCH₃), 4-methylbenzene oxide
(4-CH₃), 3-methylbenzene oxide (3-CH₃), benzene oxide (H), and
4-chlorobenzene oxide (4-Cl) (22).

spontaneously, and only acid catalysis could be detected (21). Should this isolated example prove to be typical for the K-region versus non-K-region oxides of the polycyclic, aromatic hydrocarbons presently under investigation (25), it could have considerable impact on studies of carcinogenesis. In effect, the K-region oxides would be substantially more stable than the non-K-region oxides. Thus, transport of K-region oxides to sites in the animal that are remote from the point of synthesis is much more probable, based on this criterion. Chemically, the K-region oxides will behave more like simple epoxides.

In addition to rearrangement to phenols, two other major classes of reactions are known to occur with arene oxides under physiologic conditions: hydration to dihydrodiols by epoxide hydrase and enzymatic as well as nonenzymatic addition of glutathione. Both of these reactions convert the arene oxides into compounds that appear to be innocuous to the organism. However, the reaction of an arene oxide with cellular nucleophiles other than glutathione provides a plausible explanation for the necrosis that occurs during metabolism of halobenzenes. Thus, administration of [^{14}C]bromobenzene resulted in centrilobular necrosis of liver cells; the affected cells contained chemically bound radioactivity, while the surrounding normal tissue did not (20). Thiol groups in protein were thought to be the sites of reaction. Covalent binding of arene oxides to genetic material in the cell thus becomes an attractive explanation for the carcinogenic activity of polycyclic aromatic hydrocarbons. That such binding actually occurs has been demonstrated in this volume (26).

Chemical addition of nucleophiles to benzene oxide has been examined to determine what modes of addition might be expected to occur within a living cell. Use of deuterium-labeled benzene oxide demonstrated addition could occur in a 1,2-, 1,4- or 1,6-fashion (27) [Eq. (12)]. The best nucleophiles in protic media were those that are highly polarizable, such as azide (N_3^-) and sulfides (RS^-), while ammonia (NH_3) and sodium amide ($Na^+NH_2^-$) failed to react (27, 28). These studies suggest the best cellular nucleophiles as thiols or oxygen anions for which the negative charge can be highly delocalized by resonance. Thus, thiol groups of proteins, but not the amino groups, should be expected to react with arene oxides. Both oxygen and nitrogen nucleophiles from the nucleoside bases should also react provided they are sufficiently polarizable. For arene oxides of polycyclic aromatic hydrocarbons, addition of a cellular nucleophile at any one of several ring positions well removed from the oxirane ring can be anticipated, for example, as in Eq. (13). Such a species could readily re-aromatize by loss of water, resulting in stable covalent binding of the hydrocarbon to the nucleophile. If water were the initial nucleophile, a phenol that had incorporated oxygen from water rather than from air could result. Examples of chemical

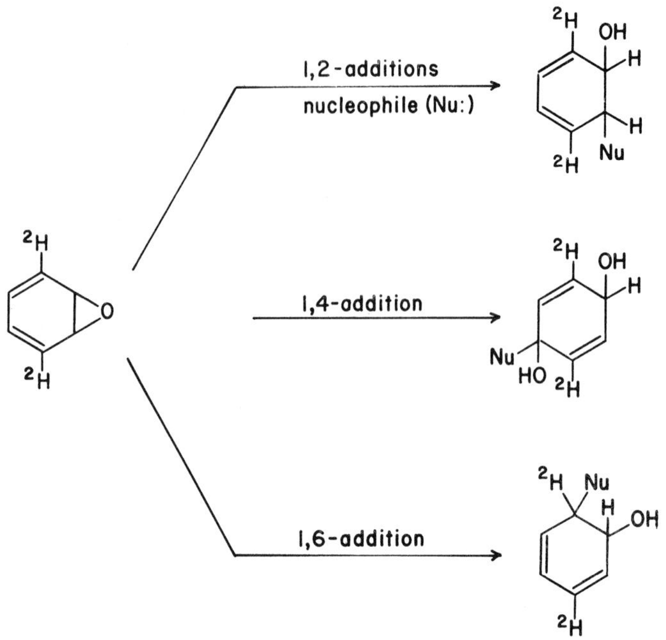

(12)

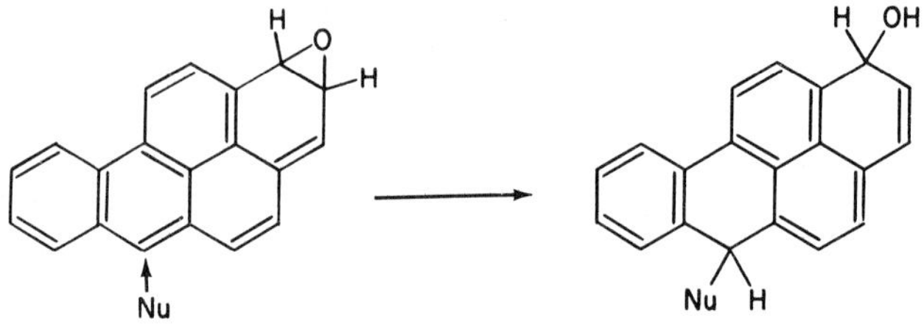

(13)

isomerizations of arene oxides to phenols in which the phenolic hydroxyl group originates from water are known for the rearrangement of 1,4-dimethylbenzene oxide (23) and of indane 8,9-oxide (24) [Eq. (14)]. Formation of a dihydrodiol by the 1,6-addition of water to indane 8,9-oxide occurs in the presence of epoxide hydrase (29).

One remaining feature of the chemistry of arene oxides must be considered. After the initial enzymatic formation of an arene oxide, chemical rearrangement to a new arene oxide might be possible. Thus, the internal oxides of naphthalene (8) and pyrene (30) rearrange to phenols [see Eq. (15)] in nonaqueous media by mechanisms that seem to require the migration of oxygen. The kinetics of isomerization of indane 8,9-oxide [Eq. (16)] are best explained by postulating such an "oxygen walk" (24) as one of the major pathways during isomerization. Several methyl-substituted benzene oxides may also undergo such migrations of oxygen (14).

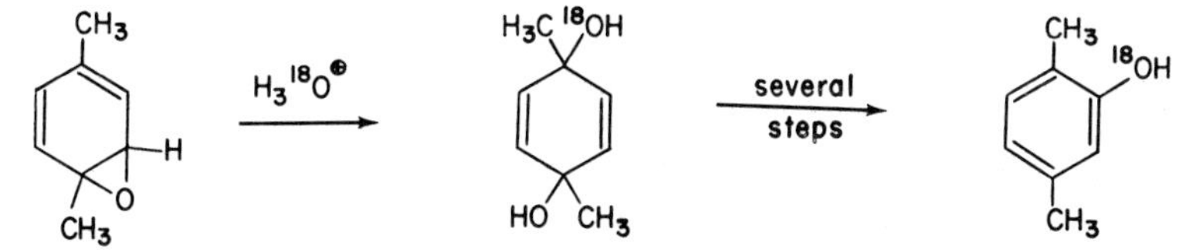

(14)

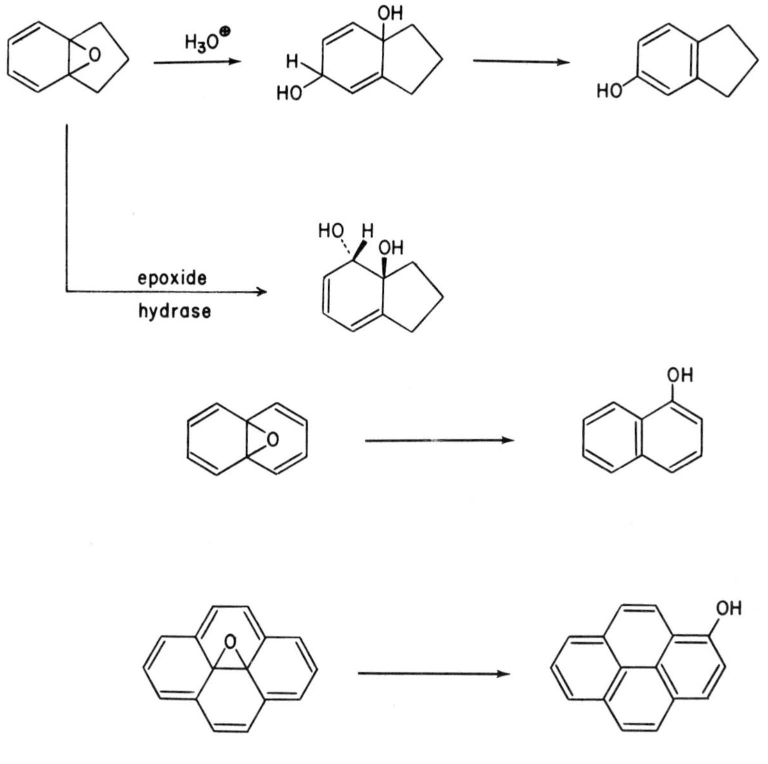

(15)

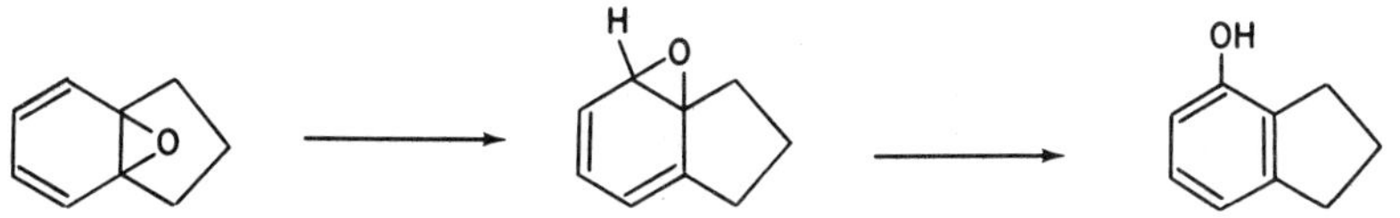

(16)

The possibility of detoxification of arene oxides in vivo through control of epoxide hydrase would be of substantial pharmacologic value. Attempts to purify this enzyme activity from liver microsomes have shown that at least two enzymes or families of enzymes are present: One has specificity for simple epoxides, and arene oxides that do not undergo valence bond isomerization with their oxepin forms (8); the other has greater specificity for benzene oxide (31), which exists in equilibrium with oxepin. In the case of simple epoxides, monosubstitution and cis-1, 2-disubstitution on the oxirane ring produce the best substrates (32). The enzyme can be highly stereospecific (33) in its hydration of some substrates, while hydration of others, such as styrene oxide, produces a racemic product. Numerous in vitro inhibitors and stimulators have been examined (32), and examples of competitive, uncompetitive, and noncompetitive inhibition have been found. The in vivo effects of some of these compounds are considered later.

Like epoxide hydrase, there appear to be several enzymes that are capable of catalyzing the addition of glutathione to simple epoxides and arene oxides. Here, however, the differences in specificity are extremely marked. While the 10, 000 X g supernatant fraction from liver shows enzymatic activity for addition of gluta-thione to practically any compound that contains the oxirane ring, the one glutathione-S-epoxide transferase that has been obtained pure shows no activity toward benzene and naphthalene oxides (34). Since glutathione readily adds to arene oxides without enzyme catal-ysis (11) and since the actual level of glutathione in the liver (20) seems the determining factor in necrosis, control of the activity of these transferase enzymes in vivo may not prove to be a useful pharmacologic tool.

ENZYMATIC CONTROL OF LEVELS AND BIOLOGIC ACTIVITY OF ARENE OXIDES

There are, in principle, several points at which control over the deleterious in vivo effects of arene oxides might be accomplished. These control points include (a) the oxidative enzymes that form arene oxides, (b) the chemical stability of the arene oxides formed, (c) the levels of glutathione in the liver, and (d) the activity of enzymes such as epoxide hydrase and glutathione-S-epoxide trans-ferase. Since the mutagenic and carcinogenic effects of arene oxides have been discussed by others in this work, only the necrotic effects of arene oxides are treated here. Studies on bromobenzene-induced necrosis (20, 35) have demonstrated that many of these control points can be influenced. Administration of bromobenzene to male Sprague-Dawley rats results in extensive centrilobular liver necrosis. When [14C]bromobenzene was used, the regions of the liver where cell death had occurred were found to contain radioactivity that was covalently bound. Most of this radioactivity is associated with protein fractions, and the binding is thought to result from the

reaction of thiol groups on these proteins with the arene oxides of
bromobenzene produced through metabolism. Treatment of the animals
with SKF-525A or piperonyl butoxide, inhibitors of drug metabolism,
blocks the covalent binding and necrosis; conversely, induction of
the drug metabolizing enzymes with phenobarbital greatly increases
the extent of binding and necrosis. These induction and inhibition
experiments clearly link the bromobenzene-induced necrosis to
metabolic activation of the bromobenzene. Compounds such as
benzene, toluene, xylenes, and naphthalene, on the other hand,
cause either minimal or no necrosis. Differences in the ability of
these substrates to induce necrosis seems best related to the stability
of the possible intermediate arene oxides toward rearrangement to
phenols. As established earlier (Fig. 1), the arene oxides from halo-
benzenes are considerably more stable than those from benzene,
toluene, or naphthalene (22). Consideration of the stabilities of
potential arene oxides could become a significant factor in design of
drugs. Administration of diethyl maleate along with bromobenzene
causes greatly increaséd amounts of necrosis. The maleate acts as a
scavenger for glutathione in the liver and greatly reduces the in vivo
levels of this thiol. Since arene oxides are also trapped by glutathione (11, 15), reduction in the level of this thiol should exacerbate
necrosis. Capability of influencing the degree of necrosis is thus
clearly established. The experiments that follow describe attempts to
modulate the adverse effects of arene oxides through control of the
enzyme epoxide hydrase.

The drug metabolizing system in mammalian liver is localized in
the endoplasmic reticulum. Recently (36), this system has been
solubilized and resolved into three mutually requisite components:
the cytochrome (a mono-oxygenase) at which oxidation of substrate
occurs, cytochrome c reductase, which supports oxidation via
electron transport, and a lipid fraction. Two forms of the oxygenase
enzyme are known. Pretreatment of the animals with the inducer
phenobarbital allows isolation of an oxygenase termed "cytochrome
P-450, " while pretreatment with 3-methylcholanthrene leads to
"cytochrome P-448. " Complete capability to oxidize xenobiotic
substrates occurs when the lipid, the cytochrome c reductase, and
either P-450 or P-448 are recombined.

Despite the instability of intermediate arene oxides, substantial
amounts of dihydrodiol and catechol metapolites can be isolated from
the urine of animals treated with appropriate aromatic hydrocarbons.
Thus, a close physical association between epoxide hydrase and the
oxygenase enzymes that produce arene oxides in the endoplasmic
reticulum seems probable. The resolved and partially purified fractions
of cytochrome P-450 and P-448 have been examined for epoxide

TABLE 1

Epoxide Hydrase Activity in Cytochrome Oxygenase
Fractions from Rat Liver (37)

| Enzyme fraction | Diol formation, nmoles/mg N/5 min | |
	[^{3}H]Styrene oxide	Naphthalene 1, 2-oxide
Cytochrome P-450	1103	810
Cytochrome P-448	943	560

TABLE 2

Formation of Metabolites from [^{14}C]Naphthalene with Reconstituted
Cytochrome P-450 and P-448 Systems in the Presence of Carrier
Naphthalene-1, 2-Oxide (37)

| Reconstituted System | Product, nmoles/nmole hemoprotein/5 min | | | |
	Naphthalene oxide	1-Naphthol	Dihydrodiol	Total Metabolites
Cytochrome P-440	1.6	3.6	3.1	8.3
Cytochrome P-450	3.0	5.2	1.9	10.1

hydrase activity (37). As shown in Table 1, the epoxide hydrase
activity toward either styrene oxide or naphthalene oxide is quite
high, especially when compared to the specific activity of ~4000
nmoles diol/mg N/5 min found for the solubilized and partially purified
hydrase preparation from guinea pig liver (38). Notably, the specific
activity of the hydrase in the P-450 fraction is higher than in the
P-448. The results are suggestive of a close association between the
hydrase and oxygenase activities, even in these solubilized preparations. With [^{14}C]naphthalene as substrate and a pool of carrier
naphthalene oxide (Table 2), the oxidizing systems reconstituted with
either P-450 or P-448 produce oxide, naphthol, and dihydrodiol. The
overall amount of metabolism with either system is about the same.
However, with P-448 the amount of radioactive oxide trapped in the
pool is reduced and the amount of radioactive diol formed is higher
relative to the results with P-450. The result is even more impressive
in light of the higher level of epoxide hydrase activity in the P-450
fraction toward added naphthalene oxide. The data can be interpreted
as indicative of a closer association between epoxide hydrase and
P-448 than between hydrase and P-450. Should this association prove
to be generally true for a variety of substrates, metabolism of aromatic

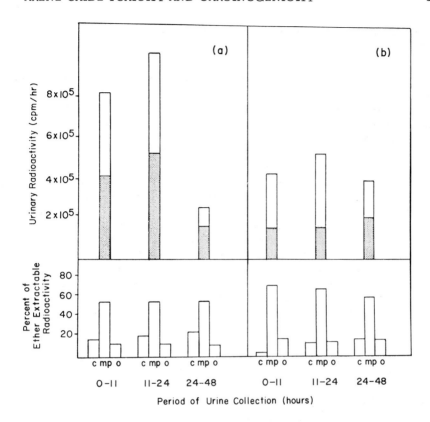

FIG. 2. Urinary metabolites from $[^{14}C]$chlorobenzene in rat: effect of cyclohexene oxide (40). Total excretion during 0-11, 11-24, and 24-28 hr periods has been presented as bar graphs in cpm urinary radioactivity/hr. The solid portion of the bars represents non-extractable radioactivity in glusulase-treated urine. The open portion represents ether-extractable radioactivity. The lower portion of the figure depicts the results of thin-layer chromatographic analysis of the ether-extractable radioactivity. The percentage of the major fractions — catechol (c), o-chlorophenol (o), and m- and p-chlorophenol (mp) — are shown. (a) Administration of $[^{14}C]$chlorobenzene; (b) administration of $[^{14}C]$chlorobenzene and cyclohexene oxide.

substrates by animals pretreated with 3-methylcholanthrene should maintain lower levels of intermediate arene oxides than those pretreated with phenobarbital due to the more efficient coupling between the oxygenase and hydrase in the P-448 system. This tighter association between epoxide hydrase and P-448 may explain in part how induction of rats with P-448 completely blocks the liver necrosis caused by bromobenzene (35). Interestingly, benzo(a)pyrene is a much better substrate for the completely reconstituted system with P-448 than with P-450 (39).

Attempts to affect the degree of liver necrosis resulting from halo-benzenes by altering the in vivo activity of epoxide hydrase have met with some difficulty. Although several compounds are known that either stimulate or inhibit epoxide hydrase in vitro (32), they are often very toxic, do not reach the liver, or affect other enzyme systems in vivo. However, the in vivo study of one of these, cyclohexene oxide, did prove rewarding (40). In vitro, cyclohexene oxide (2 mM) inhibits hydration of naphthalene oxide (2 mM) by 50-60%, while activity of the drug-metabolizing enzymes, assayed with [^{3}H]benzenesulfonanilide, remains unaffected (40). Two hours after administration of cyclohexene oxide (2.4 mM/kg body weight) to rats, the animals were sacrificed, and the activity of epoxide hydrase was measured in their livers. Rather than inhibiting epoxide hydrase, the cyclohexene oxide had slightly increased (5-10%) hydrase activity above normal controls, while decreasing the liver concentration of glutathione by 90%. The net effect should result in a substantial increase in necrosis. A small increase in hydrase activity would be substantially offset by the 90% reduction in glutathione level since the amount of catechols and dihydrodiols in the urine is small compared with mercapturic acid and mercapturic acid precursors (Fig. 2). However, co-administration of cyclohexene oxide and chlorobenzene (10 mmoles/kg body weight) resulted in a complete blockade of the necrosis caused by chloro-benzene at this dose.

Comparison of the metabolites found in the urine of animals treated with chlorobenzene versus those treated with chlorobenzene and cyclohexene oxide as a function of time (Fig. 2) indicated a marked reduction in the rate of formation of metabolites during the first 24-hr period for those animals receiving cyclohexene oxide. Ratios between the various metabolites of chlorobenzene were not substantially altered between the two sets of experiments. Apparently, the steady-state levels of chlorobenzene oxides in the liver were more important than altered rates of conversion of the oxides to stable metabolites in causing necrosis. Further study is clearly warranted.

ACKNOWLEDGMENT

The author is pleased to acknowledge the invaluable contributions of his many colleagues who have made these studies possible.

REFERENCES

1. G. Guroff, J. W. Daly, D. Jerina, J. Renson, S. Udenfriend, and B. Witkop, Hydroxulation-induced intramolecular migrations: The NIH shift, Science, 157, 1524 (1967).
2. D. M. Jerina, J. W. Daly, W. Landis, B. Witkop, and S. Udenfriend, Intramolecular migration of tritium and deuterium during nonenzymatic aromatic hydroxylation, J. Amer. Chem. Soc., 89, 3347 (1967).
3. D. M. Jerina, J. W. Daly, and B. Witkop, "The NIH Shift and the Mechanism of Enzymatic Aryl Hydroxylation, " in Biogenic Amines and Physiological Membranes in Drug Therapy, Part B (J. H. Biel and L. G. Abood, eds.), Dekker, New York, 1971, p. 413; and J. W. Daly, D. M. Jerina, and B. Witkop, Arene oxides and the NIH shift. The metabolism, toxicity, and carcinogenicity of aromatic compounds, Experientia, 28, 1129 (1972).
4. D. M. Jerina, Chemical models for the biological hydroxylation of the aromatic ring, Chemical Technol., 120 (1973).
5. D. M. Jerina, J. W. Daly, and B. Witkop, Deuterium migration during the acid-catalyzed dehydration of 6-deutero-5, 6-dihydroxy-3-chloro-1, 3-cyclohexadiene, a nonenzymatic model for the NIH shift, J. Amer. Chem. Soc., 89, 5488 (1967).
6. E. Boyland and A. A. Levi, Production of dihydroxydihydroanthracene from anthracene, Biochem. J., 29, 2679 (1935). For a current review on dihydrodiols, see Ref. 3.
7. M. S. Newman and S. Blum, A new cyclization reaction leading to epoxides of aromatic hydrocarbons, J. Amer. Chem. Soc., 86, 5598 (1964).
8. E. Vogel and H. Gunther, Benzene oxide-oxepin valence tautomerism, Angew. Chem. Intern. Ed., 6, 385 (1967).
9. For examples see R. T. Williams, Detoxification Mechanisms, 2nd ed., Chapman and Hall, London, 1959; D. V. Parke, The Biochemistry of Foreign Compounds, Pergamon, Oxford, 1968.
10. P. K. Ayengar, O. Hayaishi, M. Nakajima, and I. Tomida, Enzymatic aromatization of 3, 5-cyclohexadiene-1, 2-diol, Biochem. Biophys. Acta, 33, 111 (1959).
11. D. M. Jerina, J. Daly, B. Witkop, P. Zaltzman-Nirenberg, and S. Udenfriend, The role of arene oxide-oxepin system in the metabolism of aromatic substrates. I. In vitro conversion of benzene oxide to a permercapturic acid and a dihydrodiol, Arch. Biochem. Biophys., 128, 176 (1968).
12. D. M. Jerina, J. W. Daly, and B. Witkop, The role of arene oxide-oxepin systems in the metabolism of aromatic substrates. II. Synthesis of 3, 4-toluene-4-^{2}H oxide, J. Amer. Chem. Soc., 90, 6523 (1968).

306 D. M. JERINA

13. D. R. Boyd, J. W. Daly, and D. M. Jerina, Rearrangement 1-^{2}H and 2-^{2}H-deuteronaphthalene oxides to 1-naphthol: Mechanism of the NIH shift, Biochemistry, 11, 1961 (1972).
14. D. M. Jerina, N. Kaubisch, and J. W. Daly, Arene oxides as intermediates in the metabolism of aromatic substrates: Alkyl and oxygen migrations during isomerization alkylated arene oxides, Proc. Nat. Acad. Sci., 68, 2545 (1971); N. Kaubisch, D. M. Jerina, and J. W. Daly, Arene oxides as intermediates in the oxidative metabolism of aromatic compounds: Isomerization of methyl substituted arene oxides, Biochemistry, 11, 3050 (1972).
15. D. M. Jerina, J. W. Daly, B. Witkop, P. Zaltzman-Nirenberg, and S. Udenfriend, The role of the arene oxide-oxepin system in the metabolism of aromatic substrates. III. Formation of 1,2-naphthalene oxide from naphthalene by liver microsomes, J. Amer. Chem. Soc., 90, 6525 (1968).
16. E. Boyland, The Biological Significance of Metabolism of Polycyclic Compounds, Biochemical Society Symposia. No. 5. Biological Oxidation of Aromatic Rings, University Press, Cambridge, England, 1950, p. 40.
17. J. A. Selkirk, E. Huberman, and C. Heidelberger, An epoxide is an intermediate in the microsomal metabolism of the chemical carcinogen, dibenz[a,h]anthracene, Biochem. Biophys. Res. Commun., 43, 1010 (1971); P. L. Grover, A. Hewer, and P. Sims, Epoxides as microsomal metabolites of polycyclic hydrocarbons, FEBS Letters, 18, 76 (1971). See also the chapters by P. Sims and by C. Heidelberger in this volume.
18. E. Huberman, L. Aspiras, C. Heidelberger, P. L. Grover, and P. Sims, Mutagenicity to mammalian cells of epoxides and other derivatives of polycyclic hydrocarbons, Proc. Nat. Acad. Sci., 68, 3195 (1971).
19. B. N. Ames, P. Sims, and P. L. Grover, Epoxides of carcinogenic polycyclic hydrocarbons and frameshift mutagens, Science, 176, 47 (1972).
20. B. B. Brodie, W. D. Reid, A. K. Cho, G. Sipes, G. Krishna, and J. R. Gillette, Possible mechanism of liver necrosis caused by aromatic organic compounds, Proc. Nat. Acad. Sci., 68, 160 (1971).
21. G. J. Kasperek and T. C. Bruice, The mechanism of the aromatization of arene oxides, J. Amer. Chem. Soc., 94, 198 (1972).
22. G. J. Kasperek, T. C. Bruice, H. Yagi, and D. M. Jerina, Differentiation between the concerted and stepwise mechanisms for aromatization (NIH-shift) of arene epoxides, J. Chem. Soc. Chem. Commun. 1972, 784.
23. H. Yagi, D. M. Jerina, G. J. Kasperek, and T. C. Bruice, A novel mechanism for the NIH shift, Proc. Nat. Acad. Sci., 69, 1985 (1972).

24. P. Y. Bruice, G. J. Kasperek, T. C. Bruice, H. Yagi, and D. M. Jerina, The oxygen walk as a complementary observation to the NIH-shift, J. Amer. Chem. Soc., 95, 1673 (1973); J. G. Kasperek, P. Y. Bruice, T. C. Bruice, H. Yagi, and D. M. Jerina, The multiple pathways for the aromatization of 8, 9-indane oxide, J. Amer. Chem. Soc., 95, 6041 (1973).

25. Joint studies with Professor T. C. Bruice on the synthesis and mechanisms for rearrangement of arene oxides are in progress.

26. P. Brookes, DNA reaction of methylbenz[a]anthracene derivatives in relation to carcinogenesis by these compounds, Chapter 4.

27. A. M. Jeffrey, H. Yeh, D. M. Jerina, R. M. DeMarinis, C. H. Foster, D. E. Piccolo, and G. A. Berchtold, Stereochemical course of nucleophilic additions to arene oxides, J. Amer. Chem. Soc., (submitted).

28. R. M. DeMarinis and G. A. Berchtold, Reaction of oxepin-benzene oxide with nucleophiles, J. Amer. Chem. Soc., 91, 6252 (1969); and C. H. Foster and G. A. Berchtold, cis-1, 6-addition of methyllithium to oxepin-benzene oxide, ibid., 93, 3831 (1971).

29. J. W. Daly, D. M. Jerina, H. Ziffer, B. Witkop, F. G. Klarner, and E. Vogel, Enzymatic hydration of 8, 9-indane oxide: Homoallylic addition of water, J. Amer. Chem. Soc., 92, 702 (1970).

30. V. Boekelheide, 'Synthesis of Aromatic Molecules Bearing Substituents Within the Cavity of the Pi Electron Cloud, " Proceedings of the Robert A. Welch Foundation Conferences on Chemical Research XII Organic Synthesis (W. O. Milligan, ed.), Houston, Texas, 1969, p. 83.

31. F. Oesch, D. M. Jerina, and J. W. Daly, Substrate specificity of hepatic-epoxide hydrase in microsomes and in a purified preparation: evidence for homologous enzymes, Arch. Biochem. Biophys., 144, 253 (1971).

32. F. Oesch, N. Kaubisch, D. M. Jerina, and J. W. Daly, Hepatic epoxide hydrase: structure-activity relationships for substrates and inhibitors, Biochemistry, 10, 4858 (1971).

33. D. M. Jerina, H. Ziffer, and J. W. Daly, The role of the arene oxide-oxepin system in the metabolism of aromatic substrates. IV. Stereochemical considerations of dihydrodiol formation and dehydrogenation, J. Amer. Chem. Soc., 92, 1056 (1970).

34. W. B. Jakoby and T. A. Fjellstedt, "Epoxidases, " in The Enzymes, 3rd ed. (P. D. Boyer, ed.), Academic, New York, 1972, p. 199.

35. N. Zampaglione, D. J. Jollow, J. R. Mitchell, B. Stripp, M. Hamrick, and J. R. Gillette, Toxicity caused by drug metabolism. Role of detoxifying enzymes in bromobenzene-induced liver necrosis, J. Pharm. and Exptl. Therap., 187, 218 (1973).

36. A. Y. H. Lu, R. Kuntzman, S. West, M. Jacobson, and A. H. Conney, Reconstituted liver microsomal enzyme system that hydroxylates drugs, other foreign compounds, and endogenous substrates. II. Role of cytochrome P-450 and P-448 fractions in drug and steroid hydroxylations, J. Biol. Chem., 247, 1727 (1972).

37. F. Oesch, D. M. Jerina, J. W. Daly, A. Y. H. Lu, R. Kuntzman, and A. H. Conney, A reconstituted microsomal enzyme system that converts naphthalene to trans-1, 2-dihydroxy-1, 2-dihydronaphthalene via naphthalene-1, 2-oxide. Presence of epoxide hydrase in cytochrome P-450 and P-448 fractions, Arch. Biochem. Biophys. , 153, 62 (1972).

38. F. Oesch and J. W. Daly, Solubilization, purification, and properties of a hepatic epoxide hydrase, Biochim. Biophys. Acta, 227, 692 (1971).

39. A. Y. H. Lu and S. B. West, Reconstituted liver microsomal enzyme system that hydroxylates drugs, other foreign compounds, and endogenous substrates. III. Properties of the reconstituted 3, 4-benzpyrene hydroxylase system, Mol. Pharmacol. , 8, 490 (1972).

40. F. Oesch, D. M. Jerina, J. W. Daly, and J. M. Rice, Induction, activation, and inhibition of epoxide hydrase: An anomalous prevention of chlorobenzene-induced hepatotoxicity by an inhibitor of epoxide hydrase, Chem. -Biol. Interactions 6, 189 (1973).

Chapter 14

ARYL HYDROCARBON HYDROXYLASE: REGULATION AND ROLE
IN POLYCYCLIC HYDROCARBON ACTION

H. V. Gelboin, F. J. Wiebel, and N. Kinoshita

Chemistry Branch
National Cancer Institute
National Institutes of Health
Bethesda, Maryland

Four years ago at the Jerusalem Symposium on Chemical Carcinogenesis, the commonly held view was that polycyclic hydrocarbons
were direct-acting carcinogens. At that meeting, we presented data
showing that the microsomal hydroxylase system from rat liver catalyzes the formation of benzpyrene and DMBA metabolites that covalently bind to DNA. This and a series of other studies from our
laboratory have indicated that the polycyclic hydrocarbons are activated by the microsomal enzyme system to carcinogenic forms (1).

I will now discuss some aspects of the role of this enzyme
system in both the detoxification and the activation of polycyclic
hydrocarbons and our studies on the biologic regulation of the
enzyme system.

For millions of years organisms have lived in environments that
were often a chemical threat to their survival. Although the dangers
of the chemical environment are surely greater in our present industrial society due to our exposure to an increased amount of man-made
pollutants such as food additives, pesticides, and preservatives as
well as industrial wastes and products of combustion, there is no
doubt that the products of combustion and other foreign chemicals
such as plant toxins have been part of man's environment for aeons of
time. Thus, survival was dependent on the development of biologic
systems that could remove these chemicals effectively and safely
from the organism. One of the major mammalian systems of detoxification is the enzyme complex localized in the endoplasmic reticulum
or microsomes. This system is the important biochemical interface
between the organism and the foreign chemicals in its environment.

Thus, it is a major defense system for small foreign molecules. In one sense it may be analogous to the role of the immune system in the host defense against large foreign macromolecules.

The microsomal enzyme complex metabolizes a variety of drugs and pollutants, such as hydrocarbons and pesticides, as well as certain steroids (2-5). Conservative estimates suggest that the vast majority of foreign organic molecules metabolized by the mammalian organism are metabolized by the microsomal enzyme system. The present report is concerned with a certain class of these enzymes, the microsomal hydroxylases, and in particular, the aryl hydrocarbon hydroxylase (AHH). This enzyme system was first described in rat liver by Conney and Miller and Miller (6) and called benzpyrene hydroxylase. It was subsequently shown by histochemical methods (7) to be present in a variety of nonhepatic tissues. Subsequently, quantitative methods for the detection of the enzyme were developed and applied to nonhepatic tissues (8, 9).

Some of the characteristics of aryl hydrocarbon hydroxylase are as follows: The enzyme is present in almost all of the tissues examined in rats, hamsters, mice, and primates such as monkeys (9). It is also found in human tissues such as placenta (10) and lymphocytes (11). This enzyme, of which a key component is cytochrome P-450, has also been found in lower organisms such as fish cells, some microorganisms, and even in plant material. In higher organisms the enzyme is ubiquitous. It is thus reasonable to suggest that it is present in a wide spectrum of human tissues as it is in other species. Different tissues exhibit quite different levels of activity. The amount present in the liver is generally of an order of magnitude greater than the amount present in other tissues. Different strains of mice show specificity as to both the basal level and inducibility of the enzyme. The enzyme is highly inducible by polycyclic hydrocarbons, drugs, and other xenobiotics. Thus, when an animal is exposed to the inducer, the enzyme level will rise, in some tissues as much as 50- to 100-fold within 24 hr. The enzyme system of our concern oxygenates polycyclic hydrocarbons at a variety of positions to form epoxides, phenols, dihydrodiols, and quinones. Most of these metabolites are then conjugated to water soluble products. The enzyme system has a broad specificity for substrates as well as for the type of molecules causing the induction of the enzyme. Thus, both carcinogenic and noncarcinogenic hydrocarbons are inducers as well as substrates for the enzyme system. The enzyme system is part of the endoplasmic reticulum and includes a complex of enzymes that includes TPNH cytochrome c reductase, cytochrome P-450, cytochrome P-448, a lipid factor, and cytochrome P-450 reductase.

The enzyme system is present in at least two forms in the liver and is probably present in two forms in extrahepatic tissues. This is indicated by kinetic and spectral data and the unique susceptibility of the two forms to inhibition by 7, 8-benzoflavone (12).

Since the Jerusalem Symposium in 1968, we have developed five lines of evidence that suggest a role for the microsomal hydroxylase system in both the toxic and the carcinogenic action of polycyclic hydrocarbons. These are as follows.

1. AHH enzyme catalyzes formation of BP-DNA and BP-protein complexes (13, 14).

2. Cell AHH level parallels cell susceptibility to polycyclic hydrocarbon toxicity (15).

3. Inhibitor of AHH system prevents polycyclic hydrocarbon toxicity in HE cells (16).

4. Inhibitor of AHH system also inhibits tumorigenesis by DMBA in mouse skin (17).

5. Inhibitor of AHH system reduces the covalent binding of DMBA to DNA, RNA, and protein of mouse skin (17).

ROLE OF ARYL HYDROCARBON HYDROXYLASE IN THE BINDING OF POLYCYCLIC HYDROCARBONS TO NUCLEIC ACIDS

Polycyclic hydrocarbons are known to interact with macromolecules either through weak physical interaction (18-20) or through covalent linkage (21-23). The formation of these covalent linkages seemed to require the conversion of the relatively inert polycyclic hydrocarbons to more reactive species. An enzymatic basis for this conversion was thought likely. Since polycyclic hydrocarbons are primarily metabolized by the microsomal NADPH-requiring oxygenases, we studied the effect of enzymatically active microsomal preparations on the formation of DNA-polycyclic hydrocarbon complexes.

The formation of DNA-polycyclic hydrocarbon complexes was found in fact to be dependent on a microsome-catalyzed reaction. The requirement for the binding of [^{3}H] 3, 4-benzo(a)pyrene in microsomal preparations of rat liver is shown in Table 1. High purification of the DNA and extensive extractions of the material with organic solvents, as described elsewhere (13), indicated that the polycyclic hydrocarbon is bound to the DNA through a covalent linkage. This purified preparation and the coincidence of radioactivity from benzpyrene and the absorption of DNA are shown in Fig. 1.

Under the experimental conditions used, binding of [^{3}H] 3, 4-benzo(a)pyrene derivatives with RNA occurred at approximately the same level as the binding with DNA (13). The observations of others

TABLE 1

Requirements for [^{3}H]BP to DNA Binding^a (13)

	[^{3}H]BP to DNA Binding, % control
Complete system	100
Complete system, DNA after incubation	81-112
Complete system, [^{3}H]BP after incubation	11
Complete system, no NADPH	3
Complete system, zero time	< 1

^{a}Each flask contained in a total volume of 3.0 ml the following: 50 μmoles sodium phosphate buffer, pH 7.4; 100 μmoles ethylene-diamine-tetraacetate (EDTA); 2 mg NADPH; 2.0 mg DNA; 0.2 ml of microsomal suspension in 0.25 M sucrose; and 40 μg of [^{3}H]-labeled polycyclic hydrocarbons in 0.2 ml of ethanol (10^5 dpm per min per μg). The flasks were incubated in air at 37 °C for 14 min. Microsomes from methylcholanthrene (MC)-treated rats were used. The DNA was isolated by phenol extraction.

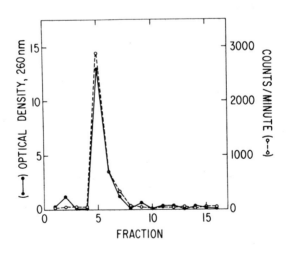

FIG. 1. Purification by phenol extraction in cesium chloride sedimentation of [^{3}H]DNA-BP complex; BP, benzo(a)pyrene (13).

have indicated that microsomal enzymes catalyze the binding of polycyclic hydrocarbons to proteins as well as to nucleic acids (14). The
nature of the reactive species formed during the hydroxylation reaction
and the site of linkage of the polycyclic hydrocarbon with the macromolecules is not known. The active forms could be carbonium ions as
well as radical cations (24, 25). Boyland (26) speculated that the ring
hydroxylation of polycyclic hydrocarbons proceeds via the formation
of highly reactive epoxides and Jerina et al. (27) have demonstrated
that an epoxide is an intermediate in the microsomal hydroxylation of
naphthalene. It is also possible that a metabolite formed by activation
of the 6-position of benzo(a)pyrene, as reported by Nagata and by T'so
in this volume, may be the intermediate bound to the DNA (28, 29). It
is likely that the microsomal enzyme system is also responsible for
the formation of covalently bound DNA polycyclic hydrocarbon complexes in vivo. The significance of the binding of polycyclic hydrocarbons to cellular constituents for the process of carcinogenesis is
not entirely clear. The binding of polycyclic hydrocarbons to both
proteins (22, 30) and DNA (21) has been implicated in carcinogenesis,
but the intimate mechanism relating this binding to transformation
has not been clarified. In either case, microsomal aryl hydrocarbon
metabolizing enzymes appear to be central in the activation of polycyclic hydrocarbons to their carcinogenic form and a central component
of the carcinogen-binding process.

ROLE OF AHH IN POLYCYCLIC TOXICITY: AHH LEVELS
PARALLEL SUSCEPTIBILITY TO TOXICITY

Earlier observations indicated that cell lines highly resistant to
the toxic effect of benzpyrene contain little or no enzyme activity(31).
We examined this more closely in collaboration with Huberman and
Sachs (15). Table 2 shows the level of enzyme in a variety of different
types of cells and their relative susceptibility to the toxic action of
benzpyrene. The toxic effect of benzpyrene and the level of AHH was
measured in identical cell cultures.

Those cells that contain very low hydroxylase activity are highly
resistant to the toxic effects of benzpyrene, whereas cells exhibiting
high enzyme activity are quite susceptible to benzpyrene toxicity.
These results were obtained with a large series of hamster or mouse
cells transformed by viruses, chemicals, or other treatments (Table 2).

In other studies (15) we found that cells that were resistant to
benzpyrene toxicity were nevertheless sensitive to the toxic effects
of a major metabolite of the enzyme system, 3-hydroxybenzo(a)-
pyrene (15). These observations suggest that the cytotoxic effects of

TABLE 2

Aryl Hydrocarbon Hydroxylase Activity and Susceptibility
to the Cytotoxic Effect of BP of
Normal and Transformed Cells (15)

Hamster cells	BP treated, $10\,\mu g/ml$,[a] % surviving colonies	Hydroxylated BP[b] $\mu g/mg$ cell protein per hour, $\times 10^3$
Normal[c]	40.5	340
SV 1	48.5	140
DMNA	77.0	8
PV 1	80.4	< 5
BP	83.0	< 5
Spont.	88.0	< 5
PV 2	96.0	< 5
SV 2	98.0	< 5
PV Cl 1	3.3	150
PV Cl 2	20.0	120
PV Cl 3	31.0	30
PV Cl 4	59.0	8
PV Cl 5	87.3	< 5
PV Cl 6	100.0	< 5
Mouse cells		
Normal	37.5	450
SV 1	33.3	180
SV 2	57.7	23
SV 3	95.2	<5
3T3	15.0	140
3T3 SV 1	40.0	58
3T3 PV	60.0	14
3T3 SV 2	82.6	<5

[a]Benzpyrene was added the day after seeding of cells, and the number of colonies was determined seven days later.

[b]Cells were exposed to benzanthracene (10 $\mu g/ml$) for 20-24 hr.

[c]Origin of cells, as given in Gelboin et al. (15).

polycyclic hydrocarbons depend on their enzymatic conversion to toxic metabolites, one of which is 3-hydroxybenzo(a)pyrene, and that the presence and level of aryl hydrocarbon hydroxylase is the major determinant for the susceptibility of cells to polycyclic hydrocarbon cytotoxicity.

INHIBITION OF POLYCYCLIC HYDROCARBON CYTOTOXICITY BY 7,8-BENZOFLAVONE, AN INHIBITOR OF ARYL HYDROCARBON HYDROXYLASE

7,8-Benzoflavone is a synthetic compound related to naturally occurring flavonoids, some of which were found to exhibit antioxidative properties (32, 33) and some of which were found to have enzyme-inducing activity (34). This compound is shown in Fig. 2. In collaboration with Diamond (16), we found that 7,8-benzoflavone inhibits the metabolism of benzo(a)pyrene in hamster embryo cell cultures (Fig. 3). Treatment of cells with 7,8-benzoflavone (0.1 μg/ml) for 18 hr reduced the appearance of water soluble metabolites of benzo(a)pyrene by 30%, and treatment with 1.0 μg/ml inhibited the metabolic conversion by more than 70%. In other experiments, 7,8-benzoflavone also inhibited the metabolism of 7,12-dimethylbenzanthracene (16).

The effect of 7,8-BF on the cytotoxicity induced by 7,12-dimethylbenz(a)anthracene is shown in Fig. 4. The growth of hamster embryo cells declines rapidly after the addition of 7,12-dimethylbenz(a)anthracene (0.1 μg/ml). However, when 7,12-dimethylbenz(a)anthracene is added in the presence of 7,8-benzoflavone (1.0 μg/ml), the rate of cell growth is restored to that of control cultures. Thus, inhibition of the metabolism of the polycyclic hydrocarbon parallels the prevention of polycyclic hydrocarbon cytotoxicity.

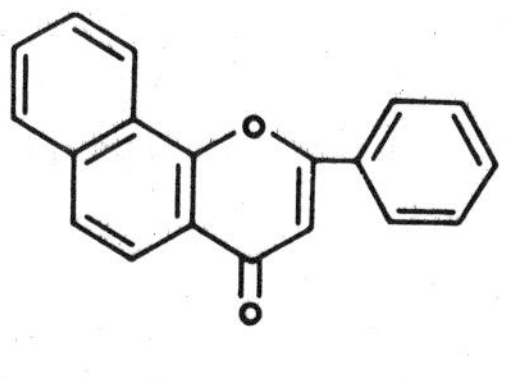

FIG. 2. Structure of 7,8-benzoflavone.

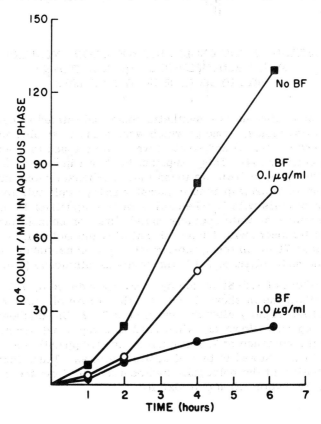

FIG. 3. Effect of 7,8-benzoflavone (BF) on the metabolism of benzo(a)pyrene (BP) (14). Secondary cultures of hamster embryo cells were treated with 7,8-benzoflavone for 18 hr. [^{3}H]BP was then added at a final concentration of 0.06 µg/ml. Aliquots of the medium were extracted with a mixture of chloroform and methanol (2:1 v/v) at times indicated and radioactivity in the aqueous phase was assayed (16).

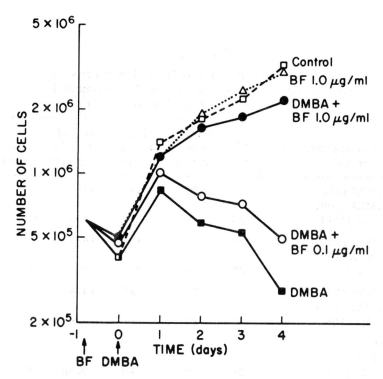

FIG. 4. Effect of 7, 8-benzoflavone (BF) on the inhibition of cell growth by DMBA (14). Hamster embryo cultures were treated with 7, 8-benzoflavone for 18 hr before addition of DMBA at a final concentration of 0.1 μg/ml. Control cultures received neither 7, 8-benzoflavone nor DMBA (16).

TUMORIGENESIS INDUCED BY A SINGLE APPLICATION OF DMBA OR BENZO(a)PYRENE: EFFECT OF 7, 8-BENZOFLAVONE

A single low dose of 100 nmole of DMBA applied to the backs of mice, followed by weekly applications of croton oil, an essentially noncarcinogenic promoting agent, produces multiple tumors on the backs of the mice. In three experiments, 20 weeks after application of DMBA, the average number of tumors per mouse ranged from about 12 to 17 (Table 3). As we have reported (17), a single simultaneous application of equimolar amounts of 7, 8-benzoflavone and DMBA inhibits tumorigenesis to a marked extent. In the three experiments shown in Table 3, the observed inhibition was 80, 55, and 74%. In contrast to the inhibition of DMBA-initiated tumorigenesis, 7, 8-

TABLE 3

Effect of 7, 8-Benzoflavone (BF) on Tumorigenesis
Initiated by a Single Application of 7, 12-Dimethyl-
benz(a)anthracene or Benzo(a)pyrene (17)[a]

Expt.	Compounds, nmole[b]	Survivors	Mice with tumors	Total no. of tumors	No. of tumors per mouse	% control
1	DMBA (100)	29	28	348	12. 0	—
	DMBA (100) + BF (100)	29	8	69	2. 4	20
2	DMBA (100)	22	22	368	16. 7	—
	DMBA (100) + BF (100)	29	23	217	7. 5	45
3	DMBA (100)	28	28	387	13. 8	—
	DMBA (100) + BF (100)	17	14	61	3. 68	26
4	BP (100)	24	8	10	0. 42	—
	BP (100) + BF (100)	26	9	10	0. 38	90
5	BP (100, twice)	28	10	20	0. 71	—
	BP (100, twice) + BF (100, twice)	28	8	35	1. 25	176
6	BP (100)	23	12	34	1. 5	—
	BP (100) + BF (100)	21	7	18	0. 9	60
7	BP (300)	23	12	27	1. 17	—
	BP (300) + BF (600)	21	10	22	1. 05	90

[a]The experiment was terminated 20 weeks after application of carcinogen with or without BF.

[b]Each compound was applied once only, except in Expt. 5, where it was applied twice. In all experiments this treatment was followed by the weekly application of 1% croton oil.

benzoflavone had little effect on benzo(a)pyrene-initiated tumorigenesis. Benzo(a)pyrene is a much weaker initiating agent than is DMBA. In three experiments, in which benzo(a)pyrene and 7,8-benzoflavone were applied once simultaneously, we observed a 40% inhibition of tumorigenesis in one experiment and essentially no inhibition in two other experiments. In another experiment in which the benzo(a)pyrene was applied twice, with a three-day interval, the 7,8-benzoflavone stimulated tumor formation by about twofold. Thus, although 7,8-benzoflavone is an effective inhibitor of DMBA initiation of tumorigenesis, it is essentially ineffective as an inhibitor of benzo(a)pyrene-initiated tumorigenesis.

TUMORIGENESIS INDUCED BY REPEATED APPLICATIONS OF DMBA OR BENZO(a)PYRENE: EFFECT OF 7,8-BENZOFLAVONE

In three experiments, tumor formation caused by the repeated application of DMBA was inhibited by 74, 69, and 30% by the simultaneous application of 7,8-benzoflavone (Table 4). The effect of 7,8-benzoflavone on benzo(a)pyrene tumorigenesis was again markedly different from its effect on DMBA tumorigenesis. In three experiments, the 7,8-benzoflavone either had no effect or markedly stimulated tumor formation by benzo(a)pyrene. In two experiments, there was a threefold and sixfold enhancement of tumor formation when 7,8-benzoflavone was applied simultaneously with the benzo(a)pyrene. 7,8-Benzoflavone alone was essentially nontumorigenic.

EFFECT OF 7,8-BENZOFLAVONE ON THE COVALENT BINDING OF DMBA AND BENZO(a)PYRENE TO MOUSE SKIN DNA, RNA, AND PROTEIN

The application of carcinogen and inhibitor in the experiments shown in Table 5 was similar to that described in the tumorigenesis experiment of Table 3. A single application of the carcinogen was applied with or without 7,8-benzoflavone. In two experiments, the 7,8-benzoflavone inhibited the binding of DMBA to all three macromolecules to about the same extent. Thus, the binding to DNA, RNA, and protein was inhibited by 59, 68, and 52%, respectively. The finding that the binding of DMBA to macromolecules was inhibited by the enzyme inhibitor suggests that enzymatic activation is a requirement for binding of DMBA to macromolecules. Similarly, the 7,8-benzoflavone inhibited the binding of benzo(a)pyrene to RNA and protein by 55 and 46%, respectively, about the same extent observed with DMBA. In marked contrast, the 7,8-benzoflavone inhibited the binding of benzo(a)pyrene to DNA by only 18%. Although the specific locus of binding of carcinogen to DNA, RNA, or protein is not known, the carcinogenic effect of the hydrocarbon most closely parallels its binding to DNA. Thus, the lack of inhibitory effect of 7, 8-benzo-flavone on benzo(a)pyrene tumorigenesis was paralleled by its relatively weak effect on the binding of benzo(a)pyrene to DNA.

TABLE 4

Effect of 7, 8-Benzoflavone (BF) on Tumorigenesis
Induced by Repeated Application of
7, 12-Dimethylbenz(a)anthracene or Benzo(a)pyrene (17)[a]

Expt.	Compounds, nmole[b]	Sur-vivors	Mice with tumors	Total no. of tumors	No. of tumors per mouse	% control
1	DMBA (100)	29	29	531	18.3	—
	DMBA (100) + BF (100)	21	14	99	4.7	20
2	DMBA (50)	27	27	505	18.7	—
	DMBA (50) + BF (50)	26	24	201	7.7	41
3	DMBA (100)	22	22	550	25.0	—
	DMBA (100) + BF (100)	21	21	360	17.1	68
4	BP (100)	29	11	15	0.5	—
	BP (100) + BF (100)	28	20	80	2.9	580
5	BP (100)	27	9	18	0.7	—
	BP (100) + BF (100)	27	20	63	2.3	328
6	BP (100)	19	16	52	2.7	—
	BP (100) + BF (100)	19	14	50	2.6	96
7	BF (100)	21	0	0	0	—

[a]The experiment was terminated 20 weeks after first application of carcinogen with or without BF.

[b]Each compound was applied twice weekly. No croton oil was applied.

TABLE 5

In vivo Binding of [³H]DMBA and [³H]Benzo(a)pyrene (BP) to Mouse Skin Macromolecules: Effect of 7,8-Benzoflavone (7,8-BF) (17)[a]

Compounds, 100 nmole of each	Time, hr	DNA μmole per mole of phosphorus	% inhibition[b]	RNA μmole per mole of phosphorus	% inibition	Protein μmole per 100 g	% inhibition
[³H]DMBA	0	0.35 ± 0.03	—	0.08 ± 0.01	—	4.51 ± 0.22	—
[³H]DMBA	24	4.60 ± 0.41	—	2.26 ± 0.02	—	15.51 ± 0.60	—
[³H]DMBA + 7,8-BF	24	2.08 ± 0.20	59	0.78 ± 0.12	68	9.78 ± 1.76	52
[³H]BP	0	0.46 ± 0.12	—	0.11 ± 0.06	—	2.56 ± 0.81	—
[³H]BP	24	1.71 ± 0.14	—	1.35 ± 0.02	—	20.19 ± 1.42	—
[³H]BP + 7,8-BF	24	1.49 ± 0.16	18	0.67 ± 0.07	55	12.05 ± 0.56	46

[a]The table represents the average of values obtained in two separate experiments in which groups of mice were treated with labeled carcinogens in a manner identical to the procedure used in the tumorigenesis experiment in which the carcinogen was applied once only. See text for details.

[b]Percentage of inhibition was calculated after zero time controls were subtracted.

MECHANISM OF REGULATION OF
ARYL HYDROCARBON HYDROXYLASE

Since the AHH enzyme system occupies a central role in xenobiotic metabolism, we are also very much concerned with its biologic
regulation. In order to study the mechanism of AHH induction, we
developed a cell culture system that offers an opportunity to study the
molecular mechanism of the induction process. The enzyme is present
and inducible in a variety of cells grown in culture. The enzyme is
present and inducible in secondary cultures of hamster, mouse, and
rat embryos as well as in several cell lines (Table 6). Certain cell
lines such as L-cells contain little or no enzyme but others such as
HeLa and mouse 3T3 are highly inducible. Figure 5 shows the kinetics
of induction with different levels of inducer ranging from 13 to 0.65 μM.
Most of the studies described here use benzanthracene as the inducer
at a level of 13 μM. This level causes no observable toxic effects on
the cells that would be reflected as changes in gross morphology.
Figure 6 shows that a single brief exposure of inducer, for as little as
2 min, is sufficient to cause induction to proceed maximally for as
much as 6 hr. Thus, the inducer is incorporated very rapidly in the
cell and a single brief exposure causes maximum induction. Figure 7
shows a more careful study of the early kinetics of induction. Upon
addition of inducer, we observe a lag of about 35 min. The level of
enzyme then rises linearly for approximately 8-16 hr, after which time
the level plateaus.

HALF-LIFE AND SUBSTRATE STABILIZATION OF THE ENZYME

Figure 8 shows an additional analysis of the half-life of this
enzyme system. When the inducer is removed or when cycloheximide
is added so that no more synthesis can occur, the enzyme decays
with a half-life of about 3-4 hr. Thus, the half-life of the enzyme is
relatively short. We also examined the effect of inducer or substrate,
they are the same in this case, on the stability of the enzyme. Figure
8 shows the half-life of the enzyme with no inducer present and in
the presence of an inhibitor of protein synthesis that would prevent
any new synthesis of enzyme. We observe a normal half-life of about
4 hr. However, if protein synthesis is inhibited to prevent any further
synthesis of enzyme and the inducer is present in the medium, there
is a significant stabilization of the enzyme system so that the decay
is reduced by more than 50%. Thus the inducer-substrate of this
enzyme system stabilizes the enzyme and is at least partially
responsible for the rise in AHH during induction. The degree of stabilization by substrate and the kinetics of induction, however,

TABLE 6

AHH Level and Inducibility in Different Cell Cultures

Experiment	Control	Induced
1. Hamster embryo (2°)	11	190
Mouse embryo (2°)	8	236
Rat embryo (2°)	30	100
2. Mouse 3T3	<4	87
Minimum deviation hepatoma HTC	<4	<4
Chinese hamster lung	<4	<4
L-Cells	<4	<4
3. HeLa	17	300

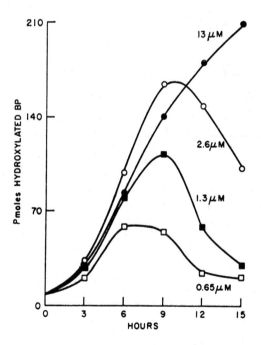

FIG. 5. Kinetics of induction of aryl hydrocarbon hydroxylase in hamster embryo cells by various levels of benz(a)anthracene.

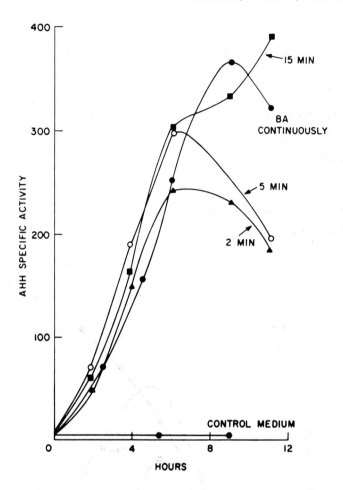

FIG. 6. Kinetics of induction of aryl hydrocarbon hydroxylase
(AHH)[1] after brief exposure to benz(a)anthracene (BA). Hamster embryo
cells were exposed to BA (13 μM) containing medium for time periods
indicated. Monolayers were then washed twice with phosphate-
buffered solution and reincubated with inducer-free growth medium.
Specific activity of aryl hydrocarbon hydroxylase is expressed by
picomoles of alkali extractable product formed per milligram protein
per 30 min.

indicate that the induction process involves processes other than
stabilization since the latter can only account for a small part of the
rise in AHH during induction.

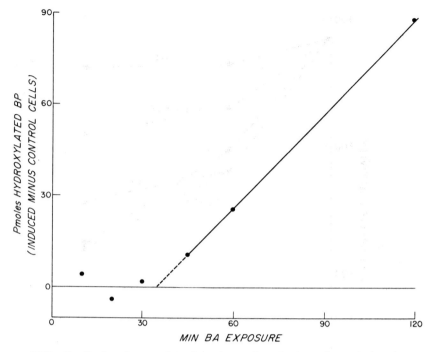

FIG. 7. Early phase of aryl hydrocarbon hydroxylase induction by benz(a)anthracene (13 μM) in hamster embryo cells (31).

MECHANISM OF INDUCTION: EFFECT OF INHIBITORS OF PROTEIN AND RNA SYNTHESIS

In early experiments we found that the simultaneous addition of either actinomycin D, an inhibitor of RNA synthesis, or cycloheximide or puromycin, both inhibitors of protein synthesis, completely block the rise of enzyme activity caused by the inducer. Thus, the rise in enzyme activity requires initially both RNA and protein synthesis. We were then able to proceed with questions relating to the temporal nature of these requirements and whether these requirements can be dissociated. Figure 9 shows the transient nature of the dependence on RNA synthesis for induction. Here the inducer was added at 0 time and the top line shows the kinetics of induction. The bottom curve shows that if actinomycin D is added simultaneously with the inducer, the induction is completely prevented. If, however, actinomycin D is added 2 hr after the inducer, the induction proceeds normally for another 5-6 hr. When actinomycin D is added earlier than 2 hr, the induction is partially inhibited. Thus, within 2 hr after the inducer

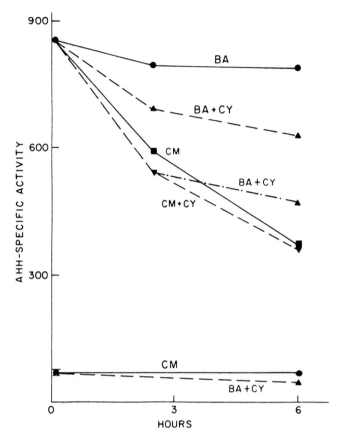

FIG. 8. The decay of aryl hydrocarbon hydroxylase activity in embryo cell cultures and the stabilization by benz(a)anthracene. Secondary cultures were exposed to benz(a)anthracene (3 μg/ml medium) for 16 hr. The medium was replaced by conditioned medium from cell cultures of the same age without any additions (= CM) or with cycloheximide (= CM + CY), benz(a)anthracene (= BA), or benz-(a)anthracene and cycloheximide (= BA + CY). The two bottom lines show the AHH activity in previously untreated cultures incubated with control medium or medium used at a final concentration of 10 μg/ml medium. Cultures were washed three times with the appropriate medium prior to the change of medium (45).

is added, the induction-specific RNA has been made and accumulated so that no RNA synthesis is needed for at least an additional 5-6 hr. Thus, in the presence of inducer the cells pass from an actinomycin D sensitive state to an actinomycin D insensitive state, which means

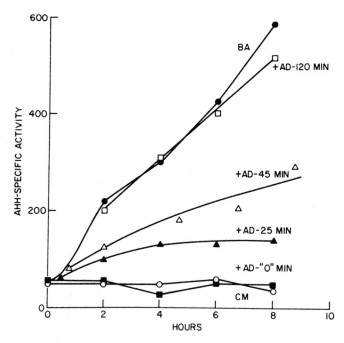

FIG. 9. Requirement of RNA synthesis for the induction of aryl hydrocarbon hydroxylase in hamster embryo cell cultures. Actinomycin D (AD) (1 µg/ml medium) was added simultaneously with, or at various times after, the inducer benz(a)anthracene (3 µg/ml medium). The base line represents aryl hydrocarbon hydroxylase (AHH) activity in cultures incubated in medium free of benz(a)anthracene (BA) or AD (= CM). (J. M. Miller and H. V. Gelboin, unpublished observations.)

that a very early step in the induction process is the production and accumulation of an induction-specific RNA. The next question we were able to ask is whether the production of this RNA requires protein synthesis, that is, is the initial step one of protein synthesis that then can effect an RNA synthesis or can the RNA be made entirely independent of protein synthesis.

Figure 10 shows the experimental approach to this question. Cells were treated with inducer and cycloheximide for 10 hr. This level of inhibitor prevents more than 95% of protein synthesis, and enzyme induction is completely prevented. At this point the cycloheximide was removed. If the induction-specific RNA was formed during this pretreatment, the cells would be insensitive to subsequent actinomycin D treatment. If the RNA had not been made, the cells would remain sensitive to actinomycin D, and actinomycin D

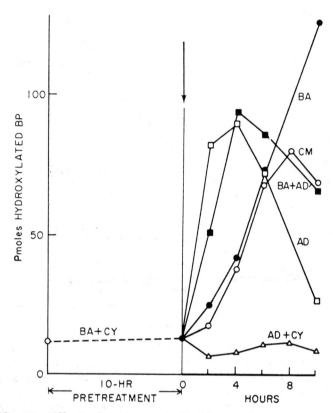

FIG. 10. Effect of actinomycin D (AD) on the induction of aryl
hydrocarbon hydroxylase in hamster embryo cells previously treated
with inducer (BA) and cycloheximide (CY). Concentrations used:
actinomycin D = 0. 40 μM ; cycloheximide = 3. 5 μM ; benz(a)-
anthracene = 13 μM (44).

would prevent induction. As is observed in Fig. 10, the cells are
completely insensitive to actinomycin D. Thus, actinomycin D does
not prevent the increase in enzyme activity after cycloheximide is
maintained in the medium. Thus, Fig. 10 shows clearly that the
initial RNA that is made is not preceded by a requirement for a protein synthesis step, but rather is independent and dissociable from
protein synthesis. Thus, we arrived at a rather important conclusion,
i. e. , the inducer is not directly and primarily stimulating protein
synthesis, but rather is initiating the synthesis of an induction-
specific RNA in the very early stages of induction. Another important
conclusion that can be drawn from Fig. 10 is that once the RNA has

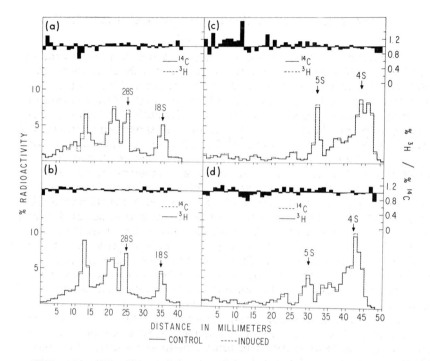

FIG. 11. Gel electrophoresis of cultured hamster embryo cell
RNA labeled during the 75-min period immediately following addition
of inducer. Four groups of three plates, each of secondary hamster
embryo cell cultures, were used. At zero time the medium on each
plate was replaced with 6 ml of fresh medium with the following additions: group 1, no BA, 12 μCi of [³H]uridine (960 μCi/μmole); group
4, 3 μg/ml of BA, 6 μCi of [¹⁴C]uridine (480 μCi/μmole). After 75
min, the cells were collected, combining groups 1 and 4 and groups
2 and 3. Extraction and electrophoresis of the RNA and sectioning
and counting of the gels are described under Materials and Methods
(17). (a) 2% acrylamide-0.5% agarose gel, groups 2 and 3. (b) 2%
acrylamide-0.5% agarose gel, groups 1 and 4. (c) 10% acrylamide
gel, groups 1 and 4 (58).

been made, the subsequent protein synthesis can proceed independent
of continuing or concomitant RNA synthesis. Thus, Fig. 10 shows
the interdependence but dissociability of the RNA and protein synthesis steps required for AHH induction.

ANALYSIS OF RNA PATTERNS DURING AHH INDUCTION

As mentioned earlier there are large changes in the patterns of synthesis of RNA in vivo. We failed to observe these changes in RNA pattern during AHH induction in cell culture. Figure 11 shows an analysis of both high and low molecular weight RNA separated by electrophoresis on polyacrylamide gels. Induction of AHH was not accompanied by changes in RNA patterns. In these experiments RNA from induced cells labeled with [^{14}C]uridine are combined with control cells labeled with [H^3]uridine. The cells are combined and extracted for RNA and analyzed. Duplicate experiments shown in Fig. 11(c) show the same experiment with the isotope labels reversed. Any significant changes in a unique RNA specific would be indicated by a change in the ratio of ^{3}H to ^{14}C and would be inverse in the reverse experiment. The results clearly show that there are no single areas of RNA that we could presently identify as associated with the induction process. Thus, although our inhibitor studies clearly indicate a requirement for an induction-specific RNA, we have been unable to isolate and identify this induction-specific RNA. This might be expected if the induction-specific RNA represents only a small fraction of the total complement of cellular RNA. These results also indicate that the gross changes in RNA observed in vivo may be related to alterations in total growth and proliferation rather than a reflection of changes in specific microsomal enzyme system.

We used another approach to characterize the nature of the induction-specific RNA. There are many indications in the literature that so-called "messenger-RNA" is packaged in the nucleolus and transported to the cytoplasm with ribosomal RNA. We developed a series of experiments to test the question as to whether the hydroxylase induction-specific RNA is either ribosomal RNA or requires ribosomal RNA synthesis and transfer in order to function in the induction process.

RELATIONSHIP OF AHH INDUCTION TO RIBOSOMAL RNA SYNTHESIS:
EFFECT OF ACTINOMYCIN D ON ARYL HYDROCARBON
HYDROXYLASE INDUCTION

In these studies, we used low concentrations of actinomycin D that preferentially inhibit the synthesis of rRNA (35-37). Figure 12 shows the time course of hydroxylase induction in JLSV 5 cells and the effect of a low dose of actinomycin D (0.1 µg/ml) on this induction. Addition of the inducer, benz(a)anthracene, to cultures of JLSV 5 cells caused a rapid increase in hydroxylase activity after a

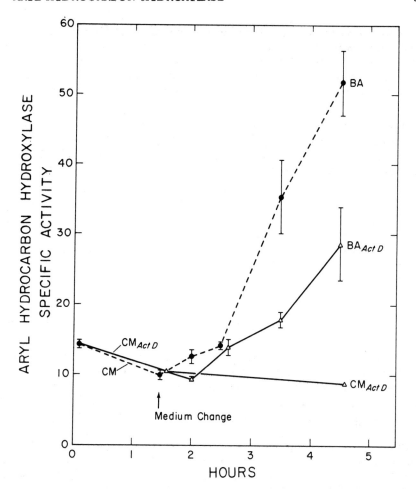

FIG. 12. Effect of a low concentration of actinomycin D (Act D) on the induction of aryl hydrocarbon hydroxylase in JLSV 5 cells. Cells were exposed to growth medium containing 0.1 μg/ml of actinomycin D (CM$_{Act\ D}$) or to fresh medium without Act D (CM) for 90 min. The medium of actinomycin D-treated cultures was then replaced by medium containing the inducer BA (2 μg/ml) and 0.1 μg/ml of actinomycin D (BA$_{Act\ d}$). The medium of control cultures was changed to inducer-containing medium (BA). At various times after treatment aryl hydrocarbon hydroxylase activity was determined in two to four cultures. The graph indicates mean and range of observed values. Aryl hydrocarbon hydroxylase activity is expressed as pico-moles of alkali extractable products formed per milligram of protein per 30 min (specific activity) (68).

lag period of 30 to 60 min. Three to four hours after inducer was
added, there was about a fivefold increase in enzyme activity. When
actinomycin D (0.10 μg/ml) was present 90 min before and during a
$3\frac{1}{2}$-hr exposure to the inducer, enzyme activity increased at a rate
that was approximately half of that in cultures exposed to inducer
only.

The period of exposure to actinomycin D prior to the addition of
inducer could be extended up to 180 min without any further reduction in the amount of induction. Thus, a significant level of aryl
hydrocarbon hydroxylase induction was observed in the presence of
a low dose of actinomycin D administered for prolonged times.

The effect of various concentrations of actinomycin D on hydroxylase induction is shown in Fig. 13. The degree to which enzyme
activity can be induced during a 3-hr period decreased linearly with
increasing actinomycin D concentrations above 0.03 μg/ml. Induction was reduced by 75% at 0.12 μg/ml of actinomycin D and was
entirely prevented by actinomycin D concentrations above 0.25 μg/ml.

EFFECT OF ACTINOMYCIN D ON RNA SYNTHESIS

The effect of low concentrations of actinomycin D on the synthesis of different fractions of RNA and their appearance in the cytoplasm
was determined in parallel to the effect of actinomycin D on hydroxylase activity. After a 90-min period of preliminary treatment with
actinomycin D, [5-^{3}H]uridine was added simultaneously with the
inducer and allowed to be incorporated for 3 hr. Figure 14 shows the
electrophoretograms of cytoplasmic RNA from control cells and cells
exposed to actinomycin D. Most striking is the almost complete
absence of labeled rRNA species (28 and 18S) in the cytoplasm of
cells treated with low concentrations of actinomycin D. Figure 13
summarizes the data on the effect of low concentrations of actinomycin D on the synthesis of cytoplasmic RNA. The incorporation of
labeled uridine into total cytoplasmic RNA synthesis is inhibited
about 60% by actinomycin D concentrations of from 0.03 to 0.12
μg/ml. Most of this inhibition is accounted for by a more than 98%
suppression in the appearance of labeled rRNA.

RNA species in the 4 to 7S region seem virtually unaffected by
low doses of actinomycin D. Incorporation of uridine into cytoplasmic heterodisperse RNA (hRNA) declines gradually at concentrations of actinomycin D above 0.03 μg/ml. Thus, the decrease in
the synthesis of this RNA fraction shows the closest correlation to
the inhibition of aryl hydrocarbon hydroxylase induction by actinomycin D.

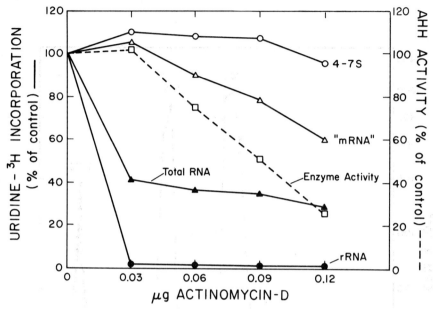

FIG. 13. Correlation of aryl hydrocarbon hydroxylase (AHH) induction and [5-³H]uridine incorporation into cytoplasmic RNA; effect of low concentrations of actinomycin D. Cultures were exposed to growth medium (5 ml) containing actinomycin D at various concentrations (0.03 to 0.12 µg/ml) or growth medium free of actinomycin D for 90 min. Then BA was added in 0.5 ml of medium to give a final 0.5 µg/ml simultaneously with 250 µCi of [5-³H]uridine. Cultures were then incubated for another 180 min. At the end of this period aryl hydrocarbon hydroxylase activity and [5-³H]uridine incorporation into RNA were measured. For fractionation of cells and separation of RNA samples on gel electrophoresis see Ref. 68. The amount of radioactivity in rRNA, low molecular weight RNA (4 to 7S) and heterodisperse RNA (hRNA) was determined from electrophoretograms as described under Methods. Enzyme activity and radioactivity in RNA fractions from actinomycin D-treated cultures are expressed as percentage of control, i.e., of corresponding activities in cultures not exposed to actinomycin D (68).

The high sensitivity of rRNA synthesis to actinomycin D can also be seen in the profile of [5-³H]uridine incorporation into nuclear RNA. (Fig. 15). The synthesis of RNA species in the ribosomal precursor region was almost completely inhibited: The 32S peak disappeared entirely, and in the 45S region only a small peak persisted and remained virtually unchanged at all actinomycin D concentrations

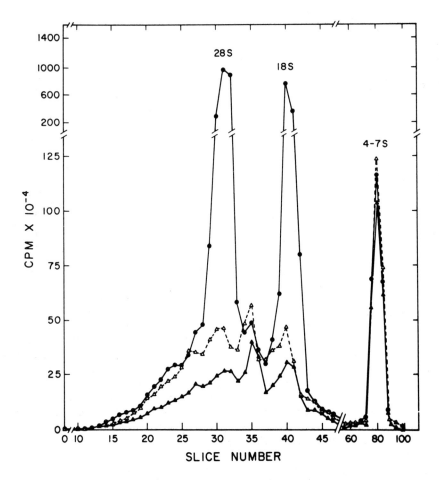

FIG. 14. Electrophoretic analysis of cytoplasmic RNA labeled in the presence of low concentrations of actinomycin D. Experimental conditions were as described in the text and the legend to Fig. 2. '————', control (no actinomycin D); Δ----Δ, 0.06 μg/ml of actinomycin D; Δ————Δ, 0.12 μg/ml of actinomycin D. The profiles of cytoplasmic RNA after treatment with 0.03 and 0.09 μg/ml follow closely the one after 0.06 μg/ml or is intermediate to those of 0.06 and 0.12 μg/ml, respectively./ Note the changes in scale on ordinate and abscissa (68).

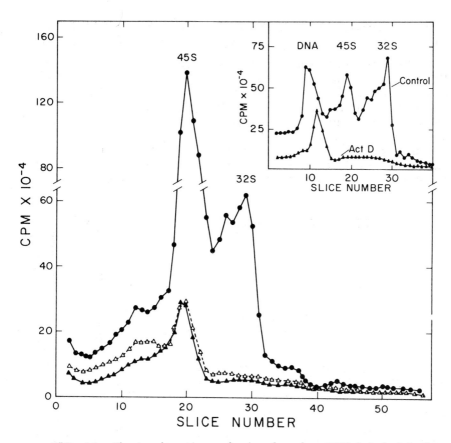

FIG. 15. Electrophoretic analysis of nuclear RNA labeled in the
presence of low concentrations of actinomycin D (Act D). •——•, control (no actinomycin D); Δ----Δ, 0.06 µg per ml of actinomycin
D; ▲——▲, 0.12 µg per ml of actinomycin D. The profiles of
nuclear RNA after treatment with 0.03 and 0.09 µg/ml of actinomycin D are very similar to those shown. RNA samples were
analyzed on composite gels (2% acrylamide, 0.5% agarose) that
were run for 90 min at 200 V and at a temperature of 12.5°C. Note
the change of scale on the ordinate. The inset shows separation of
nuclear RNA from control cultures and cultures treated with 0.12
µg/ml of actinomycin D on acrylamide gels that were run for 6 hr at
50 V and at a temperature of 12.5°C. (We thank Dr. C.W. Dingman
for suggesting this procedure.) Values represent counts per minute
per slice (68).

used. In contrast, however, the rapidly labeled heteronuclear RNA was much less sensitive to low actinomycin D concentrations.

With these electrophoretic conditions the DNA migrates in the 45S region (slice number 20). When the electrophoretic conditions were changed so that DNA was separated from the peak of 45S ribosomal precursor RNA, the actinomycin D-"resistant" labeled material was found to migrate with the DNA (see inset, Fig. 15). No peaks of radioactivity appear in the 32S or the 45S "ribosomal precursor" region in actinomycin D-treated cell preparations. Thus, the data demonstrate that maximum induction can occur when the synthesis of rRNA and its appearance in the cytoplasm are largely suppressed.

EFFECT OF CYCLOHEXIMIDE ON SYNTHESIS OF RNA AND ITS TRANSFER TO CYTOPLASM

A number of studies have shown that the inhibition of protein synthesis strongly inhibits the synthesis and maturation of rRNA (38–40). Thus, inhibition of protein synthesis by cycloheximide served as a tool for a second approach to understanding the relationship between the formation of rRNA and aryl hydrocarbon hydroxylase induction.

Cell cultures were treated with cycloheximide (10 μg/ml) for 3 hr prior to the addition of inducer in order to suppress the synthesis of rRNA and its availability in the nucleus at the onset of induction. The inducer was then added simultaneously with [5-^{3}H]uridine in the presence of cycloheximide (Fig. 15). During this period some RNA synthesis occurs. After 2 hr, total RNA synthesis was blocked for the remainder of the experiment by a high dose of actinomycin D (1 μg/ml). Two hours after the addition of the actinomycin D, the block of protein synthesis was released by removal of the cycloheximide from the medium. From that time on, the cultures continued to be exposed to both the inducer and actinomycin D-containing medium for various periods.

The 2-hr period of exposure to both cycloheximide and actinomycin D was performed for two reasons. (a) Although cycloheximide largely inhibits the appearance of ribosomal RNA in the cytoplasm, some precursor rRNA's are still synthesized and mature at a reduced rate in the nucleus (39). During the period of inhibited protein synthesis, inhibited RNA synthesis, and transfer to the cytoplasm, these ribosomal precursor RNA's are subject to degradation (39–41), so that they are less likely to be available as carriers for the induction-specific RNA when protein synthesis and subsequent rRNA transport resumes. (b) Induction of enzyme activity, if it occurred under these conditions, would give an indication of the relative stability of the induction-specific RNA formed.

The effect of cycloheximide is shown to inhibit the synthesis of total cytoplasmic RNA and its transport by about 60%. The appearance of 28S and 18S RNA in the cytoplasm is suppressed by 90% and 98%, respectively, at the time of onset of hydroxylase induction.

In contrast to rRNA, appearance of hRNA in the cytoplasm is inhibited by only 30%. The apparent increase in the cytoplasmic low molecular weight RNA (4 to 7S) might be due to the continued export of these species from the nucleus, but might also be due to an accumulation of breakdown products caused by the actinomycin D treatment (42, 43).

EFFECT OF CYCLOHEXIMIDE AND ACTINOMYCIN D ON INDUCTION OF ARYL HYDROCARBON HYDROXYLASE

A comparison of Fig. 16(a) and (b) indicates that enzyme activity can be induced although rRNA synthesis and its appearance in the cytoplasm are largely suppressed during the entire induction period. The results are consistent with the data obtained by use of low concentrations of actinomycin D. Thus, treatment with the metabolic inhibitors, cycloheximide or actinomycin D, that largely inhibit the formation of cytoplasmic rRNA does not prevent the synthesis and expression of the induction-related RNA.

The purpose of this work was to examine the role of rRNA in the transport and the expression of genetic information during enzyme induction. Our studies are based on the premise that the induction of enzyme (aryl hydrocarbon hydroxylase) activity depends on the synthesis of an RNA that is specifically involved in the formation of the induction-related protein (44). Evidence for such a requirement is derived from our previous studies (44, 45) as well as from those reported here; these studies also indicate that inhibitors of RNA synthesis, such as actinomycin D and 2-mercapto-1-(β-4-pyridethyl)-benzimidazole (46, 47), prevent the induction of aryl hydrocarbon hydroxylase activity in cells in culture (44). Inhibition of hydroxylase induction by actinomycin D has also been observed in vivo (9). Similar to actinomycin D, ultraviolet irradiation, known to severely impair DNA-template activity by thymidine-dimer formation (48), inhibits the increase in aryl hydrocarbon hydroxylase activity by interfering with some event prior to the translational steps of the induction (49, 50). The requirement of RNA synthesis for the increase in enzyme

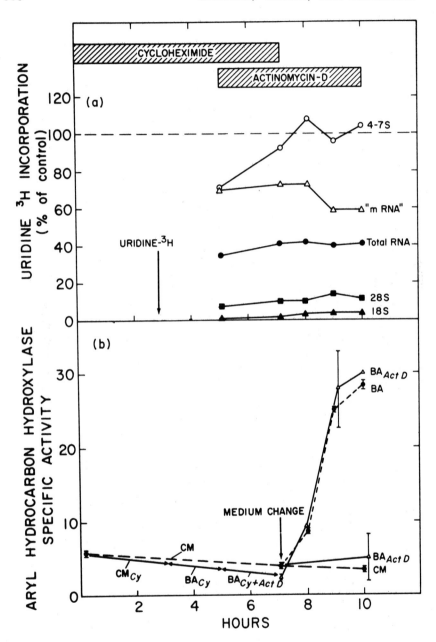

FIG. 16. Induction of aryl hydrocarbon hydroxylase and the appearance of newly labeled RNA in the cytoplasm; effect of inhibition of protein synthesis by cycloheximide. (a) Appearance of labeled

activity is not unique for this microsomal multicomponent enzyme system, but has also been found for the induction of various soluble enzymes in vivo (66) and in vitro (51-55).

The concentration of actinomycin D sufficient to prevent induction of the hydroxylase (0. 25 µg/ml) is far lower than concentrations of actinomycin D that cause a variety of effects in mammalian cells other than the inhibition of DNA-dependent RNA synthesis (43, 5 6, 57). Similarly, the "superinduction" of enzyme activity by actinomycin D at the concentrations used (0. 25 to 1. 0 µg/ml) blocks aryl hydrocarbon hydroxylase induction because of its inhibitory effect on RNA synthesis.

The nature of the induction-specific RNA is unknown. Although some changes were observed in the RNA profile during enzyme

---

RNA in the cytoplasm at 2, 4, 5, 6, and 7 hr after addition of [5-^{3}H]uridine. RNA samples were analyzed on polyacrylamide gels. Radioactivity in RNA fractions from cycloheximide-treated cultures is given as percentage of the radioactivity in corresponding fractions from control cultures (see below). (b) Aryl hydrocarbon hydroxylase activity is expressed as picomoles of alkali extractable products formed per milligram of protein per 30 min (specific activity). The experimental conditions for (a) and (b) are indicated on the top and in (b). Experimental sequence for the controls (broken lines) was as follows. Growth medium (CM, • --•) was replaced (medium change) by inducer-containing medium, 0. 3 µg/ml (BA, • ---•), or medium containing inducer and actinomycin D, 1 µg/ml (BA$_{Act D}$, Δ——Δ), or fresh growth medium (CM • ——•). The sequence of experimental conditions shown by the unbroken line was as follows. Cultures were first exposed to cycloheximide for 3 hr (CM$_{cy}$). Then inducer was added in 0. 5 ml of medium to a final 0. 3 µg/ml (BA$_{cy}$). After 2 hr, actinomycin D was added in 25 µl of ethanol to a final 1 µg/ml for another 2-hr period (BA$_{cy + Act D}$). At this point cycloheximide was removed by exchange of the medium (medium change), and cultures were exposed for various times to medium-containing inducer, 0. 3 µg/ml, and actinomycin D, 1. 0 µg/ml (BA$_{Act D}$, Δ-Δ). Another set of cultures was treated identically except that [5-^{3}H)uridine (50 µCi/ml of medium) was added simultaneously with the inducer [arrow, [^{3}H]uridine in (a)]. Control cultures were exposed to labeled uridine and inducer for 2 hr following a 3-hr period in fresh growth medium. Cycloheximide (10 µg/ml) inhibited incorporation of labeled amino acids by 95% (68).

induction in vivo, analysis by gel electrophoresis of RNA species
formed in hamster embryo cells in culture revealed no significant difference before and after exposure to inducer (58). Similar observations have been made on the hormonal induction of tyrosine aminotransferase in mammalian cells in culture (59). Several conclusions
concerning the induction-specific RNA may be drawn from the present
studies. (a) The near absence of newly formed rRNA in the nucleus
or cytoplasm during enzyme induction indicates that rRNA does not
specify the synthesis of the induction-related proteins. (b) Since
actinomycin D concentrations that inhibit induction do not affect the
synthesis of low molecular weight RNA (4 to 7S), it is unlikely that
these species comprise the induction-specific RNA. The reservation
has to be made that actinomycin D does not interfere with the exchange
of terminal nucleotides of transfer RNA (60). Furthermore, actinomycin D treatment may stimulate RNase activity (42, 43), leading to some
breakdown products of lower molecular weight, although this has only
been observed at concentrations considerably higher than those used
in the present experiment (Fig. 13). (c) The correlation of inhibition
of hydroxylase induction with the inhibition of appearance of newly
formed heterodisperse RNA in the cytoplasm suggests that the induction-
specific RNA is contained in this RNA fraction, one usually associated
with messenger function. Further experiments using ethidium bromide
(1 μg/ml), which specifically inhibits the formation of mitochondrial
RNA (61, 62), suggested that newly formed mitochondrial RNA has no
major role in the induction of this microsomal enzyme system (50).

Our present results show that inhibition of rRNA synthesis does
not prevent the newly formed informational RNA from reaching the
cytoplasmic site of protein synthesis and increasing the formation of
the induction-specific protein(s). Thus, we have been able to disso-
ciate the formation or transfer of ribosomal RNA from AHH induction.
These results suggest that the induction specific RNA for AHH induction is located in the heterodisperse "M-RNA" region.

USE OF CELL HYBRIDS FOR ANALYSIS OF AHH REGULATION
AND CONSTRUCTION OF CELLS WITH UNIQUE AHH PHENOTYPE

Cell cultures with unique aryl hydrocarbon hydroxylase activity
would be very useful from several viewpoints. They could be used
(a) to clarify and designate the role of the enzyme system in the carcinogenicity of hydrocarbons and other carcinogens metabolized by
the microsomal complex; (b) to study transformation with cells requiring either high or low enzyme levels; (c) to examine cytopharmaco-

logic events, and (d) to study the genetics and molecular biology of the regulation of the AHH enzyme system.

In this approach we studied the presence and inducibility of aryl hydrocarbon hydroxylase in intraspecific hybrids of hamster, mouse, and human cells. Hybrid cells were formed between cell lines exhibiting low or no basal and inducible AHH activity and cells with high basal activity and high inducibility. In certain cell hybrids we found a suppression of enzyme activity to a level lower than that of either parent while in hybrids of other cell lines there was an enhancement of both the basal and induced enzyme to levels higher than that in the more active parental cells.

Evidence for the Hybrid Nature of Cell Strains

The hybrid character of the colonies of the mouse cell strains, A9 and 3T3-4C2, is clear from three lines of evidence: (a) The hybrid cells grow in HAT-medium, which kills both parent strains, the HGPRT$^-$ A9 cells, and the TK$^-$ 3T3-4C2 cells; (b) since 3T3-4C2 possess only telocentric chromosomes, while the L-cell derivative, A9, has accumulated 20 meta and submetacentric chromosomes, the latter serve as markers. In most of our hybrids, about 85% of the A9 markers are present, which correlates well with the total number of chromosomes retained; (c) starch gel electrophoresis of glucose phosphate isomerase (E. C. 5. 3. 1. 9) of the A9/3T3-4C2 hybrids demonstrates not only the presence of the isozyme specific for each parent but also the appearance of an intermediate heteropolymeric "hybrid" band.

The hybrid nature of the human/human cell cross, JEG-3/VA-2, is derived from the appearance of the Y chromosome, a marker for the JEG-3 line, together with the SV$_{40}$ T-antigen from the VA-2 line, indicating the presence of both parental genomes in the hybrid strains (63).

Similar to the human hybrids, the cross between the hamster cell lines BHK and OBP was made employing a half-selective system. The TK$^-$ BHK cells were eliminated by growth in HAT medium. No revertants to HAT insensitivity were found in six dishes each sown with 1-2 × 10^6 BHK cells. The OBP parent line produced very rapidly growing colonies with distinctive swirls of radially oriented groups of cells. After fusion and growth in HAT medium — and only in fusion plates containing both parents — slower-growing colonies appeared among the OBP parental colonies, which exhibited a tangled and irregular growth pattern unlike either parent.

Suppression of AHH Activity in Hybrid Cells

Exposure to the inducer, benz(a)anthracene, for 16 hr increases
AHH activity 10- to 30-fold in both BHK and OBP cells (Table 7).
However, BHK and OBP cells differ more than 20-fold in their basal
as well as induced level of AHH activity. In eight clones of OBP/BHK
hybrid cells, both the basal and induced levels of AHH activity are
apparently suppressed to that of the low activity parent.

The kinetics of AHH induction in OBP, BHK, and OBP/BHK cells
are shown in Fig. 17. The absolute amount of AHH activity in OBP
cells increases more rapidly and for a longer time than in BHK cells

TABLE 7

Aryl Hydrocarbon Hydroxylase in Hamster OBP and BHK
Cells and Their Hybrids (7)

| Cell type | AHH specific activity[a] | | Total chromosome number[c] |
	Basal	Induced[b]	
Experiment 1			
OBP	26 2	558 ± 13	46 (41–49)
BHK	<1 -	30 ± 5	40 (37–49)
OBP/BHK - 8	<1 -	7 ± 1	—
OBP/BHK - 9	<1 -	7 ± 1	81 (73–100)
OBP/BHK - 12	<1 -	11 ± 3	78 (72–81)
OBP/BHK - 14	<1 -	6 ± 1	74 (72–95)
OBP/BHK - 16	<1 -	11 ± 3	76 (74–77)
OBP/BHK - 17	< -	10 ± 1	118 (96–151)
Experiment 2			
OBP	19	1830	—
BHK	<3	71	—
OBP/BHK - 7	<3	18	72 (68–76)
OBP/BHK - 11	<3	49	76 (68–79)

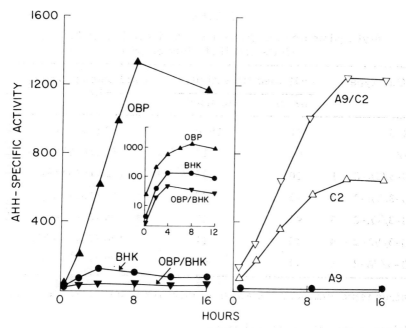

FIG. 17. Time course of induction of aryl hydrocarbon hydroxylase in hamster and mouse parental and hybrid cells. The concentration of benz(a)anthracene in the growth medium was 1.5 μg/ml for
the hamster cell lines, OBP, BHK, and their hybrid OBP/BHK, and
2.0 μg/ml for the mouse cell lines, 3T3-4C2 (= C2), A9, and their
hybrid A9/3T3-4C2 (= A9/C2). Inset presents data on the induction
time courses of the hamster cell lines on a semilogarithmic scale.
Points represent the average of duplicate plates. AHH specific
activity is given as 10^{-13} mol of alkali-extractable products formed
per mg of protein per 30 min (67).

(Fig. 17). However, as indicated by the semilogarithmic plot (inset
in Fig. 17), the increase in enzyme activity relative to the basal
level is similar in BHK and in OBP cells during the first few hours of
induction.

Suppression of basal and induced AHH activity was also observed
in hybrids of the two human cell lines, JEG-3 and VA-2 (Table 8).
JEG-3 exhibits a relatively high basal hydroxylase activity that is
induced more than 30-fold in the presence of benz(a)anthracene. In
the other parental cell, VA-2, no basal hydroxylase activity was

TABLE 8

Aryl Hydrocarbon Hydroxylase Activity in Human Parental
Cells and Their Hybrids (67)

Cell type	AHH specific activity[a]		Total chromosome[b] number
	Basal	Induced	
JEG-3	41	1500	69 (63-73)
VA-2	<5	13	77 (68-93)
JEG-3/VA-2 - 1	10	53	113 (106-119)
JEG-3/VA-2 - 2	<5	47	116 (106-126)
JEG-3/VA-2 - 3	<5	13	95 (82-104)
JEG-3/VA-2 - 4	<5	11	124 (111 - 132)
JEG-3/VA-2 - 5	<7	<7	127 (119-136)

[a]Values represent means of enzyme activities in duplicate cultures.

[b] Values represent means and ranges.

[c] Cultures were exposed to medium containing 3 μg/ml BA for 16 hr.
Serum concentration was 20% in BA- and control medium.

detectable and the induced level, although significantly increased,
was still very low. One of the JEG-3/VA-2 hybrid clones had a low
basal activity; in the others, enzyme activities were below the level
of detectability. Induced levels in the hybrids were variable but were
generally similar to the low levels found in VA-2 cells. Thus, our
results indicate that AHH activity in the hybrids OBP/BHK and JEG-3/
VA-2 more closely resembles the low activity parent.

Enhancement of AHH Activity in Hybrid Cells

Tables 9 and 10 show AHH activity in the mouse cells, 3T3-4C2
and A9, and in the hybrid strains derived from these parents. Basal
and induced AHH activities of 3T3-4C2 were relatively high and similar to those described above for OBP. Enzyme activity of 3T3-4C2
grown in medium containing BrdU (30 μg/ml) does not differ from
activity of 3T3-4C2 propagated in BrdU-free medium. No AHH activity was detectable in untreated A9 cells exposed to the inducer.
This lack of enzyme activity was found whether or not 8-azaguanine
(3 μg/ml) was in the growth medium. In contrast to the hybrids

TABLE 9

Aryl Hydrocarbon Hydroxylase Activity and Karyotype of Mouse
3T3-4C2 and A9 Cells and Their Hybrids (67)

Cell type	AHH specific activity[a]		Number of chromosomes[c]		
	Basal	Induced[b]	Total		Meta- and submetacentric
3T3-4C2 —	97	750	64	(61-68)	0	—
3T3-4C2 (BrdU)[d]	81	860	—		—	—
A9	<1	<1	56	(54-58)	20	(18-22)
A9 (8-azaguanine)	<1	<1	—		—	—
Hybrids			Expected: 120	(115-126)	20	(18-22)
			Observed:			
A9/3T3-4C2 Clone 2	67	1540	69	(58-94)	13	(9-19)
A9/3T3-4C2 Clone 5	310	2170	103	(83-112)	16	(12-22)
A9/3T3-4C2 Clone 3	410	3310	97	(85-116)	17	(11-20)
A9/3T3-4C2 Clone 7	730	3890	111	(89-118)	17	(12-21)
A9/3T3-4C2 Clone 9	710	4800	105	(91-113)	18	(15-20)

[a] For A9 cells as much as 2 mg of cellular protein was used, and for some determinations the incubation time was extended to 60 min. Specific activity is given as 10^{-3} moles of alkali extractable products formed/mg protein/30 min.

[b] Cultures were exposed to BA-containing medium (1.5 μg/ml for 16 hr).

[c] Chromosome numbers were analyzed on 20 metaphase plates. Values represent mean and ranges.

[d] Cultures were kept in media containing BrdU (30 μg/ml) and 8-azaguanine (3 μg/ml), respectively, prior to the experiment.

TABLE 10

Aryl Hydrocarbon Hydroxylase Induction in Mouse
3T3-4C2 and A9 Cells and Their Hybrids (67)

Cell type	AHH specific activity[a]		
	Basal	Induced[a]	
		6 hr	16 hr
Experiment 1			
3T3-4C2	41	420	610
A9	< 1	< 1	< 1
A9/3T3-4C2 - 4	94	800	1660
A9/3T3-4C2 - 6	212	1090	1830
A9/3T3-4C2 - 8	144	920	2120
A9/3T3-4C2 - 10	150	830	1870
Experiment 2			
3T3-4C2	45	190	424
A9/3T3-4C2 - 1	391	760	1950
A9/3T3-4C2 - 5	200	610	1250
Experiment 3			
3T3-4C2	43		779
A9	< 1		< 1
3T3-4C2 + A9	30		478

[a] Conditions as described under Table 9.

[b] 3T3-4C2 cells, A9 cells, or an equal mixture of these cell lines
were plated at a density of 10^6 cells/dish. AHH activity was determined after 5 days' growth.

described earlier, basal and inducer AHH activity in A9/3T3-4C2
hybrids was similar or higher than in the high parent, 3T3-4C2.
Clone 2 showed only a small increase in induced enzyme activity
above the parental 3T3-4C2 cells. This finding may be related to
the more extensive loss of chromosomes from this particular clone
(Table 9). As shown in Fig. 17, the time courses of induction of
3T3-4C2 and A9/3T3-4C2 were similar. The enzyme activity increases for about 12 hr and then levels off. The somewhat longer

TABLE 11

Aryl Hydrocarbon Hydroxylase Activity of in vitro
Mixtures of Cell Homogenates[a] (67)

Cell Type	AHH activity	
	Basal	Induced[b]
(a) BHK	< 1. 0	8. 0
OBP	5. 9	276. 0
BHK + OBP	3. 8 (3. 0)[c]	134. 3 (142. 0)[c]
(b) A9	< 1. 0	< 1. 0
3T3-4C	27. 0	251. 0
A9 + 3T3-4C2	16. 0 (13. 5)[c]	148. 0 (125. 5)[c]

[a] Approximately equal amounts of homogenates of BHK and OBP cells
(a) and of 3T3-4C2 and A9 cells (b) were mixed. The mixtures
were assayed for AHH activity at concentrations of cellular
protein similar to those of unmixed homogenates. Numbers
represent averages of duplicate determinations on cellular
material derived from three pooled plates. Other conditions as
in Materials and Methods.

[b] Cultures were exposed to growth medium containing benz(a)-
anthracene (1. 5 μg/ml) for 16 hr.

[c] Numbers in parentheses give averages calculated from the observed
AHH activities in unmixed homogenates.

duration of induction in these cells compared with the results shown
in Fig. 17 might be due to the higher concentration of inducer [benz-
(a)anthracene] used in this experiment.

AHH activities in A9 and 3T3-4C2 cells that were cocultivated
for five days correspond closely with activities expected from the
cell lines growing separately (Table 11). Similarly, in mixtures of
homogenates of A9 and 3T3-4C2 cells, AHH activities were almost
identical to the calculated averages of the enzyme activities in the
unmixed homogenates (Table 11). Similar results were obtained with
OBP and BHK cells (Table 11). These results suggest that the changes
in hydroxylase activity observed in the hybrids are dependent on the
fusion of cells and are not due simply to the presence of enzyme
effectors in the parental cell.

The studies show that microsomal aryl hydrocarbon hydroxylase in hybrids of parental cells differing widely in basal as well as induced activity can behave in different ways: Enzyme activity may be suppressed, as found in the BHK/OBP and JEG-3 VA-2 hybrids, and it may be greater than the level of the more active parent, as seen in the A9/3T3-4C2 hybrids. We do not know the reasons for this different behavior. The mouse hybrids differ from the others in that one parent, A9, has no detectable hydroxylase activity. It is possible that AHH activity is present in A9 cells but is too low to be detected by our assay method. It is also possible that some regulatory or structural genes of the enzyme complex are missing or defective in this cell.

The increase in basal and induced levels of enzyme activity in the A9/3T3-4C2 hybrids may be caused by one or more of a number of factors, such as potential genetic heterogeneity of the parental cells, loss of regulatory genes, activation of the L-cell genome, or complementation. An increase in activity due to some form of complementation seems likely since AHH is a membrane bound, multi-component enzyme complex. Thus, if A9 cells were defective in some of the constituents of the enzyme system but competent in other, possibly rate-limiting components in 3T3-4C2, then the addition of these elements in the hybrid could result in an enhanced enzyme activity. Complementation might also occur if the hybrid contained a larger amount of endoplasmic reticulum, which might be a limiting factor for the expression of microsomal enzymes.

Our results on the suppression of AHH activity in the OBP/BHK and JEG-3/VA-2 hybrids are similar to the observations on glycerol-3-phosphate dehydrogenase (64) and tyrosine aminotransferase (65) in hybrids of inducible and noninducible parent cells. These are compatible with the notion that a step in the process of AHH induction and formation may be under negative control. In contrast to glycerol-3-phosphate dehydrogenase and tyrosine aminotransferase (64, 65), basal and induced levels of AHH in hybrids were suppressed to a similar extent. Likewise, in the A9/3T3-4C2 hybrids baseline activity and inducibility increased coordinately. These data suggest a closely coupled control mechanism for the inducibility and the basal level of AHH activity.

Further analysis of hybrid cells may elucidate the genetic regulation of the components of this important enzyme complex and may permit the construction of hybrid cells with properties uniquely suited for the study of carcinogen, xenobiotic, and drug metabolism as well as their modes of action.

REFERENCES

1. H. V. Gelboin, N. Kinoshita, and F. J. Wiebel, Fed. Proc. 31, Fed. Amer. Soc. Exptl. Biol., 1298 (1972).
2. A. H. Conney and J. J. Burns, Science, 178, 576 (1972).
3. A. H. Conney and H. V. Gelboin, The Handbook of Drug-Induced Diseases, Chapter 10, Excerpta Medica Foundation, Amsterdam, 1970.
4. H. V. Gelboin, Advances in Cancer Research, Academic, New York, 1967.
5. J. R. Gillette, Progr. Drug Res., 6, 11 (1963).
6. A. H. Conney, E. C. Miller, and J. A. Miller, J. Biol. Chem., 228, 753 (1957).
7. L. W. Wattenberg and J. L. Leong, J. Histochem. Cytochem., 10, 412 (1962).
8. H. V. Gelboin and N. Blackburn, Cancer Res., 24, 356 (1964).
9. D. W. Nebert and H. V. Gelboin, Arch. Biochem. Biophys., 134, 76 (1969).
10. D. W. Nebert, J. Winker, and H. V. Gelboin, Cancer Res., 29, 1763 (1969).
11. J. P. Whitlock, H. L. Cooper, and H. V. Gelboin, Science, 177, 618 (1972).
12. F. J. Wiebel, J. C. Leutz, L. Diamond, and H. V. Gelboin, Arch. Biochem. Biophys., 144, 78 (1971).
13. H. V. Gelboin, Cancer Res., 29, 1272 (1969).
14. P. O. Grover and P. Sims, Biochem. J., 110, 159 (1968).
15. H. V. Gelboin, E. Huberman, and L. Sachs, Proc. Nat. Acad. Sci., 64, 1188 (1969).
16. L. Diamond and H. V. Gelboin, Science, 166, 1023 (1969).
17. N. Kinoshita and H. V. Gelboin, Proc. Nat. Acad. Sci., 69, 824 (1972).
18. E. Boyland and B. Green, Brit. J. Cancer, 16, 507 (1962).
19. A. M. Liquori, B. DeLerma, F. Ascoli, C. Botre, and M. Trasciatti, J. Mol. Biol., 5, 521 (1962).
20. P. Ts'o and P. Lu, Proc. Nat. Acad. Sci., 51, 17 (1964).
21. P. Brookes and P. D. Lawley, Nature, 202, 781 (1964).
22. C. Heidelberger and M. G. Moldenhauer, Cancer Res., 16, 442 (1956).
23. E. C. Miller, Cancer Res., 11, 100 (1951).
24. A. Dipple, P. D. Lawley, and P. Brookes, Europ. J. Cancer, 4, 493 (1968).
25. M. Wilk and W. Girke, Physicochemical Mechanisms of Carcinogenesis (E. D. Bergmann and B. Pullman, eds.), Israel Academy of Sciences and Humanities, Jerusalem, 1969, pp. 91-105.

26. E. Boyland, Symp. Biochem. Soc., 5, 50 (1950).
27. D. M. Jerina, J. W. Daly, B. Witkop, P. Zaltzman-Nirenberg, and S. Udenfriend, Biochemistry, 9, 147 (1970).
28. N. Nagata et al, Chapter 2, this volume.
29. P. O. P. Ts'o et al., Chapter 3, this volume.
30. C. Heidelberger, Cellular Comp. Physiol., 64, 129 (1964).
31. D. W. Nebert and H. V. Gelboin, J. Biol. Chem., 243, 6250 (1968).
32. W. G. Clark and T. A. Geissman, J. Pharmacol. Exptl. Therap., 95, 363 (1949).
33. R. H. Wilson and F. DeEds, J. Pharmacol. Exptl. Therap., 95, 399 (1949).
34. L. W. Wattenberg and J. L. Leong, Cancer Res., 30, 1922 (1970).
35. R. P. Perry, Proc. Nat. Acad. Sci., 48, 2179 (1962).
36. W. K. Roberts and J. F. E. Newman, J. Mol. Biol., 20, 63 (1966).
37. S. Penman, C. Vesco, and M. Penman, J. Mol. Biol., 34, 49 (1968).
38. H. L. Ennis, Mol. Pharmacol., 2, 543 (1966).
39. M. Willems, M. Penman, and S. Penman, J. Cell Biol., 41, 177 (1969).
40. M. Muramatsu, N. Shimada, and T. Higashinakagawa, J. Mol. Biol., 53, 91 (1970).
41. S. Penman, J. Mol. Biol., 17, 117 (1966).
42. H. Harris, Nature, 202, 1301 (1964).
43. G. A. Stewart and E. Farber, J. Biol. Chem., 243, 4479 (1968).
44. D. W. Nebert and H. V. Gelboin, J. Biol. Chem., 245, 160 (1970).
45. H. V. Gelboin and F. J. Wiebel, Ann N. Y. Acad. Sci., 179, 529 (1971).
46. R. A. Bucknall and S. B. Carter, Nature, 213, 1099 (1967).
47. J. J. Skehel, A. J. Hay, D. C. Burke, and L. N. Cartwright, Biochim. Biophys. Acta, 142, 430 (1967).
48. F. J. Wiebel and H. V. Gelboin, unpublished results.
49. A. Wacker, H. Delweg, and D. Weinblum, Naturwissenschaften, 47, 477 (1960).
50. F. J. Wiebel, E. J. Matthews, and H. V. Gelboin, Latin American Symposium, Protein Synthesis and Nucleic Acids, La Plata, Argentina, 1972.
51. B. R. McAuslan, Virology, 21, 383 (1963).
52. H. C. Pitot, C. Peraino, C. Lamar, Jr, and A. L. Kennan, Proc. Nat. Acad. Sci., 54, 845 (1965).
53. G. M. Tomkins, E. B. Thompson, S. Hayashi, T. Gelehrter, D. Granner, and B. Peterkofsky, Cold Spring Harbor Symp. Quant. Biol., 31, 349 (1966).
54. B. W. O'Malley, Biochemistry, 6, 2546 (1967).
55. A. A. Moscona, M. H. Moscona, and N. Saenz, Proc. Nat. Acad. Sci., 61, 160 (1968).

56. J. Laszlo, D. S. Miller, K. S. McCarty, and P. Hochstein, Science, 51, 1007 (1966).
57. G. R. Honig and M. Rabinovitz, J. Biol. Chem., 241, 1681 (1966).
58. L. R. Younger, R. Salomon, R. W. Wilson, A. C. Peacock, and H. V. Gelboin, Mol. Pharmacol., 4, 452 (1972).
59. T. D. Gelehrter and G. M. Tomkins, J. Mol. Biol., 29, 59 (1967).
60. R. M. Franklin, Biochim. Biophys. Acta, 72, 555 (1963).
61. E. Zylber, C. Vesco, and S. Penman, J. Mol. Biol., 44, 195 (1969).
62. R. Leibowitz, J. Cell Biol., 51, 116 (1971).
63. P. O. Kohler, H. J. Ruder, and H. G. Coon, in preparation.
64. R. L. Davidson and P. Benda, Proc. Nat. Acad. Sci., 67, 1870 (1970).
65. J. A. Schneider and M. C. Weiss, Proc. Nat. Acad. Sci., 68, 127 (1971).
66. L. D. Garren, R. R. Howell, G. M. Tomkins, and R. M. Cocco, Proc. Nat. Acad. Sci., 52, 1121 (1964).
67. F. J. Wiebel, H. V. Gelboin, and H. V. Coon, Proc. Nat. Acad. Sci., 69, 3580 (1972).
68. F. J. Wiebel, E. J. Matthews, and H. V. Gelboin, J. Biol. Chem., 247, 4711 (1972).

Chapter 15

FACTORS INFLUENCING BENZO(a)PYRENE METABOLISM
IN ANIMALS AND MAN

A. H. Conney

Department of Biochemistry and Drug Metabolism
Hoffmann-La Roche Inc.
Nutley, New Jersey

People are exposed to polycyclic hydrocarbons, nitrosamines, aflatoxins, and many other chemical carcinogens in their environment, and factors that inhibit or stimulate the metabolism of these substances may influence the formation of human cancers. Enzymes that N-demethylate aminoazo dyes, hydroxylate benzo(a)pyrene (BP), and N-demethylate dimethylnitrosamine are present in human liver (1, 2), and an enzyme that hydroxylates BP is present in human skin (3-5), placenta (6-8), and in lymphocytes (9). The presence of carcinogen-metabolizing enzymes in human tissues points out a need to study the factors that influence the activity of these enzymes in man and to determine the relationship between the levels of carcinogen-metabolizing enzymes and the induction of cancer in humans that are exposed to chemical carcinogens. The present report describes some of our studies on factors influencing the metabolism of BP in animals and in man.

STIMULATION OF BENZO(a)PYRENE METABOLISM IN THE RAT

More than 15 years ago, studies in the laboratory of J.A. and E.C. Miller demonstrated that the administration to rats of BP or other polycyclic hydrocarbons induced the synthesis of an enzyme system in liver microsomes that hydroxylated BP (Fig. 1) (10). The induction of BP-hydroxylase occurred not only in the liver, but also in several other organs of the rat, such as the gastrointestinal tract, lung, kidney, skin and placenta (7, 11-15). The increased level of BP-hydroxylase activity in rats was reflected in vivo by enhanced metabolism of BP, decreased blood and tissue concentrations of this carcinogen, and enhanced biliary excretion of its metabolites (16-18).

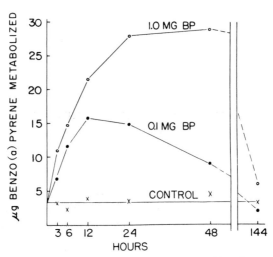

FIG. 1. The metabolism of benzo(a)pyrene (BP) by rat livers
obtained at various times after a single intraperitoneal injection of
BP. Fifty milligrams of liver was added per flask; the incubation
time was 12 min. Each value represents the average from two livers
(10).

3-Methylcholanthrene, 7,12-dimethylbenz(a)anthracene, and BP are
potent stimulators of hepatic BP-hydroxylase activity, and treatment
of rats with these compounds enhanced the metabolism of intraven-
ously administered [^{3}H]BP and decreased the fat concentration of this
hydrocarbon (Table 1). Pretreatment of rats with pyrene or anthracene
had little or no stimulatory effect on hepatic microsomal hydroxylase
activity or on the in vivo metabolism of [^{3}H]BP. Pretreatment of rats
with phenobarbital, a compound with a small stimulatory effect on
hepatic BP-hydroxylase activity, did not stimulate the in vivo
metabolism of [^{3}H]BP. Since the primary route for the elimination of
BP metabolites in rats is excretion into the bile, we investigated the
effects of enzyme inducers on the biliary excretion of BP metabolites.
Pretreatment of rats with BP for two days prior to the intravenous
injection of [^{14}C]BP stimulated the excretion of metabolites of [^{14}C]BP
into the bile (Figs. 2 and 3) (17). Seven minutes after the intravenous
injection of 300 μg of [^{14}C]BP, the concentration of radioactive BP
metabolites in the bile of pretreated rats was about 20-fold higher
than the concentration of [^{14}C]BP metabolites in the bile of control
rats (Fig. 3). The concentration of radioactive BP metabolites in the
bile of control rats reached a maximum 45 min after the injection of
[^{14}C]BP and then decreased slowly, with an initial $t\frac{1}{2}$ of about 90
min. The concentration of radioactive BP metabolites in the bile of

TABLE 1

Effect of Pretreatment of Rats with Polycyclic Hydrocarbons
or Phenobarbital on the Metabolism of Tritiated Benzo(a)pyrene (BP)[a]

Experiment	Pretreatment	Concentration of [³H]BP in:	
		Blood, ng/ml	Fat, ng/g
1	Control	2. 6 ± 0. 2	21. 6 ± 6. 6
	BP	0. 4 ± 0. 1	4. 1 ± 0. 8
2	Control	2. 9 ± 0. 3	15. 0 ± 3. 5
	MC	0. 5 ± 0. 0	4. 3 ± 0. 7
	DMBA	0. 7 ± 0. 1	5. 4 ± 0. 6
	Pyrene	2. 5 ± 0. 1	18. 9 ± 0. 7
	Anthracene	2. 3 ± 0. 3	16. 9 ± 2. 5
3	Control	2. 5 ± 0. 2	14. 4 ± 1. 4
	Phenobarbital	2. 3 ± 0. 2	18. 1 ± 1. 8

[a] Female rats weighing 175 to 185 g were treated orally with 20 mg/kg
of BP once daily for two days. An equimolar amount of MC, DMBA,
pyrene, or anthracene was administered in Experiment 2. In Experiment 3, rats were given i. p. injections of 37 mg/kg of sodium
phenobarbital twice daily for four days. The day after the last dose
of polycyclic hydrocarbon or phenobarbital, rats were given i. v.
injections of 10 µg of [³H]BP, and the animals were killed 45 min
later. The data represent the mean ± S. E. from three to six values
(16).

pretreated rats reached a maximum 15 min after the injection and then
decreased, with an initial $t_{\frac{1}{2}}$ of about 27 min. The $t_{\frac{1}{2}}$ for the disappearance of radioactive metabolites in bile increased with time and
was about 2 hr in control and pretreated rats 3 hr after the injection
of [¹⁴C]BP.

The stimulatory effect of BP on its own metabolism is also illustrated by the decreased tissue concentration of this compound that
occurs when it is administered chronically. At 24 hr after a single
oral dose of 1 mg of [³H]BP to adult rats, the concentration of this
hydrocarbon in fat was 249 ng/gm, whereas 24 hr after seven daily
doses of [³H]BP its concentration in fat was only 24 ng/gm (16).

Inhibitors of microsomal enzymatic activity, such as carbon
tetrachloride, β-diethylaminoethyl diphenylpropylacetate (SKF 525-A),
and the pesticide synergist, piperonyl butoxide, inhibited the in vivo

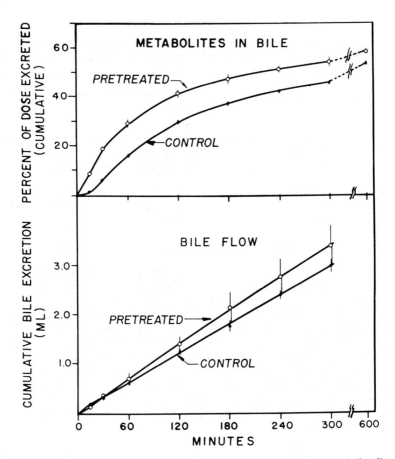

FIG. 2. Effect of benzo(a)pyrene (BP) pretreatment on bile flow
and the cumulative excretion of [^{14}C]BP metabolites in the bile of rats
given i. v. injections of 300 μg of [^{14}C]BP. Rats were treated orally
with 20 mg/kg of BP once daily for two days. The following day,
300 μg of [8, 9-^{14}C]benzo(a)pyrene was injected i. v., and radioactivity
in the bile was quantified. All of the radioactivity excreted represented BP metabolites. Each value represents the average and S. E.
from three rats (17).

metabolism of BP and potentiated the acute toxicity of this polycyclic
hydrocarbon in rodents (18-21). Studies to determine the effects of
piperonyl butoxide on microsomal enzymatic function in man revealed
that the administration of a high dose — relative to possible human
exposure during its use as a pesticide synergist — did not influence
the metabolism of antipyrine (22). Interestingly, nickel carbonyl

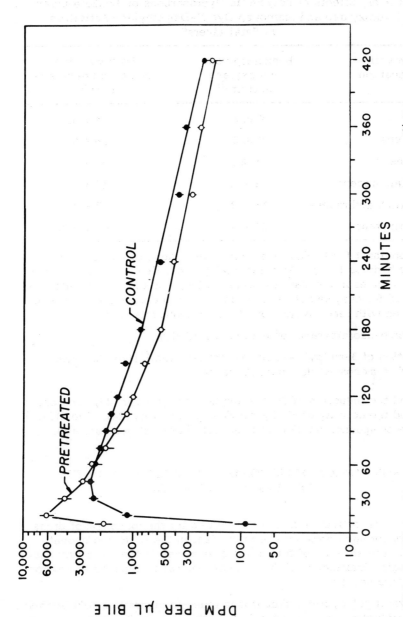

FIG. 3.   Effect of benzo(a)pyrene (BP) pretreatment on the concentration of [^{14}C]BP metabolites in the bile of rats given i.v. injections of 300 μg of [^{14}C]BP.   Rats were treated orally with 20 mg/kg of BP once daily for two days. The following day, 300 μg of [8, 9-^{14}C]benzo(a)pyrene was injected i.v., and radioactivity in the bile was quantified.   Each value represents the average and S.E. from the three rats described in Fig. 2 (17).

TABLE 2

Stimulatory Effects of Polycyclic Hydrocarbons on Benzo(a)pyrene
Hydroxylase and Aminoazo Dye N-Demethylase Activities
in Fetal Livers[a]

Polycyclic hydrocarbon	Benzo(a)pyrene hydroxylase activity[b]	Aminoazo dye N-demethylase activity[c]
Control	< 0. 2	13 ± 0. 1
Anthracene	< 0. 2	16 ± 0. 6
Chrysene	6 ± 1	30 ± 0. 7
Benz(a)anthracene	12 ± 2	29 ± 5. 0
Dibenz(a, h)anthracene	15 ± 2	59 ± 4. 0
Benzo(a)pyrene	20 ± 4	45 ± 5. 0

[a] Rats pregnant for 19 days were given injections of 60 mg of polycyclic hydrocarbon per kilogram orally and killed 24 hr later. Fetal
livers from each pregnant rat were pooled, and the homogenate was
assayed for enzyme activity. Each value represents the mean ± S. E.
obtained with fetal livers from three pregnant rats (61).

[b] Hydroxybenzo(a)pyrene formed (μg/g liver/hr).

[c] Formation of 3-methyl-4-aminoazobenzene (μg/g liver/hr) from 3-
methyl-4-monomethylaminoazobenzene.

inhibited the induction of BP-hydroxylase in the liver (23), and ozone
inhibited the activity of BP-hydroxylase in the lung (24). The effects
of these compounds on BP carcinogenesis have not been studied.

STIMULATION OF BENZO(a)PYRENE METABOLISM IN THE
FETUS AND PREGNANT RAT

Enzymes in liver microsomes required for the oxidation of drugs
and other foreign compounds are deficient in the fetus and neonate
(25-27). The absence of this group of enzymes in the fetus may have
toxicologic significance if the pregnant animal is exposed to environmental carcinogens.

Several polycyclic hydrocarbons found in cigarette smoke increase
the hydroxylation of BP and the N-demethylation of 3-methyl-4-mono-
methylaminoazobenzene (3-methyl-MAB) by fetal liver (Table 2).

TABLE 3

Effects of Various Doses of Benzo(a)pyrene (BP) on BP Hydroxylase
Activity in Placenta and in Maternal and Fetal Livers[a]

Daily dose of BP, mg/kg	BP hydroxylase activity[b]		
	Maternal liver	Placenta	Fetal liver
0	35 ± 6	< 0. 2	< 0. 2
0. 1	35 ± 6	< 0. 2	< 0. 2
0. 5	71 ± 10	0. 4 ± 0. 0	< 0. 2
1. 0	93 ± 21	1. 7 ± 0. 1	< 0. 2
10. 0	1841 ± 105	3. 5 ± 0. 2	28 ± 9
20. 0	1812 ± 141	4. 5 ± 0. 3	52 ± 17
80. 0	2187 ± 189	5. 0 ± 2. 0	85 ± 20

[a] Rats pregnant for 16 days were given oral injections, for three days,
of various doses of BP dissolved in dimethyl sulfoxide. Control rats
received only dimethyl sulfoxide. The rats were killed 24 hr after
the last dose. Enzyme activity was determined for maternal liver,
pooled placentas, and pooled livers of fetuses from each rat. The
values indicate the mean ± S. E. from four pregnant rats (61).

Dibenz(a, h)anthracene and BP were the most potent stimulators tested,
but benz(a)anthracene and chrysene also exerted strong enzyme-
inducing effects. Administration of as little as 0. 5 to 1. 0 mg of BP
per kilogram once daily for three days increased BP-hydroxylase activity in placenta and maternal liver (Table 3), but detectable hydroxylase
activity in fetal liver was observed only after the dose of BP had been
increased to 10 mg/kg.

Studies were initiated to determine whether enzyme induction
enhanced the in vivo metabolism of BP in pregnant rats and whether
pretreatment with an enzyme inducer prior to administration of [^{3}H]BP
could decrease the concentration of this carcinogen in the fetus. Rats
pregnant for 16 days were given oral injections of 20 mg of nonradioactive BP per kilogram for three days. Twenty-four hours after the last
dose, the rats were given 20 mg of [^{3}H]BP per kilogram orally and killed
2 hr later. The concentrations of [^{3}H]BP in the fetus, placenta, and
maternal lung were markedly lower, and the concentrations of metabolites of [^{3}H]BP higher if pregnant animals had been pretreated with BP.
Indeed, enzyme induction increased the ratios of the concentrations
of [^{3}H]BP metabolites to those of [^{3}H]BP by 84-, 19-, and 185-fold in
the fetus, placenta, and maternal lung, respectively (Table 4).

TABLE 4

Effect of Enzyme Induction in Pregnant Rats
on the Metabolism of [³H]BP In Vivo[a]

Tissue	Pretreatment	[³H]BP, ng/g	[³H]BP metabolites, ng equivalents/g	Ratio of [³H]BP metabolites to [³H]BP
Fetus	Control	657 ± 115	525 ± 49	0.80
	BP	11 ± 2	742 ± 113	67
Placenta	Control	1994 ± 266	364 ± 78	0.18
	BP	253 ± 29	851 ± 138	3.4
Maternal lung	Control	4129 ± 652	93 ± 47	0.02
	BP	353 ± 36	1315 ± 216	3.7

[a] Rats pregnant for 16 days were given oral injections of 20 mg of nonradioactive benzo(a)pyrene (BP) per kilogram once daily for three days. Twenty-four hours after the last dose, the rats were given an oral dose of 20 mg of [³H]BP per kilogram and were killed two hours later. The tissue concentrations of unchanged [³H]BP and its radioactive metabolites were measured in each of four rats. Each value represents the mean ± S.E. (61).

EFFECT OF ENZYME INDUCTION ON CHEMICAL CARCINOGENESIS IN ANIMALS

Treatment of rodents with inducers of microsomal hydroxylases provided protection from the carcinogenic effects of BP (28), 7,12-dimethylbenz(a)anthracene (29-33), N-2-fluorenylacetamide (34), 4-dimethylaminostilbene (35), urethane (36), aflatoxin (37), diethylnitrosamine (38), and aminoazo dyes (34, 39, 40). Although these studies suggest that the induction of hydroxylating enzymes inhibits the formation of cancer by several unrelated carcinogens, further work is required to evaluate the effects of enzyme induction on chemical carcinogenesis under varying conditions. These studies are important because of observations indicating that metabolites of polycyclic hydrocarbons and other carcinogens may account for their carcinogenicity (41-43). Reactive intermediates — perhaps epoxides — capable of interacting with DNA or other macromolecules are formed during the aromatic hydroxylation of polycyclic hydrocarbons (44-46), and hydroxylated metabolites of BP are more cytotoxic than BP in tissue culture. In agreement with these observations, BP was more toxic to cells that possessed high BP-hydroxylase activity than to cells with low enzymatic activity (41, 47-50).

BENZO(a)PYRENE METABOLISM IN MAN

Benzo(a)pyrene Metabolism by Human Liver

Biopsy samples of human liver were obtained during abdominal surgery, and the BP-hydroxylase activities of the liver homogenates were measured (1). Benzo(a)pyrene hydroxylation by human liver was proportional to the amount of tissue in the range from 0.5 to 10 mg of wet weight liver, and a twofold variation in hepatic BP-hydroxylase activity was observed in the four subjects studied (Fig. 4). Ninety percent of the BP-hydroxylase activity was in the microsomal fraction of liver homogenate. High enzymatic activity was observed when BP was incubated with human liver microsomes and NADPH, whereas low activity was found when NADH was substituted for NADPH.

Benzo(a)pyrene Metabolism by Human Placenta

Because the results of animal studies suggested that high levels of microsomal hydroxylase activity inhibited the carcinogenicity of several chemical carcinogens, we initiated studies to determine the levels of carcinogen-metabolizing enzymes in the human population and to determine whether chronic exposure of people to environmental inducers such as polycyclic hydrocarbons would increase the level of these enzymes. Since many polycyclic hydrocarbons are present in cigarette smoke, we studied the effect of cigarette smoking on BP-hydroxylase activity in the placenta — a readily obtainable human tissue (Table 5) (6, 7). Among nonsmokers, a trace of enzymatic activity was found in only two; no activity was found in the rest. In contrast, in women who smoked 10-40 cigarettes a day, BP-hydroxylase was found in all of the placentas obtained. A similar stimulatory effect of cigarette smoking on BP-hydroxylase activity in human placenta was observed by Nebert and his associates (8). Among the subjects in our study who smoked 15-20 cigarettes daily, placental BP-hydroxylase activity varied more than 70-fold (Table 6). This variability in the induction of BP-hydroxylase activity in cigarette smokers may be the reason some people develop cancer when exposed to cigarette smoke or other carcinogens whereas others do not.

Since the administration of polycyclic aromatic hydrocarbons to rats induced aminoazo dye N-demethylase activity in nonhepatic tissues (51), we studied the oxidative N-demethylation of

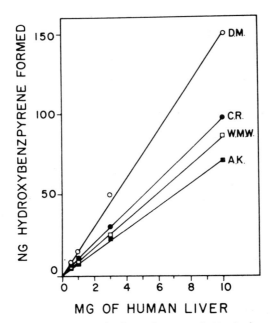

FIG. 4. Benzo(a)pyrene hydroxylase activity in human liver. Various amounts of human liver homogenate were incubated for 15 min with benzo(a)pyrene and a NADPH-generating system (1).

TABLE 5

Effect of Cigarette Smoking on Benzo(a)pyrene Hydroxylase Activity in Human Placenta[a]

Group	N	Hydroxybenzo(a)pyrene formed by placenta, ng/gm/hr
Nonsmokers	30	< 100
Nonsmokers	2	174 (128–220)
Smokers	37	5270 (240–23,200)

[a] Homogenate equivalent to 100 mg of placenta was incubated with 50 μg of benzo(a)pyrene and an NADPH-generating system for 15 min. The cigarette smokers consumed 10–40 cigarettes daily during pregnancy. The average enzyme activity and range are given (7, 62).

3-methyl-4-monomethylaminoazobenzene to 3-methyl-4-aminoazo-benzene by human placentas from smokers and nonsmokers (7). Little or no aminoazo dye N-demethylase activity was found in placentas

TABLE 6

Variability in the Induction of Benzo(a)pyrene
Hydroxylase Activity in Human Placenta[a]

Subject	Hydroxybenzo(a)pyrene formed by placenta, ng/gm/hr
L. B.	240
G. A.	260
P. C.	547
C. G.	643
A. T.	1, 269
J. K.	1, 317
L. C.	1, 860
C. J.	4, 289
E. R.	4, 390
D. B.	5, 267
D. A.	15, 181
H. J.	16, 524
M. N.	17, 100

[a] All subjects in this study were Caucasians, and all smoked 15-20 cigarettes daily during pregnancy. Variability in benzo(a)pyrene hydroxylase activity was not related to medication taken during or prior to delivery (7, 62).

of nonsmokers, but enzyme activity was found in all of the placentas obtained from cigarette smokers (Table 7).

We determined the effects of cigarette smoke on the activity of BP-hydroxylase in lung and in several other tissues of the pregnant rat. Cigarette smoke stimulated BP-hydroxylase activity in the lung, placenta, intestine, and maternal liver (Table 8) (52). Increased activity was also present in fetal liver, indicating that enzyme inducers in cigarette smoke pass the placenta and reach the fetus.

Several polycyclic aromatic hydrocarbons that are present in cigarette smoke were tested as possible inducers of BP-hydroxylase activity in rat placenta. An oral dose of 20 mg/kg of BP, benz(a)-anthracene, dibenz(a, h)anthracene, 3, 4-benzofluorene, anthracene, pyrene, fluoranthene, perylene, or phenanthrene was administered to

364

A. H. CONNEY

TABLE 7

Effect of Cigarette Smoking on Aminoazo Dye
N-Demethylase Activity in Human Placenta[a]

Subjects	Number of subjects	3-Methyl-AB formed, μg/g/hr
Nonsmokers	17	< 1
Smokers	17	6 (1-21)

[a] Homogenate equivalent to 400 mg of placenta was incubated with
150 μg of 3-methyl-4-monomethylaminoazobenzene for 30 min in
the presence of a NADPH-generating system. Formation of 3-methyl-
4-aminoazobenzene (3-methyl-AB) was measured. The cigarette
smokers consumed 10-40 cigarettes daily during pregnancy. The
average N-demethylase activity and range are given (7).

TABLE 8

Effect of Cigarette Smoke on Benzo(a)pyrene Hydroxylase
Activity in Various Organs from Pregnant Rats[a]

Organ	Hydroxybenzo(a)pyrene formed, ng/gm/hour		Increase in enzyme activity, %
	Control	Smoke exposed	
Lung	584 ± 116	7,644 ± 1,108	1,200
Placenta	136 ± 28	676 ± 60	400
Intestine	9,396 ± 2,024	20,368 ± 5,956	120
Maternal liver	40,988 ± 632	91,276 ± 5,852	120
Fetal liver	484 ± 72	1,112 ± 104	130

[a] Rats pregnant for 17 days and weighing 225-250 g were placed in a
chamber and exposed to cigarette smoke for 5 hr each day for three
days, with a 1-hr rest period between each hourly exposure. Various
organs were examined for benzo(a)pyrene hydroxylase activity. Each
value represents the mean ± S.E. (52).

rats pregnant for 18 days, and BP-hydroxylase activity in the placenta
was measured 24 hr later. All of the polycyclic hydrocarbons tested
induced BP-hydroxylase activity (Table 9), and benz(a)anthracene
was the most potent inducer. The oral administration of as little as
0.1-0.5 mg/kg of BP to rats was sufficient to stimulate BP-hydroxylase
activity in the placenta (7). In contrast to the results of studies with

TABLE 9

Effect of Polycyclic Hydrocarbons Present in Cigarette Smoke
on Benzo(a)pyrene Hydroxylase Activity in Rat Placenta[a]

Polycyclic hydrocarbon administered	Hydroxybenzo(a)pyrene formed, ng/g/hr
Control	218 ± 81
Benz(a)anthracene	4034 ± 519
Dibenz(a, h)anthracene	3577 ± 494
Benzo(a)pyrene	3543 ± 114
Chrysene	3267 ± 147
3, 4-Benzofluorene	1939 ± 98
Anthracene	1377 ± 346
Pyrene	1232 ± 203
Fluoranthene	1123 ± 129
Perylene	805 ± 159
Phenanthrene	721 ± 155

[a] Rats pregnant for 18 days were given 40 mg/kg of polycyclic hydrocarbon orally. Placentas were assayed for benzo(a)pyrene hydroxylase activity 24 hr later. Each value represents the mean ± S. E. from three rats (7).

polycyclic hydrocarbons, the chronic administration of nicotine or phenobarbital to pregnant rats did not stimulate placental BP-hydroxylase activity.

Benzo(a)pyrene Metabolism by Human Skin

Variability in the basal activity and in the induction of BP-hydroxylase activity in placenta, skin, or other human tissues in culture may indicate genetic differences in the levels of carcinogen-metabolizing enzymes and in the inducibility of these enzymes in different people. Initial studies to determine the feasibility of a tissue-culture approach to this problem have been encouraging. BP was metabolized by human skin, and benz(a)anthracene — a polycyclic hydrocarbon in cigarette smoke — induced BP-hydroxylase activity in tissue cultures of human skin (Fig. 5) (3-5).

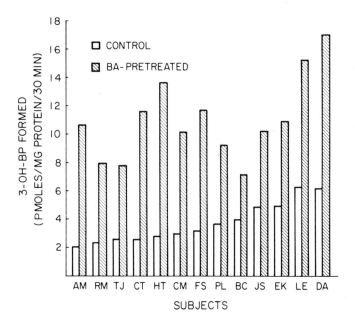

FIG. 5. Induction of benzo(a)pyrene (BP) hydroxylase activity
in tissue cultures of human foreskin. Infants were circumcised two
to four days after birth. Minced foreskin was incubated for 16 hr in
tissue-culture medium, in the presence or absence of 10 μM benz(a)-
anthracene (BA). The skins were then homogenized, and BP-
hydroxylase activity was determined by incubating foreskin homogenates with BP and a NADPH-generating system. Formation of metabolites with the same fluorescent properties as 3-hydroxybenzo(a)-
pyrene (3-OH-BP) was measured (4, 5).

Thirteen foreskins were each divided into two pieces, minced
and incubated for 16 hr with tissue-culture medium in the presence
or absence of benz(a)anthracene as an inducer. Following incubation,
the BP-hydroxylase activity of each cultured foreskin was determined,
and the results are presented in the order of increasing basal activity
(Fig. 5). The skins incubated in control medium showed the presence
of BP-hydroxylase, and there was a threefold variation in activity in
the skins of different individuals. BP-Hydroxylase was inducible in
skin cultured in the presence of benz(a)anthracene. The ratio of
hydroxylase activity in benz(a)anthracene-pretreated skin to that in
skin from control medium varied from 1.78 in subject BC to 5.30 in
subject AM. The average induction of BP-hydroxylase in the 13
subjects studied was 3.2-fold.

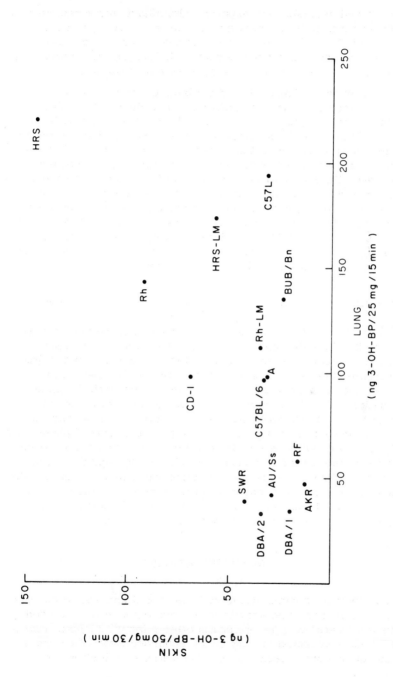

FIG. 6. Relationship between skin and lung benzo(a)pyrene (BP) hydroxylase activities in various strains of mice. Homogenates of skin and lung were incubated with BP, and the formation of metabolites with the same fluorescent properties as 3-hydroxybenzo(a)pyrene (3-OH-BP) was measured (53).

Skin BP-hydroxylase, like hepatic hydroxylase, has a requirement
for NADPH and molecular oxygen, and the hydroxylation proceeds
optimally at pH 7.4. Exposure of the enzyme to carbon monoxide
resulted in a marked inhibition of activity, indicating the involvement
of cytochrome P-450 or P-448 in the hydroxylation reaction.

The differences in basal BP-hydroxylase activity in the skin of
different individuals and the variability in the inducibility of this
enzyme in different people led us to ask whether the levels of BP-
hydroxylase in skin were correlated with the levels of this enzyme in
liver, lung, or other tissues. There was a 10- to 15-fold difference
in the concentrations of BP-hydroxylase in the skins of 15 strains of
mice. Although the levels of BP-hydroxylase in the skins of various
strains of mice did not parallel the levels of BP-hydroxylase in the
liver or kidney, there was a positive correlation (p < 0.05) between
the activities of BP-hydroxylase in the skins and lungs of the various
strains of mice (Fig. 6) (53). Additional studies are necessary to
determine whether the concentration of BP-hydroxylase in human skin
parallels the concentration of this enzyme in the lung.

Drug Metabolism as an Index of Carcinogen Metabolism in Man

A safe drug that is metabolized by the same enzyme system that
metabolizes BP or another carcinogen would be useful since such a
drug could be administered to humans and the metabolism of the drug
(as measured by blood-level determinations) could be used as an
index of carcinogen metabolism in man. Since phenacetin is oxida-
tively metabolized by liver microsomes and the metabolism of this
drug and of BP is stimulated by polycyclic hydrocarbons, we studied
the effect of cigarette smoking on the in vivo metabolism of phenacetin
in man (54). The blood levels of phenacetin were considerably lower
in cigarette smokers than in nonsmokers (Table 10), and the ratios
of the concentrations of N-acetyl-p-aminophenol (the major metabolite
of phenacetin) to those of phenacetin were increased in the cigarette
smokers. Additional work is needed to determine whether the metabolism of phenacetin parallels the metabolism of BP in man.

CONCLUDING REMARKS

Benzo(a)pyrene is metabolized by hepatic and nonhepatic enzymes
in animals and in man. The activity of BP-hydroxylase is increased
when rats are treated with BP or certain other polycyclic hydrocarbons,
and this effect is reflected in vivo by an enhanced metabolism and a
decreased tissue concentration of BP. Conversely, inhibitors of

TABLE 10

Plasma Levels of Phenacetin in Cigarette Smokers and Nonsmokers
at Various Intervals after the Oral Administration
of 900 mg of Phenacetin[a]

| Subjects | Hours after phenacetin administration | | | |
| | 1 | 2 | $3\frac{1}{2}$ | 5 |
	Phenacetin in plasma, μg/ml			
Nonsmokers	0.81 ± 0.20	2.24 ± 0.73	0.39 ± 0.13	0.12 ± 0.04
Smokers	0.33 ± 0.23	0.48 ± 0.28	0.09 ± 0.04	0.02 ± 0.01

[a] Each value represents the mean ± S. E. for nine subjects (54).

microsomal hydroxylation inhibit the in vivo metabolism of BP. Many
factors influence the activity of enzymes that metabolize drugs (55-58),
and it is likely that these same factors influence the metabolism of BP
and other carci nogens. Studies in man indicate widely different rates
of drug metabolism in different individuals, and one person may
metabolize a drug tenfold faster than another person (59, 60). It is
likely that similar variability occurs for the in vivo metabolism of
chemical carcinogens in man. Although our current knowledge indicates that high levels of microsomal hydroxylating enzymes protect
animals from the carcinogenicity of polycyclic hydrocarbons and
several unrelated chemicals, further research is needed to more completely determine how changes in carcinogen metabolism influence
tumorigenesis.

The presence of BP-hydroxylase in human liver, skin, and placenta
was demonstrated, and we showed that cigarette smokers have higher
levels of BP-hydroxylase in their placentas (obtained after normal
deliveries) than nonsmokers. In addition, BP-hydroxylase was induced
in tissue culture of human skin. Considerable variability in basal
BP-hydroxylase activity was found among different individuals, as
well as variability in the induction of the enzyme. Further investigations are needed to determine whether individual differences in the
amounts of carcinogen-metabolizing enzymes and variability in the
induction of these enzymes can explain why some individuals are more
susceptible than others to the action of chemical carcinogens in the
environment.

ACKNOWLEDGMENT

I thank Ms. MaryAnn Sadvary for her excellent assistance in the preparation of this manuscript.

NOTE

1. The rate of decrease in the concentration of BP metabolites in bile changes with time. The initial $t_{\frac{1}{2}}$ for the studies described in Fig. 3 is defined as the time required to decrease the maximum concentration of BP metabolites in the bile by 50%.

REFERENCES

1. R. Kuntzman, L. C. Mark, M. Jacobson, W. Levin, and A. H. Conney, Metabolism of drugs and carcinogens by human liver enzymes, J. Pharmacol. Exptl. Therap., 152, 151 (1966).
2. R. Montesano and P. N. Magee, Metabolism of dimethylnitrosamine by human liver slices in vitro, Nature, 228, 173 (1970).
3. A. H. Conney, A. P. Alvares, W. Levin, and A. Kappas, Induction of benzo(a)pyrene hydroxylase in human skin culture, Pharmacologist, 13, 244 (1971).
4. W. Levin, A. H. Conney, A. P. Alvares, I. Merkatz, and A. Kappas, Induction of benzo(a)pyrene hydroxylase in human skin, Science, 176, 419 (1972).
5. A. P. Alvares, A. Kappas, W. Levin, and A. H. Conney, Inducibility of benzo(a)pyrene hydroxylase in human skin by polycyclic hydrocarbons, Clinical Pharmacol. Therap., 14, 30 (1973).
6. R. M. Welch, Y. E. Harrison, A. H. Conney, P. J. Poppers, and M. Finster, Cigarette smoking: stimulatory effect on metabolism of 3, 4-benzpyrene by enzymes in human placenta, Science, 160, 541 (1968).
7. R. M. Welch, Y. E. Harrison, B. W. Gommi, P. J. Poppers, M. Finster, and A. H. Conney, Stimulatory effect of cigarette smoking on the hydroxylation of 3, 4-benzpyrene and the N-demethylation of 3-methyl-4-monomethylaminoazobenzene by enzymes in human placenta, Clinical Pharmacol. Therap., 10, 100 (1969).

8. D. W. Nebert, J. Winker, and H. V. Gelboin, Aryl hydrocarbon hydroxylase activity in human placenta from cigarette smoking and nonsmoking women, Cancer Res., 29, 1763 (1969).
9. J. P. Whitlock, Jr., H. L. Cooper, and H. V. Gelboin, Aryl Hydrocarbon (benzopyrene) hydroxylase is stimulated in human lymphocytes by mitogens and benz[a]anthracene, Science, 177, 618 (1972)..
10. A. H. Conney, E. C. Miller, and J. A. Miller, Substrate-induced synthesis and other properties of benzpyrene hydroxylase in rat liver, J. Biol. Chem., 228, 753 (1957).
11. L. W. Wattenberg and J. L. Leong, Histochemical demonstration of reduced pyridine nucleotide-dependent polycyclic hydrocarbon-metabolizing systems, J. Histochem. Cytochem., 10, 412 (1962).
12. L. W. Wattenberg, J. L. Leong, and P. L. Strand, Benzpyrene hydroxylase activity in the gastrointestinal tract, Cancer Res., 22, 1120 (1962).
13. H. V. Gelboin and N. R. Blackburn, The stimulatory effect of 3-methylcholanthrene on benzpyrene hydroxylase activity in several rat tissues: Inhibition by actinomycin D and puromycin, Cancer Res., 24, 356 (1964).
14. D. W. Nebert and H. V. Gelboin, The in vivo and in vitro induction of aryl hydrocarbon hydroxylase in mammalian cells of different species, tissues, strains and development of hormonal states, Arch. Biochem. Biophys., 134, 76 (1969).
15. E. Schlede and A. H. Conney, Induction of benzo(a)pyrene hydroxylase activity in rat skin, Life Sci., 9, Part II, 1295 (1970).
16. E. Schlede, R. Kuntzman, S. Haber, and A. H. Conney, Effect of enzyme induction on the metabolism and tissue distribution of benzo(a)pyrene, Cancer Res., 30, 2893 (1970).
17. E. Schlede, R. Kuntzman, and A. H. Conney, Stimulatory effect of benzo(a)pyrene and phenobarbital pretreatment on the biliary excretion of benzo(a)pyrene metabolites in the rat, Cancer Res., 30, 2898 (1970).
18. W. G. Levine, The role of microsomal drug-metabolizing enzymes in the biliary excretion of 3,4-benzpyrene in the rat, J. Pharmacol. Exptl. Therap., 175, 301 (1970).
19. P. Kotin, H. L. Falk, and A. Miller, Effect of carbon tetrachloride intoxication on metabolism of benzo(a)pyrene in rats and mice, J. Natl. Cancer Inst., 28, 725 (1962).
20. S. S. Epstein, J. Andrea, P. Clapp, and D. Mackintosh, Enhancement by piperonyl butoxide of acute toxicity due to freons, benzo(a)pyrene, and griseofulvin in infant mice, Toxicol. Appl. Pharmacol., 11, 442 (1967).
21. S. S. Epstein, S. Joshi, J. Andrea, P. Clapp, H. Falk, and N. Mantel, Synergistic toxicity and carcinogenicity of freons and piperonyl butoxide, Nature, 214, 526 (1967).

22. A. H. Conney, R. Chang, W. Levin, and A. Garbut, Effects of piperonyl butoxide on drug and carcinogen metabolism in rodents and man, Environ. Health, 24, 97 (1972).

23. F. W. Sunderman, Jr., Inhibition of induction of benzpyrene hydroxylase by nickel carbonyl, Cancer Res., 27, 950 (1967).

24. M. S. Palmer, D. H. Swanson, and D. L. Coffin, Effect of ozone on benzpyrene hydroxylase activity in the syrian golden hamster, Cancer Res., 31, 730 (1971).

25. W. R. Jondorf, R. P. Maickel, and B. B. Brodie, Inability of newborn mice and guinea pigs to metabolize drugs, Biochem. Pharmacol., 1, 352 (1958).

26. J. R. Fouts and R. H. Adamson, Drug metabolism in the newborn rabbit, Science, 129, 897 (1959).

27. E. Bresnick and J. G. Stevenson, Microsomal N-demethylase activity in developing rat liver after administration of 3-methylcholanthrene, Biochem. Pharmacol., 17, 1815 (1968).

28. L. W. Wattenberg and J. L. Leong, Inhibition of the carcinogenic action of benzo(a)pyrene by flavones, Cancer Res., 30, 1922 (1970).

29. C. Huggins, L. Grand, and R. Fukunishi, Aromatic influences on the yields of mammary cancers following administration of 7, 12-dimethylbenz(a)anthracene, Proc. Nat. Acad. Sci., 51, 737 (1964).

30. C. Huggins and J. Pataki, Aromatic azo derivatives preventing mammary cancer and adrenal injury from 7, 12-dimethylbenz(a)-anthracene, Proc. Nat. Acad. Sci., 53, 791 (1965).

31. D. N. Wheatley, Enhancement and inhibition of the induction by 7, 12-dimethylbenz(a)anthracene of mammary tumours in female Sprague-Dawley rats, Brit. J. Cancer, 22, 787 (1968).

32. L. W. Wattenberg and J. L. Leong, Inhibition of the carcinogenic action of 7, 12-dimethylbenz(a)anthracene by beta-naphthoflavone, Proc. Soc. Exptl. Biol. N. Y., 128, 940 (1968).

33. K. Kovacs and A. Somogyi, Suppression by spironolactone of 7, 12-dimethylbenz(a)anthracene-induced mammary tumors, Europ. J. Cancer, 6, 195 (1970).

34. E. C. Miller, J. A. Miller, R. R. Brown, and J. C. MacDonald, On the protective action of certain polycyclic aromatic hydrocarbons against carcinogenesis by aminoazo dyes and 2-acetylaminofluorene, Cancer Res., 18, 469 (1958).

35. H. N. Tawfic, Studies on ear duct tumors in rats. II. Inhibitory effect of methylcholanthrene and 1, 2-benzanthracene on tumor formation by 4-dimethylaminostilbene, Acta Pathol. Japon., 15, 255 (1965).

36. R. S. Yamamoto, J. H. Weisburger, and E. K. Weisburger, Controlling factors in urethane carcinogenesis in mice: effect of enzyme inducers and metabolic inhibitors, Cancer Res., 31, 483 (1971).

37. A. E. M. McLean and A. Marshall, Reduced carcinogenic effects of aflatoxin in rats given phenobarbitone, Brit. J. Exptl. Pathol., 52, 322 (1971).

38. W. Kunz, G. Schaude, and C. Thomas, Die beeinflussung der nitrosamincarcinogenese durch phenobarbital und halogenkohlenwasserstoffe, Z. Krebsforsch., 72, 291 (1969).

39. H. L. Richardson, A. R. Stier, and E. Borsos-Nachtnebel, Liver tumor inhibition and adrenal histologic responses in rats to which 3'-methyl-4-dimethylaminoazobenzene and 20-methylcholanthrene were simultaneously administered, Cancer Res., 12, 356 (1952).

40. R. J. Meechan, D. E. McCafferty, and R. S. Jones, 3-Methylcholanthrene as an inhibitor of hepatic cancer induced by 3'-methyl-4-dimethylaminoazobenzene in the diet of the rat: A determination of the time relationships, Cancer Res., 13, 802 (1953).

41. H. V. Gelboin and F. J. Wiebel, Studies on the mechanism of aryl hydrocarbon hydroxylase induction and its role in cytotoxicity and tumorigenicity, Ann. N. Y. Acad. Sci., 179, 529 (1971).

42. P. L. Grover, P. Sims, E. Huberman, H. Marquardt, T. Kuroko, and C. Heidelberger, In vitro transformation of rodent cells by K-region derivatives of polycyclic hydrocarbons, Proc. Nat. Acad. Sci., 68, 1098 (1971).

43. J. A. Miller and E. C. Miller, Chemical carcinogenesis: Mechanisms and approaches to its control, J. Natl. Cancer Inst., 47, V-XIV (September 1971).

44. H. V. Gelboin, A microsome-dependent binding of benzo(a)pyrene to DNA, Cancer Res., 29, 1272 (1969).

45. J. K. Selkirk, E. Huberman, and C. Heidelberger, An epoxide is an intermediate in the microsomal metabolism of the chemical carcinogen, dibenz(a, h)anthracene, Biochem. Biophys. Res. Commun., 43, 1010 (1971).

46. S. Udenfriend, Arene oxide intermediates in enzymatic hydroxylation and their significance with respect to drug toxicity, Ann. N. Y. Acad. Sci., 179, 295 (1971).

47. H. V. Gelboin, E. Huberman, and L. Sachs, Enzyme hydroxylation of benzpyrene and its relationship to cytotoxicity, Proc. Nat. Acad. Sci., 64, 1188 (1969).

48. L. Diamond and H. V. Gelboin, Alpha-naphthoflavone: An inhibitor of hydrocarbon cytotoxicity and microsomal hydroxylase, Science, 166, 1023 (1969).

49. G. A. Belitskii, Iu. M. Vasil'ev, O. Iu. Ivanova, N. A. Lavrova, E. L. Progozhina, N. L. Samoilina, A. A. Stavrovskaya, A. Ya. Khesina, and L. M. Shabad, Metabolism of benzo(a)pyrene by cells of different mammals in vitro and toxic effect of polycyclic hydrocarbons on the cells, Vop. Onkol., 16, 53 (1970).

50. L. Diamond and H. F. Clark, Comparative studies on the interaction of benzo(a)pyrene with cells derived from poikilothermic and homeothermic vertebrates. I. Metabolism of benzo(a)pyrene, J. Nat. Cancer Inst., 45, 1005 (1970).

51. A. G. Gilman and A. H. Conney, The induction of aminoazo dye N-demethylase in nonhepatic tissues by 3-methylcholanthrene, Biochem. Pharmacol., 12, 591 (1963).

52. R. M. Welch, A. Loh, and A. H. Conney, Cigarette smoke: stimulatory effect on metabolism of 3, 4-benzpyrene by enzymes in rat lung, Life Sci., 10, 215 (1971).

53. A. Somogyi, R. Kuntzman, and A. H. Conney, unpublished observations, 1972.

54. E. J. Pantuck, R. Kuntzman, and A. H. Conney, Decreased plasma levels of phenacetin in cigarette smokers, Science, 175, 1248 (1972).

55. A. H. Conney and J. J. Burns, Factors influencing drug metabolism, Advan. Pharmacol., 1, 31 (1962).

56. J. R. Gillette, Metabolism of drugs and other foreign compounds by enzymatic mechanisms, Progr. Drug Res., 6, 11 (1963).

57. A. H. Conney, Pharmacological implications of microsomal enzyme induction, Pharmacol. Rev., 19, 317 (1967).

58. A. H. Conney and J. J. Burns, Metabolic interactions among environmental chemicals and drugs, Science, 178, 576 (1972).

59. E. S. Vesell, G. T. Passananti, F. E. Greene, and J. G. Page, Genetic control of drug levels and of the induction of drug-metabolizing enzymes in man: Individual variability in the extent of allopurinol and nortriptyline inhibition of drug metabolism, Ann. N. Y. Acad. Sci., 179, 752 (1971).

60. B. Alexanderson, D. A. P. Evans, and F. Sjöqvist, Steady-state plasma levels of nortriptyline in twins: Influence of genetic factors and drug therapy, Brit. Med. J., 1969-4, 764.

61. R. M. Welch, B. Gommi, A. P. Alvares, and A. H. Conney, Effect of enzyme induction on the metabolism of benzo(a)pyrene and 3'-methyl-4-monomethylaminoazobenzene in the pregnant and fetal rat, Cancer Res., 32, 973 (1972).

62. A. H. Conney, R. Welch, R. Kuntzman, R. Chang, M. Jacobson, A. D. Munro-Faure, A. W. Peck, A. Bye, A. Poland, P. J. Poppers, M. Finster, and J. A. Wolff, Effects of environmental chemicals on the metabolism of drugs, carcinogens and normal body constituents in man, Ann. N. Y. Acad. Sci., 179, 155 (1971).

Chapter 16

THEORETICAL CALCULATION OF THE REACTIVITY OF ADENINE AND GUANINE TOWARD ALKYLATION

Alberte Pullman

Institut de Biologie Physico-Chimique
Fondation Edmond de Rothschild
Paris, France

In connection with the curious results concerning the displacement of the major site of alkylation of biologic purines and pyrimidines as a function of the nature of the base investigated (e. g., N_1 or N_3 in adenine but N_7 or O_6 in guanine) or of the solvent used (alkylation by 7-bromomethylbenzanthracene of N_7 of guanine in dimethylacetamide but of its NH_2 group in water), I would like to draw attention to a particularly promising new theoretical approach to this problem.

This approach is based on the study of the <u>molecular potential</u> seen by an approaching reagent. The knowledge of a <u>molecular wavefunction</u> allows the accurate calculation of the electrostatic potential $V_{(r_i)}$ created in the neighboring space by the nuclear charges and the electronic distribution. The interaction energy between the molecular distribution and an external point charge q placed at point i is $qV_{(r_i)}$. Taking q as a unit positive charge, the interaction potential can be used for studying proton affinities and, hopefully, electrophilic attack (1-3).

In fact, recent detailed investigations using nucleic acid bases to solve this very problem give extremely promising results.

Thus, e. g., isopotential maps for an approaching unit positive charge in the molecular plane account remarkably for the different principal alkylation sites in adenine and guanine (1), and they are the first to do so unambiguously. Figure 1 presents such a map for adenine (2) as constructed with an <u>ab initio</u> wavefunction for this base. It clearly shows that the strongest attraction toward an external positive charge occurs with N_1 and N_7. The NH and CH regions, as well as the in-plane approach to the amino group, are repulsive. <u>Ab initio</u> results are

A. PULLMAN

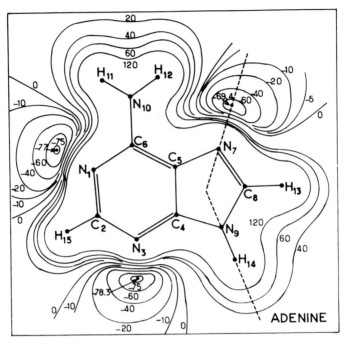

FIG. 1. Electrostatic molecular potential energy map for adenine
in the ring plane (ab initio data). Energies are given in kilocalories
per mole.

not yet available for guanine, but the maps obtained for the two bases
by the CNDO/2 method, although less reliable on the absolute scale,
show without any possible doubt the reasons for the difference in behavior between the two compounds (Fig. 2). They show again the characteristic potential wells facing N_1 and N_3 of adenine, with a smaller
similar region near N_7, while in guanine the only attractive region is
the neighborhood of N_7 and O_6. We hope to resolve this broad attractive region by more refined calculations.

Moreover a particularly significant result in connection with the
experimental findings presented here concerning the displacement of
the site of attack of 7-BrMeBA from N_7 of guanine to its N_{10} (amino
nitrogen) when passing from an organic solvent to water is observed
when the isopotential curves are constructed for an approach of the
positive charge in a plane perpendicular to the plane of the base.
Figure 3 presents such a potential energy map, constructed with the
ab initio wavefunction for adenine in the plane perpendicular to the
ring and passing through N_{10}, C_6, and N_3. It is seen that for such
an approach, although the maximum attraction is toward N_3, a

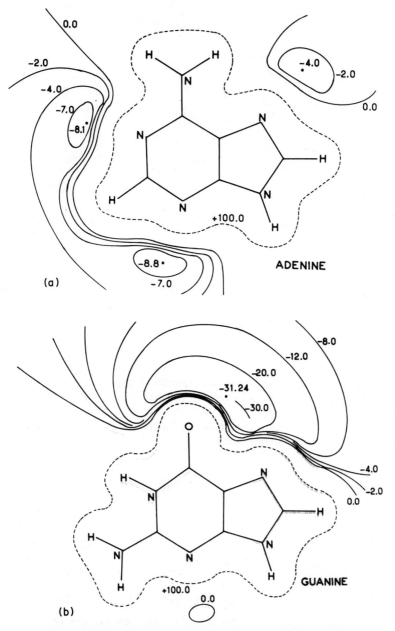

FIG. 2. Electrostatic molecular potential energy maps for (a) adenine and (b) guanine in the ring plane (CNDO/2 data). Energies are given in kilocalories per mole.

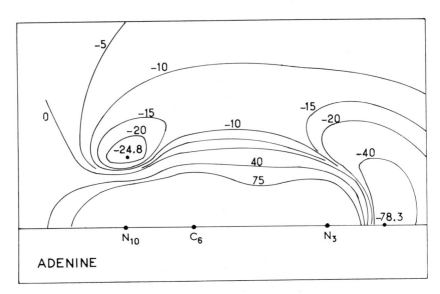

FIG. 3. Electrostatic molecular potential energy map for adenine in the plane perpendicular to the plane of the ring and passing through N_{10} (amino nitrogen), C_6, and N_3 (ab initio data). Energies are given in kilocalories per mole.

secondary attractive pole is located above the amino nitrogen. Thus it appears that for an appropriate geometrical arrangement of the partners, which could probably be obtained by the stacking of 7-BrMeBA and the bases in water, an attack of the electrophilic agent upon the amine group becomes feasible. This type of theoretical result suggests the possible mechanism of the reaction.

REFERENCES

For more details see

1. Cl. Giessner-Prettre and A. Pullman, Compt. Rend., 272, 750 (1972); Theoret. Chim. Acta, 25, 83 (1972).
2. R. Bonaccorsi, A. Pullman, E. Scrocco, and J. Tomasi, Theoret. Chim. Acta, 24, 51 (1972).
3. A. Pullman, Fortschr. Chem. Forsch., 31, 45 (1972).

For similar studies for the peptide bond see (4) and (5).

4. R. Bonaccorsi, A. Pullman, E. Scrocco, and J. Tomasi, Chem. Phys. Letters, 12, 622 (1972).
5. B. Mély and A. Pullman, Compt. Rend., 274, 1371 (1972).

III
DNA REPAIR PROCESS
IN
MAMMALIAN CELLS

Chapter 17

DNA SYNTHESIS BY ALKYLATED CELLS

Dominic Scudiero and Bernard Strauss

Department of Microbiology
The University of Chicago
Chicago, Illinois

DNA synthesis by HEp.2 cells treated with the mutagenic alkylating agent methyl methanesulfonate (MMS) has the following characteristics (1):

1. DNA made immediately after treatment of cells with lethal concentrations (50% survival) of MMS is formed by semi-conservative synthesis, but the newly synthesized DNA is not replicated.

2. DNA repair processes (non-semi-conservative replication) occur after treatment of HEp 2 cells with MMS.

3. In contrast with the DNA made immediately after treatment (characteristic 1), the DNA that is synthesized after a period of incubation following treatment replicates. It was therefore concluded that the DNA that is formed before repair has been completed is not replicated (1).

These experiments did not indicate the nature of the abnormality that kept the DNA formed after alkylation from replicating. Two alternate hypotheses are possible: either (a) there is some defect produced in the replication machinery, or (b) a defect in the DNA template prevents replication. For example, alkylation might produce some abnormality in the cells that prevents the completion of the first S period after treatment, or prevents the cells from entering G_2 or M or from dividing and entering a second S period. However, Plant and Roberts (2) and Myers and Strauss (3) have shown that the first cell cycle following methylation is completed and that the second S period actually begins in some cells. It is, therefore, reasonable to look for an abnormality in the DNA made after alkylation that might prevent its replication. Since the DNA formed after repair has occurred does replicate, it is reasonable to assume that the lesion is in DNA itself.

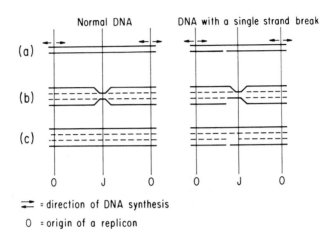

FIG. 1. Effect of a single strand break on the replication of DNA.

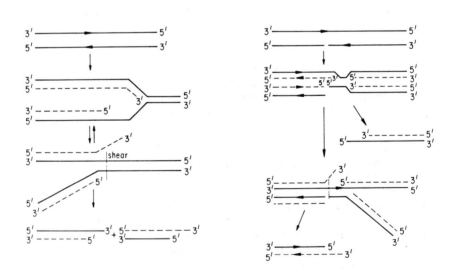

FIG. 2. Origin of regions of single strandedness in DNA.
(a) Normal DNA template: replication with the formation of "D" loops.
(b) DNA template with a strand break.

Our experiments are based on the following assumptions:

1. It is likely that DNA synthesis in mammalian cells occurs simul-
    taneously from numerous starting points and in two directions as
    first suggested by Huberman and Riggs (4).

2. MMS-induced lesions block DNA synthesis directed by the strand
    in which the lesion occurs. Since we have been unable to detect
    abnormal initiation events at MMS-induced lesions in HEp 2 cells,
    we suppose that DNA replication does not occur between the site
    of the lesion and the end of the particular replicon in which the
    lesion occurs (Fig. 1). The rate of DNA synthesis in alkylated
    cells should then depend on the number of lesions and the average
    length of each replicon.

3. Finally, we assume that DNA synthesis from a damaged template
    results in the production of chromatid breaks and that the chromo-
    some pieces produced will be lost or misdistributed at cell division
    and therefore will not replicate normally at the next S period (5).

These assumptions lead to the prediction that DNA synthesis in
cells with unrepaired, MMS-induced lesions should result in the production of a variety of DNA fragments with single stranded regions
(Fig. 2). These single stranded regions might result from at least two
processes:

1. DNA synthesis is discontinuous (6) and synthesis along both
    strands need not proceed simultaneously. The observation of the
    formation of "D" loops (7) in mitochondrial DNA synthesis implies
    that similar discontinuities may occur in chromosomal DNA syn-
    thesis. Slowing the rate of DNA synthesis, by whatever mechanism,
    might increase the lifetime of such single stranded regions.

2. If DNA synthesis does "jump" from the point of an MMS-induced
    lesion to the adjoining replicon, then single-stranded pieces of
    both "old" and "newly synthesized" DNA might be generated
    (Fig. 2). Although the presence of regions of single strandedness
    in normal DNA synthesis has been reported by a number of investi-
    gators (8-10), cells treated with MMS should produce DNA's par-
    ticularly rich in such fragments.

We used columns of benzoylated naphthoylated DEAE cellulose
(BNC, Gerhard Schlesinger Co.) to find DNA with single stranded regions
(11-13). Hydroxyapatite columns (HA, Biogel Corp.) were prepared and
used as described by Bernardi (14) to recognize DNA with regions of
double strandedness. Exonuclease I was obtained from Dr. Nicholas
Cozzarelli and Neurospora nuclease was prepared and used as described
by Rabin et al. (15) for the digestion of single stranded regions except
that the phosphocellulose column purification was omitted. HEp 2 cells

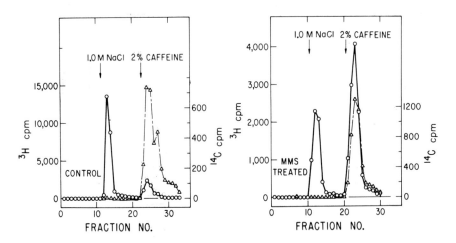

FIG. 3. Chromatography of lysates of control and alkylated cells on benzoylated naphthoylated DEAE cellulose. Cells were treated with 2.5 mM MMS for 1 hr. The MMS was removed and the cultures were incubated for 2 hr with [^{3}H]TdR (10 μCi/ml; 3 Ci/mM). The cells were collected and lysed, the sheared lysate was then passed through the column and eluted in stepwise fashion as indicated. Circles, ^{3}H-labeled sample; triangles, ^{14}C-labeled denatured DNA co-chromatographed as a control.

were grown and the DNA was prepared as previously described (1). Methyl methanesulfonate (MMS, Eastman Organic Chemicals) was vacuum distilled before use. The details of our methodology will be presented elsewhere (21).

RESULTS

Double stranded DNA elutes from BNC columns on washing with 1 M NaCl; DNA with single stranded regions is eluted only when the column is washed with caffeine. The required concentration of caffeine is dependent on the proportion of single stranded regions in the molecule (11, 12). It will be convenient throughout this paper to refer to the radioactive label with the properties of DNA containing single stranded regions as "DNA$_{ss}$" determined in BNC chromatography.

HEp 2 cells were alkylated by treatment with 2.5 mM MMS for 1 hr; the cells were then washed and incubated with [^{3}H] thymidine for 120 min. The cells were lysed; the lysate was then sheared by passing it through a 20-gauge needle five times. A lysate from control, nonalkylated cells was prepared in the same way. The lysates were then applied

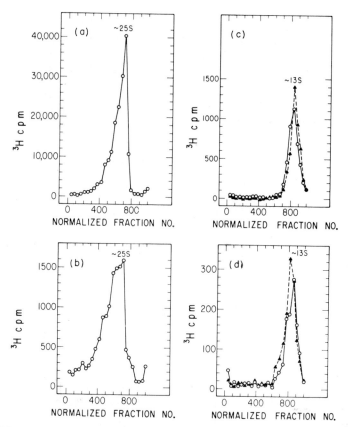

FIG. 4. Neutral sucrose gradient centrifugation of DNA fragments.
(a) Control, phenol-extracted DNA labeled with [^{3}H] TdR for 30 min
and sheared. Centrifugation of samples before chromatography on BNC.
(b) As in (a) except from cultures treated with 2.5 mM MMS for one hour
before the addition of [^{3}H] TdR. (c) BNC-caffeine eluate of control
samples. Duplicate runs shown. (d) As in (c) but from BNC-caffeine
eluates of MMS-treated samples. All samples were centrifuged in 1 M
NaCl plus 0.05 M tris through a 5-20% neutral sucrose gradient for
240 min at 25,000 rpm in the Beckman L2 centrifuge.

to separate BNC columns along with denatured [^{14}C]-labeled DNA added
as a control. We found (Fig. 3) that a greater proportion of the label
from alkylated cells required caffeine for elution, although both control and treated preparations contain some DNA$_{ss}$. Equivalent results
were obtained when purified DNA preparations were used instead of
cell lysates. The difference in the relative amounts of DNA$_{ss}$ from
alkylated and control cultures was less drastic with shorter periods
of labeling (see Table 7, Fig. 7). We know that the synthesis of

TABLE 1

Effect of Shearing[a]

Treatment	Shearing	Total cpm added	Total cpm recovered	% recovered activity eluting from BNC	
				1.0 M NaCl	2% caffeine
Control	Unsheared	8250	7274	16	82
Control	20 gauge needle: 5 times	8250	7580	42	56
Control	30 sec sonication	8250	8438	38	60
MMS (2.5 mM)	Unsheared	1850	1560	7	88
MMS (2.5 mM)	20 gauge needle: 5 times	1850	1510	8	89
MMS (2.5 mM)	30 sec sonication	1850	1642	10	88

[a]HEp 2 cells were treated for 1 hr with MMS. The MMS was removed and the cells were incubated for 30 min with [^{3}H] TdR (10 μCi/ml; 17 Ci/mM). The cells were lysed and phenol-extracted DNA was applied to the column as shown.

TABLE 2

Performance of the BNC Columns[a]

Sample	% recovered activity eluting from BNC			
	1.0 M NaCl		2.0% caffeine	
	^{3}H	^{14}C	^{3}H	^{14}C
Control—phenol-extracted DNA + [^{14}C] heat-denatured DNA	42	2	56	96
a. 1.0 M NaCl eluate from control eluted from second BNC	85	0	10	0
b. 2.0% caffeine eluate from control eluted from second BNC	9	0	88	100
2.5 mM MMS—phenol-extracted DNA + [^{14}C] heat-denatured DNA	8	0.2	90	99
a. 1.0 M NaCl eluate from MMS eluted from second BNC	80	0	15	0
b. 2.0% caffeine eluate from MMS eluted from second BNC	7	0	86	100
Heat denatured [^{14}C] HEp 2 DNA	—	0.6	—	99
Heat denatured [^{3}H] HEp 2 DNA	0.2	—	99	—

[a]DNA was labeled and prepared as described in footnote a to Table 1. Percent inhibition of uptake due to MMS treatment: 22%.

DNA$_{ss}$ occurs in the nucleus because we observe this material in DNA preparations from isolated nuclei. The nuclei in such preparations were isolated by lysis of the cells with the detergent NP-40 (Shell Oil Co., N.Y.) followed by differential centrifugation and appeared free of cytoplasmic contamination as determined by microscopic examination.

DNA from control cultures behaved as though it contained a higher proportion of DNA$_{ss}$ if it were passed through the BNC column without previous shearing (Table 1). Shearing reduced the yield of DNA$_{ss}$ from controls but not from alkylated cells. After shearing, the average size of the DNA from both control and alkylated cultures was about the same: 25 S as determined in a neutral sucrose gradient (Fig. 4), corresponding

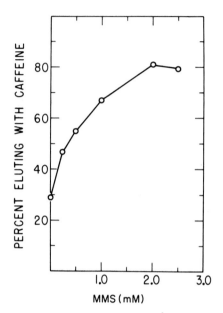

FIG. 5. Formation of DNA$_{SS}$ after treatment of HEp 2 cells with different concentrations of MMS. Cells were treated with MMS for 1 hr and then incubated for 2 hr with [^{3}H]TdR (10 μCi/ml; 3 Ci/mM) before isolation of the DNA and chromatography on BNC.

to a molecular weight (16) of about 1.2 × 10^7. All of our subsequent experiments were done with DNA sheared by passing it through a 20-gauge needle five times.

The DNA retained by BNC because it is partially denatured behaves consistently on passage through a second BNC column (Table 2). However a small proportion of native DNA (i. e., DNA that is washed through an initial BNC column with 1 M NaCl) always adheres to BNC and requires caffeine for elution. Our values for the amount of DNA$_{SS}$ from control and treated cell preparations may therefore be high by this factor.

The proportion of DNA$_{SS}$ is a function of the dose of MMS to which the cells are exposed (Fig. 5). Cells were treated with MMS and were then labeled by incubation with [^{3}H]TdR for 120 min before harvesting. The proportion of DNA$_{SS}$ isolated in the newly synthesized DNA increased from about 30 to 80% with increasing doses of MMS.

In order to study the structure of DNA$_{SS}$, caffeine eluates were dialyzed and the caffeine-free material was tested by sucrose gradient centrifugation, HA chromatography, and BNC chromatography after

TABLE 3

Adsorption of BNC Eluates on Hydroxyapatite[a]

Sample	Total pm added	Total cpm recovered	% recovered activity eluting from hydroxyapatite	
			0.18 M KPO$_4$	0.28 M KPO$_4$
1.0 M NaCl eluate from BNC of control cells	6000	5913	6	88
2.0% caffeine eluate from BNC of control cells	6600	6682	10	86
1.0 M NaCl eluate from BNC of 2.5 mM MMS-treated cells	1280	1054	6	82
2.0% caffeine eluate from BNC of 2.5 mM MMS-treated cells	1748	1260	24	64
HEp 2 [^{14}C] heat-denatured DNA	3045	2875	90	7

[a]DNA was prepared as described in footnote a to Table 1. Percent inhibition of [^{3}H] TdR uptake due to the MMS treatment: 22%

nuclease treatment. We wanted to obtain additional evidence for the presence of single stranded regions and to determine the relative extent of such regions in samples from control and alkylated cells.

The fragments eluted from BNC with caffeine sedimented through neutral sucrose gradients with S values of 13 for both control and alkylated cell preparations (Fig. 4). An S value of 13 was also obtained on alkaline sucrose sedimentation. This gives a molecular weight, using the Studier (16) equations, of 1.8×10^6 for native and 8.9×10^5 for denatured DNA. Since the DNA put onto BNC had an average molecular weight of 1.2×10^7, we suspect that fragmentation occurs during chromatography and subsequent handling. The DNA$_{ss}$ adsorbs to hydroxyapatite as though it contained double stranded regions since most

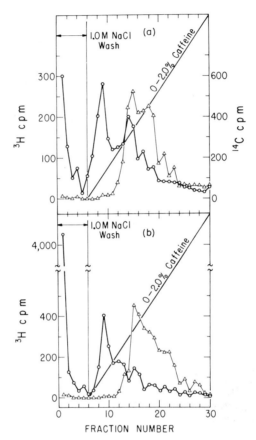

FIG. 6. Caffeine gradient elution of BNC columns. (a) Elution of purified DNA isolated from a culture treated with 2.5 mM MMS for 1 hr and then incubated 2 hr with $[^3H]$ TdR (10 µCi/ml; 3 Ci/mM). (b) Elution of DNA prepared from a control culture. Triangles indicate the elution pattern of denatured $[^{14}C]$ DNA added as a marker.

of it requires 0.28 M phosphate for elution. However, about one-fourth of the newly labeled DNA_{SS} from alkylated cells is eluted with 0.18 M phosphate, indicating that it is completely denatured (Table 3). These data are consistent with the results of caffeine gradient elution experiments (Fig. 6). Although the BNC elution profiles of DNA from alkylated and control cells are qualitatively similar, the alkylated cells do have more of a component that elutes with caffeine at the position of completely denatured DNA.

The structure of DNA_{SS} can also be determined by nuclease treatment and chromatography. Digestion with a single strand specific nuclease should convert the fragments into double stranded molecules and the percentage of radioactivity released as acid soluble should indicate the relative proportion of single strandedness.

The results of treating the dialyzed caffeine eluate of the BNC columns with nuclease are dramatic (Table 4). DNA_{ss} was converted by Neurospora nuclease into fragments that pass through BNC with the properties of native DNA. Similar results were obtained with exonuclease I. Although DNA_{ss} from both control and alkylated cells was converted into mostly native material by exonuclease treatment, there is a major difference between the two preparations. DNA from alkylated cells yields a much higher proportion of acid soluble fragments after nuclease treatment than does the DNA_{ss} from control cells. The amount of DNA from control cells that binds to BNC after nuclease treatment is about equal to the proportion of native DNA (DNA eluted from BNC with 1 M NaCl) that binds to BNC. A larger portion of the DNA_{ss} from alkylated cells still requires caffeine elution from BNC even after nuclease treatment. We have no explanation for this nuclease resistant fraction unless some of the single stranded ends "fold back" to give nuclease resistant, double stranded regions.

The experiments described so far examine the properties of newly synthesized DNA formed after alkylation of the cells. In order to examine the properties of the bulk of the DNA, we labeled cells by incubation for 42 hr with [^{3}H]TdR and then treated with MMS for 1 hr before harvest. Even after this short period of incubation with MMS, there was an excess of DNA_{ss} in the treated sample, although the difference between control and treated samples was less than when "newly synthesized" DNA was studied (Table 5). We also assayed the nuclease susceptibility of the bulk of the DNA as compared with newly synthesized DNA (Table 6). Cultures were labeled for 24 hr with [^{14}C]TdR, the isotope was washed out, the cultures were treated for 1 hr with MMS (2.5 mM), and then incubated 30 min with [^{3}H]TdR.[*] The DNA_{ss} was isolated by passage through BNC as usual, dialyzed, and treated with exonuclease I.

There is a significant amount of DNA made acid soluble by exonuclease treatment, but it is only in the "newly synthesized" DNA that there is a difference in the amount of acid soluble radioactivity produced by treatment of alkylated and control DNA_{ss} fragments with nuclease.

---

[*] This experiment has been repeated with an 18 hour chase period in non-radioactive medium intervening between labeling with (^{14}C)TdR and the MMS treatment and (^{3}H)TdR label. We obtained very similar results even with this modification.

TABLE 4

Effect of Nuclease Treatment[a]

Sample	Total cpm added	Total cpm recovered	% acid soluble cpm	% recovered activity eluting from BNC	
				1.0 M NaCl	2% caffeine
Control	55,850	48,770		42	56
2.5 mM MMS	16,088	14,730		8	90
Control caffeine eluate	3,145	2,517	0.72	9	88
MMS-caffeine eluate	1,752	1,193	1.2	7	86
Control caffeine eluate + E. coli exonuclease I	2,135	1,847	12	78	20
MMS-caffeine eluate + E. coli exonuclease I	1,130	931	26	73	20
Control caffeine eluate + Neurospora nuclease	20,450	17,848	7	89	10
MMS-caffeine eluate + Neurospora nuclease	1,845	1,577	24	80	19

[a]HEp 2 DNA was labeled as described in footnote a to Table 1. The cells were incubated with exonuclease I for 1.5 hr at 37°C and with Neurospora nuclease for 2 hr at 37°C under conditions where denatured DNA was completely digested.

TABLE 5

Bulk Labeled DNA[a]

Treatment	Total cpm added	Total cpm recovered	% recovered activity eluting from BNC	
			1.0 M NcCl	2% caffeine
Control	27,400	22,818	72	28
2.5 mM MMS	26,500	24,304	57	43

[a] HEp-2 cells were labeled by 42 hr incubation with [^{3}H]TdR (10 μCi/mM). The isotope was washed out and the cells were incubated with MMS. The cells were harvested immediately after 1 hr of incubation with alkylating agent.

TABLE 6

Nuclease Treatment of Doubly Labeled DNA

Sample	Total acid soluble cpm		Total recovered cpm		% of recovered cpm made acid soluble	
	[^{3}H]	[^{14}C]	[^{3}H]	[^{14}C]	[^{3}H]	[^{14}C]
2% caffeine eluate from control + Exo 1	943	77	8346	1057	11	7
2% caffeine eluate from MMS-treated + Exo 1	591	50	1827	776	32	6
2% caffeine eluate from control	71	11	7952	982	0.9	1.1
2% caffeine eluate from MMS-treated	21	6	1954	835	1.1	0.7

[a] HEp-2 cells were incubated with [^{14}C]TdR (0.3 μCi/ml; 54.8 mCi/mM) for 24 hr. The isotope was washed out and the cells were treated for 1 hr with 2.5 mM MMS. Both treated and control cultures were then incubated with [^{3}H]TdR (10 μCi/ml; 17 Ci/mM) for 30 min. Cultures were harvested and the DNA was prepared as described in footnote to Table 1. Nuclease treatment was as described in the footnote to Table 4.

TABLE 7

Characteristics of DNA Isolated from Cultures
Continuously Incubated with [^{3}H]TdR[a]

Treatment	Time of labeling	% recovered activity eluting from BNC	
		1.0 M NaCl	2% caffeine
Control	42 hr	72	28
	4 hr	70	29
	2 hr	68	30
	30 min (confluent culture)	63	36
	30 min	42	56
	10 min	9	90
2.5 mM MMS	42 hr	57	43
	4 hr	41	58
	2 hr	15	84
	30 min (confluent culture)	20	77
	30 min	8	89
	10 min	9	87

[a] HEp-2 cells were incubated with [^{3}H]TdR (10 μCi/ml; 17 Ci/mM except at 42 hr, where 3 Ci/mM) for the indicated times after treatment. DNA was isolated as described in footnote (a) to Table 1.

We observed differences in the proportion of DNA$_{ss}$ obtained from alkylated cultures incubated with [^{3}H]TdR for different periods of time (Table 7). Almost all of the newly formed DNA obtained from cultures incubated for 10 min with [^{3}H]TdR behaved as though it had single stranded regions regardless of whether control or alkylated cells were studied. However, after a 4-hr incubation time, 70% of the DNA formed by control cells chromatographed with the characteristics of native DNA. Similar results were obtained when cells were given a 10- or 30-min pulse of [^{3}H]TdR after treatment and then incubated before harvest for varying periods of time in the absence of isotope (Fig. 7). Incubation of such pulse-labeled cultures for increasing periods of time resulted in a reduction of the amount of DNA$_{ss}$ found in both control and alkylated cultures although the DNA from alkylated cells never attained as much native character as did the DNA from control cells. The observation that the amount of DNA$_{ss}$ is at a maximum immediately after the incorporation of label indicates that this material does not arise as a result of the degradation of DNA. As might be expected from previous results (1), cells treated with MMS and then incubated with [^{3}H]TdR added 24 hr after alkylation, incorporated the isotope into DNA, which behaved on BNC chromatography as though it were mostly double stranded.

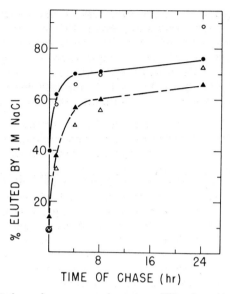

FIG. 7. Pulse chase experiments. HEp-2 cultures were treated with 2.5 mM MMS for 1 hr and then incubated either 10 min (open circles or triangles) or 30 min (closed circles or triangles) with [^{3}H]TdR (10 μCi/ml; 17 Ci/mM). The isotope was washed out and the cultures were incubated for the period indicated before harvest. Triangles: cultures treated with MMS; circles: control cultures.

DISCUSSION

The DNA made by HEp-2 cells contains extensive regions of single strandedness. Although there is no qualitative difference between the DNA from control and alkylated cells, there are important quantitative distinctions. DNA$_{ss}$ made early after alkylation contains single stranded regions at more frequent intervals than does DNA$_{ss}$ from control cells. As shown by Schlegel and Thomas (12, Fig. 6), shearing of DNA should not generate pieces devoid of single stranded regions unless these are sparsely distributed. Because shearing DNA from control cells to the same size as that from alkylated cells (Fig. 4) reduced the amount of DNA$_{ss}$ in the control (Table 1), we conclude that such single stranded regions occur less frequently along the length of newly synthesized control DNA as compared with that from alkylated cells.

The average amount of single strandedness per DNA fragment is also larger in fragments from alkylated cells. After elution from BNC

with caffeine, the fragments from both control and alkylated cell
DNA preparations are the same size, about 13S in both neutral and
alkaline sucrose gradients, which corresponds with a native molecu-
lar weight of about 1.8×10^6 and a single stranded weight of 8.9×10^5 (2.7×10^3 nucleotide pairs) (16). Nuclease digestion resulted
in the removal of $0.24 \times 5.4 \times 10^3 = 1300$ nucleotides from alkylated
fragments and $0.07 \times 5.4 \times 10^3 = 380$ nucleotides from controls.

Although completely specific for single-stranded DNA, our
exonuclease preparation contains some endonuclease activity.
We are therefore unable to distinguish structures of the type
$\overline{\text{--------------}}$ from $\text{--------} \quad \overline{\text{-------}}$.
Between 17 and 24% of the BNC caffeine eluate of DNA prep-
arations is completely single stranded (0.24 of recovered activ-
ity $\times 0.72$ recovered) since it elutes from hydroxyapatite with
0.18 M phosphate (Table 3). All of this material should be nuclease
susceptible, but, in addition, a proportion of the radioactivity must
be in single stranded regions covalently bonded to regions of native
DNA since nuclease treatment increases the proportion of labeled
DNA behaving as native on BNC columns from 7 to 80% (Table 4).
The totally single stranded DNA fragments found in BNC eluates of
DNA from alkylated cultures may be produced by shear of DNA_{SS}
structures.

There are at least two possible artifacts that prevent our understanding the complete structure of the DNA_{SS} fragments. First, most
of our experiments visualize DNA synthesized after alkylation. If
pieces of newly synthesized DNA covalently linked to previously
formed DNA were removed from the "old" DNA by shear or nuclease
treatment, this "old," unlabeled DNA would become invisible.
Second, we do not know the limits of resolution of the BNC column.
Iyer and Rupp (11) found that $[^{22}P]DNA$, when digested with λ exonuclease so that 1.9% of the molecule became acid soluble, was
retained by BNC column. This corresponds to a single stranded run
of about 760 nucleotides from each 5' end of the molecule. However,
the elution curve reported by Iyer and Rupp (11) implies that this is
not the lower limit of the column. One may assume that a run of 380
single stranded nucleotides would be retained. At the other end of
the scale, mature λ DNA with two single stranded ends of 14 nucleotides each passes through the column as though it were double
stranded (13). BNC can therefore distinguish runs of somewhere between 14 and 380 or more nucleotides. The column would adsorb
smaller pieces than the 1300 nucleotide single stranded runs from
alkylated cells, but the calculated 380 nucleotide single strand runs

observed in the DNA fragments from control cells may be near the limits of resolution of the column. The significant difference between DNA from control and alkylated cells may therefore be the relative length rather than the frequency of occurrence of single stranded regions.

These results are not unique to damage induced by MMS since we have demonstrated that over 90% of the DNA synthesized in the presence of the inhibitor, hyroxyurea, is retained by a BNC column. We therefore suppose that any treatment that slows down the rate of DNA synthesis will, necessarily, increase the time during which single stranded intermediates are present. It is unlikely that methylation per se acts as a block to DNA synthesis (at least methylation at the 7 position of guanine, which is the major stable reaction product of MMS alkylation) since DNA with attached methyl groups replicates normally in bacteria (17) and since HeLa cells treated with N-methyl-N-nitrosourea show no depression in the rate or extent of DNA synthesis when treated before the first S period with concentrations of alkylating agent that have a severe inhibiting effect in the second S period (2). Treatment with MMS does affect the amount, but not the timing, of HEp-2 DNA synthesis in the first S period (3), indicating the formation of some additional lesion. Our previous results (18) indicate that this lesion is either an apurinic site or a single strand break.

These observations are related to the phenomenon of post-replication repair as discussed by Rupp and Howard Flanders (19). The disappearance of the single stranded regions is most likely a part of DNA synthesis since it is seen in both alkylated and control cells and since most of the DNA synthesized after alkylation is made by semi-conservative replication (1). Furthermore, the correspondence between the properties of DNA_{ss} in control and alkylated cells makes it seem likely that the "filling in" of the gaps in the DNA made by damaged cells may occur by a process no different from that of ordinary replication except for the possibility of an unusual strand being used as a template. Postreplication repair might be more in the nature of a "copy choice" replication than a recombinational repair. This agrees with the observations of Lehmann (20) who did observe postreplication repair in mammalian cells without recombination and fits our observation that the presence of hydroxyurea, an inhibitor of normal DNA synthesis but not of repair synthesis, leads to an accumulation of DNA_{ss}.

SUMMARY

DNA synthesized by HEp-2 cells treated with methyl methane-sulfonate contains regions of single strandedness. DNA with such single stranded regions adsorbs to columns of benzoylated naphthoylated DEAE cellulose and is only eluted when the columns are washed with caffeine. DNA fragments with such single stranded regions are converted to purely double stranded fragments by treatment with exonuclease. The fragments produced by alkylated cells are qualitatively similar to those produced by control cells given a pulse of radioactivity but differ in both their relative number and in the extent of the regions of single strandedness. The single stranded regions from both control and alkylated cells are gradually converted to purely double stranded DNA although the conversion occurs more slowly in alkylated cells. We conclude that the fragments arise in the course of normal DNA synthesis but have a longer lifetime when DNA synthesis is delayed by a methyl methanesulfonate-induced lesion. The disappearance of the single stranded regions from the newly synthesized DNA formed by alkylated cells is probably a reflection of the processes of postreplication repair.

ACKNOWLEDGMENT

This work was supported in part by grants from the National Institutes of Health (GM 07816) and the National Science Foundation (GB 29491X1).

REFERENCES

1. M. Coyle, M. McMahon, and B. Strauss, Failure of alkylated HEp.2 cells to replicate newly synthesized DNA, Mutation Res., 12, 427-440 (1971).
2. J.E. Plant and J.J. Roberts, A novel mechanism for the inhibition of DNA synthesis following methylation: The effect of N-methyl-N-nitrosourea on HeLa cells, Chem.-Biol. Interactions, 3, 337-342 (1971).
3. T.L. Myers and B.S. Strauss, Effect of methyl methanesulfonate on synchronized cultures of HEp.2 cells, Nature New Biol., 230, 143-144 (1971).

4. J.A. Huberman and A.D. Riggs, On the mechanism of DNA repli-cation in mammalian chromosomes, J. Mol. Biol., 32, 327-341 (1968).

5. B. Strauss, M. Coyle, M. McMahon, K. Kato, and M. Dolyniuk, "DNA Synthesis, Repair and Chromosome Breaks in Eucaryotic Cells," in Molecular and Cellular Repair Processes (R.F. Beers, R.M. Herriot, and R.C. Tilghman, eds.), Johns Hopkins University Press, Baltimore, Md., 1972, pp. 111-124.

6. R. Okazaki, T. Okazaki, K. Sakabe, K. Sugimoto, R. Kainuma, A. Sugino, and N. Iwatsuki, In vivo mechanisms of DNA chain growth, Cold Spring Harbor Symp. Quant. Biol., 33, 129-142 (1968).

7. D.L. Robberson, H. Kasamatsu, and J. Vinograd, Replication of mitochondrial DNA. Circular replicative intermediates in mouse L cells, Proc. Nat. Acad. Sci., 69, 737-741 (1972).

8. M. Oishi, Studies of DNA replication in vivo, II. Evidence for the second intermediate, Proc. Nat. Acad. Sci., 60, 691-698 (1968).

9. J. Wolfson and D. Dressler, Regions of single-stranded DNA in the growing points of replicating bacteriophage T7 chromo-somes, Proc. Nat. Acad. Sci., 69, 2682-2686 (1972).

10. R.B. Painter and A. Schaefer, State of newly synthesized HeLa DNA, Nature, 221, 1215-1217 (1969).

11. V.N. Iyer and W.D. Rupp, Usefulness of benzoylated naphthoy-lated DEAE-cellulose to distinguish and fractionate double-stranded DNA bearing different extents of single-stranded regions, Biochim. Biophys. Acta, 228, 117-126 (1971).

12. R.A. Schlegel and C.A. Thomas, Some special structural features of intracellular bacteriophage T7 concatemers, J. Mol. Biol., 68, 319-345 (1972).

13. J.A. Kiger and R.L. Sinsheimer, Vegetative lambda DNA. IV. Fractionation of replicating lambda DNA on benzoylated naphthoylated DEAE cellulose, J. Mol. Biol., 40, 467-490 (1969).

14. G. Bernardi, "Chromatography of Nucleic Acids on Hydroxylapa-tite Columns," Methods in Enzymology, Vol. 21 (L. Grossman and K. Moldave, eds.), Academic, New York, 1970, pp. 95-139.

15. E.Z. Rabin, B. Preiss, and M.J. Fraser, A nuclease from Neurospora crassa conidia specific for single-stranded nucleic acids, Preparative Biochem., 1, 283-307 (1971).

16. F.W. Studier, Sedimentation studies of the size and shape of DNA, J. Mol. Biol., 11, 373-390 (1965).

17. L. Prakash and B. Strauss, Repair of alkylation damage: Stability of methyl groups in Bacillus subtilis treated with methyl methane-sulfonate, J. Bacteriol., 102, 760-766 (1970).

18. B. Strauss and T. Hill, The intermediate in the degradation of DNA alkylated by a monofunctional alkylating agent, Biochim. Biophys. Acta, 213, 14-25 (1970).
19. W. D. Rupp and P. Howard-Flanders, Discontinuities in the DNA synthesized in an excision-defective strain of Escherichia coli following ultraviolet irradiation, J. Mol. Biol., 31, 291-304 (1968).
20. A. R. Lehman, Postreplication repair of DNA in ultraviolet-irradiated mammalian cells, J. Mol. Biol., 66, 319-337 (1972).
21. D. Scudiero and B. Strauss, J. Mol. Biol., in press.

Chapter 18

DNA REPAIR AND ALKYLATION-INDUCED TOXIC, MUTAGENIC, AND CYTOLOGICAL EFFECTS IN MAMMALIAN CELLS

J. J. Roberts, J. E. Sturrock,[*] and K. N. Ward

Chester Beatty Research Institute
Institute of Cancer Research
Royal Cancer Hospital
Buckinghamshire, England

INTRODUCTION

There are many indications that the mammalian cell recognizes and removes damage to its DNA which occurs as a consequence of treatment with a variety of chemical agents. Moreover there appear to be two distinct mechanisms by which this repair of mammalian cell DNA can be achieved. In one, referred to as excision or "cut and patch" repair, the chemical lesion in the DNA is recognized by a complex enzyme system that first excises the modified base from the DNA, degrades the DNA, and then resynthesizes a section in order to reconstitute the original DNA strand, which is then joined to the pre-existing DNA. Evidence for this form of repair has come from measurements of the loss of mutagen-induced substituents on DNA (1, 2) and from the detection of non-semiconservative DNA synthesis, sometimes just called "repair synthesis" in alkylated cells (3,4). The uptake of [³H]TdR into cells that are not in the DNA synthetic phase of the cell cycle (S), which is referred to as unscheduled DNA synthesis, may be another indication of non-semiconservative DNA synthesis (5, 6).

However, differences in the sensitivity of various cell types to a particular chemical agent cannot be accounted for by differences in manifestations of this form of DNA repair (7-9). This fact, combined with the results of other studies that have been concerned with the mechanism of action of diverse alkylating agents, has indicated that

---

[*]Present address: Division of Anaesthesia, Clinical Research Centre, Northwick Park Hospital, Harrow, Middlesex, England.

the mammalian cell possesses another method for recognizing and eliminating or circumventing damage to its DNA. This mechanism seems to be analogous to that found to occur in certain excision-defective strains of bacteria for repairing UV-irradiation damage. In this form of repair, a DNA polymerase bypasses a lesion so as to produce a gap in the newly synthesized daughter DNA strand, and this gap can subsequently be filled either by the insertion of bases or by the insertion of a segment of DNA by a mechanism akin to recombination (21).

It has therefore become a question of considerable interest whether these so-called DNA repair processes restore the original DNA base sequence or only restore the DNA template sufficiently for DNA replication to occur and for the cell to survive, but with its DNA still modified so as to lead to subsequent base sequence errors during DNA transcription and hence to mutations. Such a possibility might indicate that the cellular response subsequent to DNA damage may be of more importance in determining the mutational effect of an agent than the original modification to DNA.

In order to examine this possibility we first established that caffeine interfered with the repair of alkylated DNA in mammalian cells and then examined the effect of caffeine on the frequency of mutation to 8-azaguanine resistance (10) produced by N-methyl-N-nitrosourea. If an error-prone mechanism were to be inhibited by caffeine, then one might expect to observe a reduction in the mutation frequency for a given number of survivors. Reasoning such as this led Witkin and Farquharson (11) to conclude that postreplication repair of UV damage in the E. coli excision defective strain Hcr⁻ led to the formation of mutations since treatment with UV light and the repair inhibitor caffeine was found to decrease the mutation frequency in the survivors. It was suggested that caffeine produced these effects by inhibiting the exr⁺ gene product. If, on the other hand, caffeine does not decrease the mutation frequency, then it can be argued that mutations arise in mammalian cells as a consequence of inadequate repair of damage to DNA. Our results support this interpretation. We have further used this mutation system to ascertain whether mutations are related to either the level of reaction with DNA or the nature of the products of reaction with DNA. Again our results indicate that mutation correlates with the cytotoxic action of these agents and therefore that lethal and mutational damage to DNA are manifestations of the same phenomena.

EVIDENCE FOR POSTREPLICATION REPAIR OF ALKYLATED
DNA IN HAMSTER CELLS

The evidence for the existence of a DNA repair mechanism, other than excision repair, which can be inhibited by posttreatment incubation of alkylated mammalian cells in medium containing caffeine, has come from a comparison of the mechanism of alkylation-induced cell death, arising from effects on DNA synthesis, in HeLa and Chinese hamster cells. Two vital points that should emerge from the following discussion are firstly that there are important differences in the time course of inhibition of DNA synthesis by sulfur mustard as compared with methylating agents in both HeLa and hamster cells, and secondly there is an essential difference in the response of HeLa cells, when compared with Chinese hamster cells, to the effects of alkylation as far as cell cycle progression is concerned.

Effects of Alkylation on DNA Synthesis in Mammalian Cells

HeLa Cells

Sulfur Mustard and Half Sulfur Mustard. The cell-killing action of either sulfur mustard or half sulfur mustard is a consequence of their ability to react with DNA and thereby produce an immediate block to the replication of DNA. As a result of this inhibition in the rate of DNA synthesis, cells become blocked in the S phase of the cell cycle, and, thereafter, exhibit a mitotic delay. After treatment with low concentrations of these agents, however, cells eventually escape the S phase block, and those that do so, after entering the following S phase in the next cell cycle, show no repetition of this phenomenon (12) (Figs. 1 and 2). These effects of sulfur mustard or half sulfur mustard on cell progression imply that the damage that resulted in the block to DNA synthesis has been repaired by the end of the extended S phase of the cell cycle.

Methylating Agents. In contrast to these effects of sulfur mustard and half sulfur mustard, monofunctional methylating agents such as N-methyl-N-nitrosourea (MNU) or methyl methanesulfonate (MMS), at comparable toxic concentrations to those used with the sulfur agents, do not induce an immediate block to DNA replication in HeLa cells. Cells in the G_1 phase of the cell cycle treated with MNU show no marked modification, either in the time of onset or in the rate of DNA synthesis, and, unlike sulfur mustard-treated cells, they divide without delay (13). However, in the following cell cycle one observes a clear dose-dependent depression in the rate of DNA synthesis that is accompanied by an extension of this second S phase after treatment. Alternatively cells can be said to be blocked in this S phase, and this

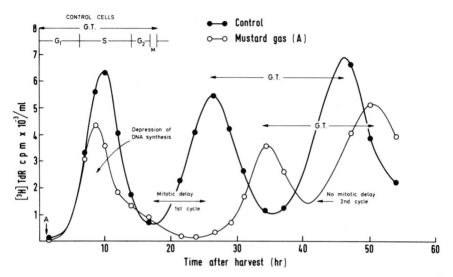

FIG. 1. The effect of mustard gas (sulfur mustard) on DNA synthesis in synchronous HeLa cells. Mitotic cells were harvested from
monolayer cultures and placed in stirred suspension culture at an
initial cell density of approximately 1×10^5 cells/ml. Mustard gas
(0.075 µg/ml) was added at time A and the effects on DNA synthesis
determined at various times thereafter by measuring the uptake of
[^{3}H]TdR (0.5 µCi/ml; 20-30 mCi/mmole) into DNA (cold trichloracetic
acid insoluble material) in a 1-ml aliquot of the culture during 20 min.

will therefore lead to a commensurate mitotic delay in this second
cell cycle (Figs. 3 and 4). These observations indicate that damage
to DNA, such as single-strand breaks, is introduced into DNA by a
time-dependent process. Two possible mechanisms exist for the
production of such damage. The first is suggested by the known
consequences of alkylation of DNA. The predominant reactions of
all alkylating agents with DNA are on the N-7 position of guanine
(approximately 60-80%) and the N-3 position of adenine (approximately 10%). These alkyl purines are known to be lost hydrolytically
from DNA and the apurinic acid thus produced can undergo main chain
scission to produce breaks in the DNA (14). However there are several
facts that militate against this mechanism for the production of DNA
synthesis-blocking damage in HeLa cell DNA by MNU or MMS. While
the proportions of the major products formed by alkylation of DNA by
MNU and MMS are essentially the same (Table 1), nevertheless at
concentrations of these compounds that are equitoxic to HeLa cells,
the actual extents of overall reaction are vastly different. Cellular
DNA is methylated by MMS nearly twenty times more than by MNU

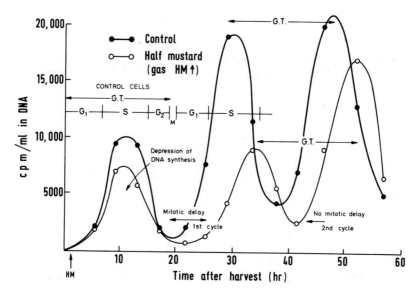

FIG. 2. The effect of half sulfur mustard on DNA synthesis in synchronous HeLa cells. The conditions are as described in Fig. 1.

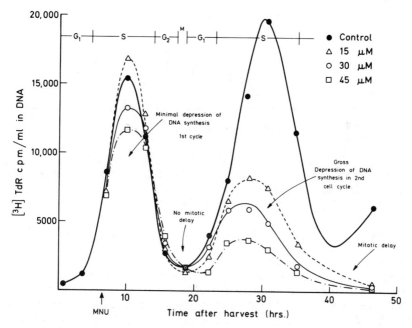

FIG. 3. The effect of N-methyl-N-nitrosourea (MNU) on DNA synthesis in synchronous HeLa cells. The conditions were as described in Fig. 1. The experiment shows minimal effects on DNA synthesis and cell division in the first cycle but marked effects on DNA synthesis in the second cycle, when a block to mitosis results.

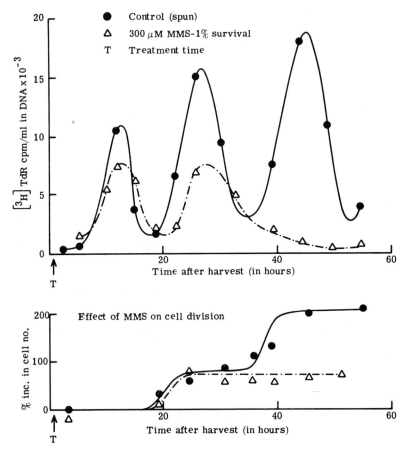

FIG. 4. The effect of methyl methanesulfonate (MMS) on DNA synthesis in synchronous HeLa cells. The conditions are as described in Fig. 1. The experiment shows essentially the same effect found after MNU treatment of HeLa cells in Fig. 3.

(Fig. 5) (8). Both agents produce a greater inhibition of DNA synthesis in the cell cycle following treatment (Figs. 3 and 4) (16), which means that this effect cannot be due to the chemical production of breaks in DNA in both instances. Therefore the damage that constitutes a subsequent block to DNA synthesis is introduced during replication on a methylated DNA template. The fact that cells treated with MNU during the G_2 phase of the cell cycle only show a similar depression in the next but one S phase, i.e., when the cells have had an opportunity to replicate their DNA, supports this hypothesis (13).

TABLE 1

PRINCIPAL PRODUCTS OF DNA BASE METHYLATION   (LAWLEY 1971/2)

	7-METHYL-GUANINE	3-METHYL-ADENINE	0-6-METHYL-GUANINE	3-METHYL-CYTOSINE	1-METHYL-ADENINE
MNNG	70	10	6	2	1
MNU	60	7.0	6.5	3	2
MMS	80	9.0	0.3	0.7	1.3

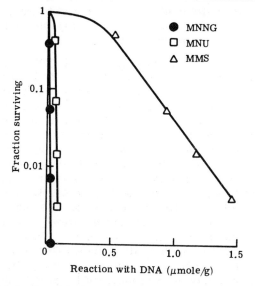

FIG. 5. Relationship between methylation of DNA and effects on HeLa cell survival of three methylating agents radioactively labeled on their methyl groups. Mass cultures of HeLa cells were treated with appropriate concentrations of the agents for 1 hr. Suitable aliquots were then diluted and plated for the determination of the effects on colony-forming ability (cell survival). The remaining cells were then harvested, the DNA isolated, and its specific activity determined (8). The effect of a given concentration of any agent on cell survival was then plotted against the reaction with DNA in micromoles per gram.

Despite the proportions of the major products of DNA alkylation by MMS or MNU being essentially similar, nevertheless there exist clear differences in the proportions of some of the minor products of DNA alkylation by these compounds. Thus the proportion of O-6 methylguanine formed by MNU is 20 times that formed by MMS (Table 1)

(15). This could well indicate that replication of methylated DNA containing O-6 methylguanine residues produces lesions in DNA that subsequently block DNA synthesis in HeLa cells.

Chinese hamster V79-379A Cells

Sulfur Mustard and Half Sulfur Mustard. The effects of these agents are essentially the same as described for HeLa cells. They induce an immediate block to DNA synthesis with the same subsequent effects on cell progression. However superimposed upon these effects is a dose-dependent delay in the time of the peak rate of DNA synthesis following treatment during the G_1 phase of the cell cycle (28). Hamster cells exhibit this response to treatment by all alkylating agents so far examined, and the possible significance of this delay is discussed more fully later.

Methylating Agents. The consequences of methylation of hamster cells are superficially similar to those in HeLa cells in that there is little or no depression of overall DNA synthesis during the cell cycle in which treatment occurs, but there is a more marked depression in the rate of DNA synthesis in the following cell cycle. In addition we observed the alkylation-induced displacement of the S phase referred to above [Figs. 6(a) and (b)]. However it seems that the potential lesion that is produced by replication of MNU-methylated DNA is recognized by a repair mechanism in these cells and eliminated before its effects are manifest during the next round of DNA synthesis. This follows from the fact that MNU is far less toxic to hamster cells than to HeLa cells. At equivalent toxic concentrations of MNU, hamster cell DNA is alkylated more than 20 times that of HeLa cell DNA (8). Hence hamster cells can repair MNU-damaged DNA more effectively than can HeLa cells, either by removing alkyl groups before DNA is replicated or alternatively by postreplication repair of gaps in DNA by the mechanisms referred to earlier (17, 18). The former possibility is unlikely since there are several indications that both cell lines possess equal excision repair potential. Thus we failed to detect differences in the initial proportions of DNA alkylation products or in the loss of labeled alkyl groups from DNA (19) or any difference in extent of alkylation-induced repair replication non-semiconservative DNA synthesis) as between HeLa and hamster cells. We therefore favor the operation of a postreplication repair mechanism in hamster cells, a mechanism that is deficient in HeLa cells, to account for these differences in drug sensitivity. Some recent results on the effects of posttreatment incubation of alkylated cells in caffeine have lent considerable support to the above interpretation.

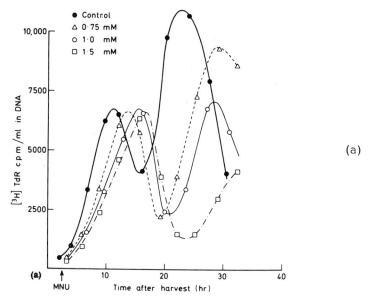

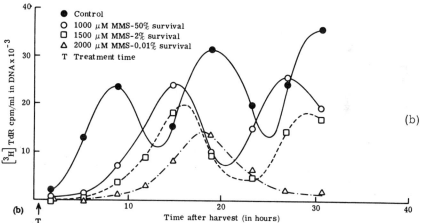

FIG. 6. The effect of: (a) N-methyl-N-nitrosourea and (b) methyl methanesulfonate on DNA synthesis in synchronous Chinese hamster V79-379A cells. The conditions were as described in Fig. 1. The experiments show: (1) the lack of effect on overall DNA synthesis with MNU or the lowest concentration of MMS during the first cell cycle, (2) the dose-dependent displacement of the S phase, and (3) the greater depression of DNA synthesis at all concentrations in the second cycle.

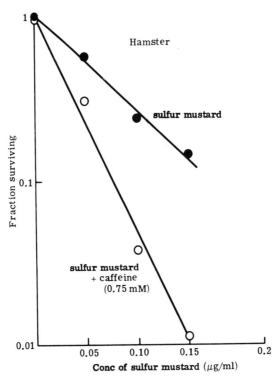

FIG. 7. The effect on cell survival of posttreatment incubation in caffeine of sulfur mustard-treated Chinese hamster cells. Sulfur mustard-treated suspension cultures were diluted and remained in a medium containing caffeine (0.75 mM) for seven days.

EVIDENCE FOR THE INHIBITION OF POSTREPLICATION REPAIR OF ALKYLATED DNA IN HAMSTER CELLS BY CAFFEINE

Caffeine has long been known to inhibit excision repair of UV-induced thymine dimers in micro-organisms (20). There is more recent evidence to suggest that it can also interfere with postreplication repair in excision defective bacteria (2, 11). The ability of caffeine to interfere with dark repair of UV damage in Chinese hamster cells has been extensively studied by Rauth and his co-workers (22-24) and recently Fujiwara and Kondo (25) have adduced evidence that it can interfere with the postreplication sealing of UV-induced daughter strand gaps in mouse L cells. During the course of our work, Walker and Reid (26) have described the potentiation of the lethal effects of some alkylating agents in mouse L cells by means of caffeine.

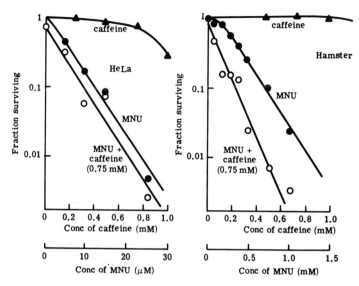

FIG. 8. The effect on cell survival of posttreatment incubation
in caffeine of N-methyl-N-nitrosourea-treated (a) HeLa cells or
(b) Chinese hamster V79-379A cells. MNU-treated suspension cultures
were plated 1 hr later into medium with (o) or without (●) added
caffeine. The effect on the colony-forming ability of HeLa or hamster
cells growing continuously in different concentrations of caffeine is
also shown (▲). The experiments show (1) the sensitization of
hamster cells but not HeLa cells to MNU by posttreatment incubation
in caffeine and (2) the greater toxic effect of caffeine in HeLa cells
as compared with hamster cells.

We have now found that posttreatment incubation of Chinese hamster cells in caffeine produces a marked potentiation of the lethal effects of either sulfur mustard or N-methyl-N-nitrosourea (Figs. 7 and 8).
There are essentially five separate lines of evidence that support the
contention that this sensitization is mediated by interference with a
DNA-repairing system in these cells and that it is most probably a
postreplication type of repair, rather than excision repair, that is
being inhibited.

1. HeLa cells cannot be similarly sensitized to the effects of these
    alkylating agents by caffeine (Fig. 8), except when it is used at
    very high, toxic concentrations, when the possible role of syn-
    ergism cannot readily be assessed. This is consistent with our
    earlier postulate that HeLa cells are deficient in their ability to
    undergo postreplication repair and with the findings of Wilkinson
    et al. (27) who failed to sensitize HeLa cells to UV irradiation.

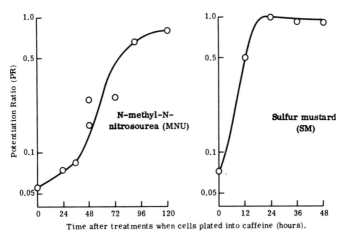

$$P.R. = \frac{\% \text{ survival of treated cells plated into caffeine}}{\% \text{ survival of treated cells plated in medium}}$$

FIG. 9. The effect of caffeine posttreatment on N-methyl-N-nitrosourea or sulfur mustard-induced toxicity in Chinese hamster cells. Control and treated suspension cultures were diluted and plated into medium with or without added caffeine (0.75 mM) at various times after addition of the agents. The potentiation ratio was obtained as the ratio of the survival of treated cells plated into caffeine-containing medium to the survival of treated cells plated into medium without caffeine.

2. Caffeine did not inhibit non-semiconservative DNA synthesis (thought to be associated with excision repair), which is produced in response to treatment of either hamster or HeLa cells with these alkylating agents. Clearly caffeine could be affecting later stages of the excision repair process, such as a ligase action, but there is no evidence to support this possibility at present.

3. Considerable support for the proposed mechanism of caffeine action came from a study of the length of time when the lethal effects of treatment with MNU or sulfur mustard could still be potentiated by incubation of Chinese hamster cells in caffeine. The ability of caffeine to sensitize sulfur mustard-treated cells only persisted for some 20 hr after addition of the alkylating agent; thereafter caffeine addition produced no increase in toxicity (Fig. 9). This is consistent with the previously stated view that repair of sulfur mustard-induced damage was completed by the end of the first S phase after treatment. The sulfur mustard-induced cross-links in DNA inhibit the rate of DNA replication and thus cells become delayed in their passage through the S

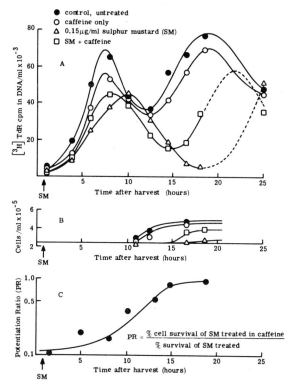

FIG. 10. The influence of caffeine on sulfur mustard-induced effects on (a) DNA synthesis, (b) cell division, and (c) cell survival, in synchronous Chinese hamster cells. (A) The sulfur mustard-induced delay in the S phase was reversed when treated cells were subsequently grown in caffeine. Caffeine alone had no effect on cell progression but seemed to cause some slight depression of DNA synthesis. (B) The above effects of caffeine on the progression of sulfur mustard-treated cells was reflected by the subsequent time of cell division of treated cells. (C) The effect on cell survival of plating treated cells into caffeine confirmed that potentiation of sulfur mustard damage by caffeine occurred only during the first S phase.

phase. This delay permits postreplication repair of any new lesions produced by replication past other monofunctional reaction products in the DNA, and this type of repair will be complete by the time the blockage due to cross-links is finally circumvented, possibly by an excision-repair mechanism (see Fig. 1).

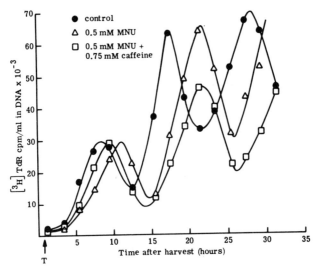

FIG. 11. The influence of caffeine on N-methyl-N-nitrosourea (MNU)-induced effects on DNA synthesis in synchronous Chinese hamster cells. Subsequent growth of MNU-treated cells in caffeine partially reversed the MNU-induced delay in the S phase and produced a greater depression in DNA synthesis in the following cell cycle as a consequence of the inhibition of repair of damage to the DNA.

MNU-treated cells, on the other hand, were still sensitized by subsequent plating into caffeine for at least 48 hr after treatment (Fig. 9). This potentiating effect of caffeine could also be seen in the growth of suspension cultures of MNU-treated hamster cells to which caffeine had been added for various periods of time. Caffeine alone did not affect the growth rate of hamster cells, but it greatly influenced the growth of MNU-treated cells when it was added at any time up to 48 hr after MNU treatment. The protracted ability of caffeine to sensitize MNU-treated cells would be anticipated on the basis of the postulated mechanism of action of MNU. Successive rounds of DNA replication on a methylated template introduces lesions in DNA that will be subject to caffeine-sensitive repair. This process can continue until such time as the methyl groups in DNA have been lost, either by enzymic excision or chemical hydrolysis. The toxic consequences of this process will be diluted by successive cell divisions.

4. Possibly the strongest support for the existence of a caffeine-sensitive postreplication repair mechanism in Chinese hamster cells came from a study of the effects of caffeine on cell cycle

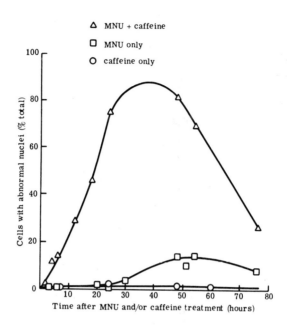

FIG. 12. The effect of caffeine on the time course of MNU-induced chromosomal damage to Chinese hamster cells. Replicate asynchronous cultures of Chinese hamster cells were treated with MNU (0.5 mM), caffeine (0.75 mM), or a combination of the two. At various times thereafter metaphase chromosomes were examined for abnormalities. Caffeine decreased the time of appearance of MNU-induced chromosomal damage and greatly increased the number of cells showing damage.

progression following MNU treatment. As found for HeLa cells, MNU or MMS treatment in the G_1 phase of the cell cycle of synchronized hamster cells did not, at low concentrations, depress the overall extent of DNA synthesis but did, as mentioned earlier, produce a dose-dependent delay in the peak of the S phase [Figs. 6(a)-(b)]. We postulated that this delay was a manifestation of a postreplication DNA repair process (28). Posttreatment incubation in caffeine of either sulfur mustard or MNU-treated synchronized hamster cells had the effect of reversing this alkylation-induced delay in the peak of the S phase (Figs. 10 and 11). It therefore seems reasonable to suppose that this reversal is in some way associated with the inhibition of repair of DNA lesions by caffeine in these cells (15).

5. Our last finding, which indicates the role of caffeine on DNA repair, is illustrated in Fig. 12, which shows that caffeine not

only decreases the time of appearance of chromosome aberrations produced by MNU but also produces a profound increase
in their number, which is directly related to the increased
cytotoxic effect of a combination of MNU and caffeine. The
chromosome aberrations can be regarded as an amplification of
unrepaired lesions in the DNA. The time of appearance of these
aberrations confirms that DNA damage is introduced during the
first S phase after treatment, which would produce gross chromosomal modifications at the following mitosis if not repaired.

Thus there is a considerable body of evidence to indicate that
caffeine can sensitize cells by inhibiting a DNA repair process.
Moreover from the arguments outlined above, it would follow that
while both HeLa and hamster cells possess the ability to carry out
excision repair (8, 9), it is only hamster cells that possess a marked
capacity for postreplication repair of DNA lesions, and it is this
repair that is subject to inhibition by caffeine. In other words, our
particular strain of HeLa cells could be regarded as comparable with
$Hcr^+ rec^-$ repair deficient bacterial mutants, while the Chinese
hamster cell line could be considered equivalent to the $Hcr^+ rec^+$
wild type.

EFFECTS OF CAFFEINE ON MNU-INDUCED MUTATIONS TO
8-AZAGUANINE RESISTANCE IN HAMSTER CELLS

We may now proceed to ask the question how does this postreplication damage to DNA and its repairability influence mutations
in mammalian cells induced by these various agents? For these
studies we have chosen to use the well-defined mutation to 8-
azaguanine resistance in Chinese hamster V79-379A cells as developed by Chu and Malling (10). The ability of MNU to increase
the mutation frequency per 10^5 survivors of 8-azaguanine resistance
in Chinese hamster cells is shown in Table 2, as is the further
increase in mutation frequency in cells treated with these same
concentrations of MNU and subsequently incubated in medium containing caffeine before addition of the selective agent 8-azaguanine.
The mutation frequency induced by MNU or MNU in conjunction with
caffeine can be plotted against the corresponding cell survival under
these conditions, as illustrated in Fig. 13, to show that mutation frequency is directly related to cell survival. The conclusion to be drawn
from these experiments is that caffeine inhibits the repair of damage
to DNA that is potentially lethal and also potentially mutagenic to
cells. This may mean that the repair system itself is not prone to
producing errors in the DNA, which can themselves lead to mutations.
It has been argued in this paper that caffeine inhibits a postreplica-

TABLE 2

Effect of Caffeine on N-Methyl-N-Nitrosourea (MNU)-induced

Mutation Frequency

Concn. of MNU (mM)	Treatment	Survival %	Mutation frequency per 10^5 survivors
0.5	No caffeine	36	25
0.5	With caffeine (0.75mM, 48 hrs)	8	150
1.0	No caffeine	7.4	140
1.0	With caffeine (0.75mM, 48 hrs)	0.28	945

tion type of DNA repair in mammalian cells. We may therefore conclude that postreplication repair in mammalian cells occurs by an
error-free mechanism. Our findings therefore differ from those found
in a microbial system, where caffeine inhibition of postreplication
repair results in a decreased mutation frequency (11). However, the
above argument only applies if it is the initial damage in the DNA
which is responsible for the mutations and not, as in this case, when
it is likely to be the secondary lesions in the DNA which are caused
when DNA replication proceeds past substituents on the DNA and
which are the true lethal and mutagenic events in the DNA (Fig. 16).

COMPARISON OF THE MUTAGENIC PROPERTIES OF MMS, MNU, AND MNNG IN HAMSTER CELLS

It may be recalled that MNU, MNNG, and MMS react with DNA
to give predominantly N-7 methylguanine (Table 1). The proportions
of the minor products of DNA reaction differ as between these compounds (15), and it is the ability of MNU to react at the extranuclear
O-6 position of guanine which is thought by Loveless (29) to be
associated with its higher mutagenic effect on T2 bacteriophage as
compared with MMS. We have therefore extended our mutational
studies using mammalian cells in culture in order to answer two
further related questions. Firstly, is the induced mutation frequency
directly related to the extent of methylation of DNA and, secondly,
does the induced mutation frequency correlate with the chemical
nature of the products of reaction?

The three methylating agents react with Chinese hamster cell
DNA to essentially the same extent at equitoxic concentrations (Fig.
14) despite the fact that vastly different concentrations of these

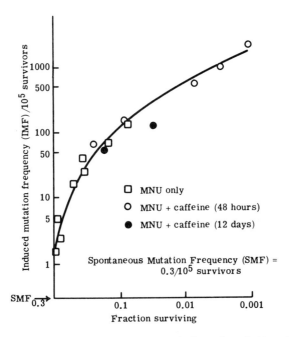

FIG. 13. The relationship between induced mutation frequency
and cell survival. Chinese hamster cells were treated with various
concentrations of MNU and, after 1 hr, plated into medium with or
without added caffeine (0.75 mM) for the determination of cell survival, and into other plates (10^5 cells/plates), with or without
added caffeine (0.75 mM), before addition of 8-azaguanine (10 µg/ml)
48 hr later for the determination of induced mutation frequency (IMF).
(Forty-eight hours was in general found to be the optimum expression
time in these experiments and those shown in Fig. 15. The spontaneous mutation frequency was less than 1 in 10^5 cells under these conditions but could be as high as 2 in 10^5 with a 24 hr expression time.)
Replicate mutation and survival plates were also treated with caffeine
for 48 hr only. Mutant 8-azaguanine resistant colonies were scored
after 12 days. The IMF per 10^5 survivors was then plotted against
cell survival for any given concentration of MNU or for any given
posttreatment condition.

agents are required to achieve a given level of reaction (8). It is
evident from Fig. 15 that equitoxic concentrations, which therefore
mean essentially equal extents of DNA reaction, of these methylating
agents have very similar effects on the induced mutation frequency.
The data would not indicate that the ability to react with the O-6
position of guanine, as in the case of the two nitroso compounds (15),
confers any markedly enhanced mutagenic activity in this mammalian
cell system.

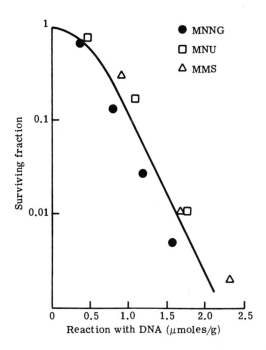

FIG. 14. The relationship between methylation of DNA and effects on Chinese hamster cell survival of three methylating agents. The values were determined as in Fig. 5. The best line through the points was drawn by eye.

CONCLUSIONS: POSTREPLICATION DAMAGE TO DNA AS THE
MECHANISM OF BOTH METHYLATION-INDUCED CELL DEATH
AND MUTATION IN MAMMALIAN CELLS

Figure 15 indicates that the relationship between mutation frequency and reaction with DNA is complex. Mutation is not directly related to DNA reaction but shows a logarithmic increase with linear increase in DNA reaction. If the mutation frequency were to be plotted on a linear rather than a logarithmic scale, then mutation frequency would show a biphasic relationship with dose of agent, or with DNA reaction, since with these compounds and at these concentrations, reaction with DNA is directly related to dose. One cannot reconcile this relationship with the concept of mutation by these agents as being point mutations arising as a consequence of errors in base pairing. In this mammaliam cell system, mutation frequency is related to the effect of agents on cell survival, and since we have

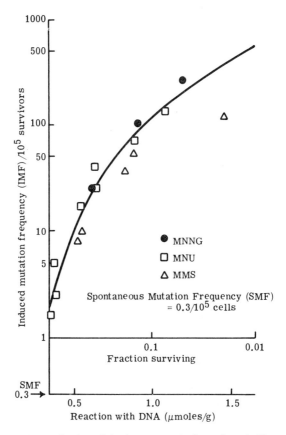

FIG. 15. The relationship between induced mutation frequency
and cell survival following methylation. The induced mutation frequency per 10⁵ survivors determined as for Fig. 13 was plotted
against colony-forming ability for various concentrations of MNNG (●)
MNU (□), and MMS (△). The line through the points was fitted by
eye and was the same as that, also fitted by eye, shown in Fig. 13.
The values for the extent of DNA reaction at any given survival was
obtained from the relationship shown in Fig. 14 between cell survival
and DNA reaction.

argued that the lethal effect of these agents is a consequence of the
secondary damage introduced during replication of DNA on a methylated
DNA template, then it follows that this same damage must also be
mutagenic. The ability of caffeine to increase mutations at the same
time as it increases lethality further establishes that mutation is the
result of inadequate repair of this secondary damage. This concept
for the mechanism of mutagenesis by alkylating agents in mammalian

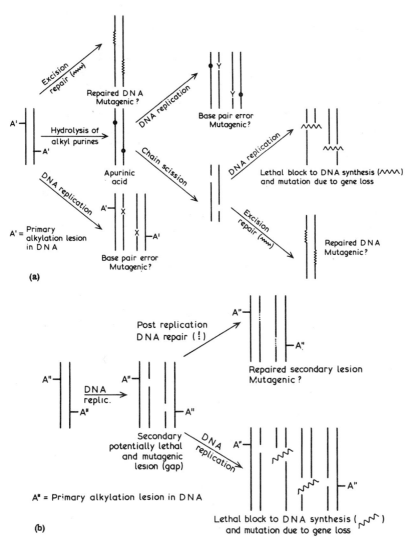

FIG. 16. Schemes showing how the alkylation of DNA and its subsequent repair could result in lethal or mutational damage to mammalian cells. (a) The effects of alkyl groups (A') in DNA, which can (1) be repaired by an excision mechanism (∿) which itself may produce errors leading to mutations; (2) undergo hydrolytic loss (if alkylated purines) to give apurinic sites (●), which can then either mispair on further DNA replication (- Y -) and yield mutations, or undergo a further chemical change to produce chain breaks (14). These breaks in DNA can presumably then either be repaired by an

cells, different from conventional ideas of mispairing, is necessary
to explain not only the dose relationship discussed above but also
the very high mutation frequency as compared with that found in
microbial systems. It further follows, since replication of DNA is
required to produce this lethal and mutational damage to DNA, that
cell division must take place before a mutation can occur. It may be
particularly relevant, therefore, that cell division is also required for
the malignant transformation of cells in vitro by chemical agents (30).
The various possible mechanisms by which alkylated mammalian DNA
can be damaged, which might result in mutations either by lack of
repair or faulty repair as discussed in this paper, are depicted schematically in Figs. 16(a) and (b).

A corollary to this finding of the relationship between cell
survival and induced mutation frequency would be that cells that are
more sensitive to a particular agent might also be more readily
mutated. HeLa cells have been found to be much more toxically
affected by MNU and MNNG than are Chinese hamster cells (Figs.
5 and 14), although the sensitivity to MMS is much the same in the
two cell lines. Clearly a knowledge of the induced mutation frequency in HeLa cells by these agents would help to clarify the
mechanism of mutation in mammalian cells. If the same relationship
between cell survival and mutation as found in hamster cells exists
for HeLa cells then agents such as the nitroso compounds MNU and
MNNG would be particularly mutagenic for this cell type. Should
cells in vivo exhibit similar differences in their sensitivity to these
nitroso compounds one would have an explanation for the carcinogenic
specificity of these compounds.

excision mechanism ($\mathcal{W}$), with possible mutagenic consequences, or,
if this DNA is used a template for further DNA replication, lead to
lethal damage and mutation due to gene loss; (3) they can lead to
base mispairing (-X-), and therefore possibly mutations when the
DNA replicates. (b) The effect of alkyl groups (A'') in DNA which
result in secondary lesions (gaps?) when DNA replicates. These
gaps may then be repaired (···) by a postreplication repair mechanism
that could itself produce errors leading to mutations. Further DNA
replication on a DNA template containing these secondary lesions
could result in a lethal block to DNA synthesis ($\mathcal{W}$) and mutations
due to gene loss. This latter mechanism is favored for the production of mutations in mammalian cells by methylating agents.

REFERENCES

1. A.R. Crathorn and J.J. Roberts, Mechanism of the cytotoxic action of alkylating agents on mammalian cells and evidence for the removal of alkylated groups from deoxyribonucleic acid, Nature, 211, 150 (1966).

2. B.D. Reid and I.G. Walker, The response of mammalian cells to alkylating agents, II. On the mechanism of removal of sulphur-mustard-induced cross-links, Biochim. Biophys. Acta, 179, 179 (1969).

3. J.J. Roberts, A.R. Crathorn, and T.P. Brent, Repair of alkylated DNA in mammalian cells, Nature, 218, 970 (1968).

4. S.R. Ayad, M. Fox, and B.W. Fox, Non-semiconservative incorporation of labelled 5-bromo-2'-deoxyuridine in lymphoma cells treated with low doses of methyl methanesulphonate, Mutation Res., 8, 639 (1969).

5. G.M. Hahn, S.J. Yang, and V. Parker, Repair of sub lethal damage and unscheduled DNA synthesis in mammalian cells treated with monofunctional alkylating agents, Nature, 220, 1142 (1968).

6. M.W. Lieberman, R.N. Baney, R.E. Lee, S. Sell, and E. Farber, Studies on DNA repair in human lymphocytes treated with proximate carcinogens and alkylating agents, Cancer Res., 31, 1307 (1971).

7. C.R. Ball and J.J. Roberts, DNA repair after mustard gas alkylation by sensitive and resistant Yoshida sarcoma cells in vitro, Chem.-Biol. Interactions, 2, 21 (1970/71).

8. J.J. Roberts, J.M. Pascoe, J.E. Plant, J.E. Sturrock, and A.R. Crathorn, Quantitative aspects of the repair of alkylated DNA in cultured mammalian cells. I. The effect on HeLa and Chinese hamster cell curvival of alkylation of cellular macromolecules, Chem.-Biol. Interactions, 3, 29 (1971/72).

9. J.J. Roberts, J.M. Pascoe, B. Smith, and A.R. Crathorn, Quantitative aspects of the repair of alkylated DNA in cultured mammalian cells. II. Non-semiconservative DNA synthesis ('repair synthesis') in HeLa and Chinese hamster cells following treatment with alkylating agents, Chem.-Biol. Interactions, 3, 49 (1971/72).

10. E.H.Y. Chu and H.V. Malling, Mammalian cell genetics. II. Chemical induction of specific locus mutations in Chinese hamster cells in vitro, Proc. Nat. Acad. Sci., 61, 1306 (1968).

11. E.M. Witkin and E.L. Farquharson, "Enhancement and Diminution of Ultraviolet Light-Initiated Mutagenesis by Post-Treatment with Caffeine in Escherichia coli," Mutation as Cellular Process, Ciba Foundation Symposium, Churchill, London, 1969, p. 36.

12. J.J. Roberts, T.P. Brent, and A.R. Crathorn, Evidence for the inactivation and repair of the mammalian DNA template after alkylation by mustard gas and half mustard gas, Europ. J. Cancer, 7, 515 (1971).
13. J.E. Plant and J.J. Roberts, A novel mechanism for the inhibition of DNA synthesis following methylation: The effect of N-methyl-N-nitrosourea on HeLa cells, Chem.-Biol. Interactions, 3, 337 (1971/72).
14. P.D. Lawley, Effects of some chemical mutagens and carcinogens on nucleic acids, Progr. Nucleic Acid Res. Mol. Biol., 5, 89 (1968).
15. P.D. Lawley and S.A. Shah, Reaction of alkylating mutagens and carcinogens with nucleic acids: detection and estimation of a small extent of methylation at O-6 of guanine in DNA by methyl methanesulphonate in vitro, Chem.-Biol. Interactions, 5, 286 (1972/73).
16. J.E. Plant and J.J. Roberts, unpublished results; J.E. Plant, Ph.D. Thesis, London University, 1972.
17. A.R. Lehmann, Post-replication repair of DNA in ultraviolet-irradiated mammalian cells, J. Mol. Biol., 66, 319 (1972).
18. P. Howard-Flanders and W.D. Rupp, Recombinational repair in UV-radiated Escherichia coli in molecular and cellular repair processes, Johns Hopkins Med. J., Suppl. I, 212 (1972).
19. J.M. Pascoe and J.J. Roberts, unpublished results; J.M. Pascoe, Ph.D. Thesis, London University, 1972.
20. E.M. Witkin, Post-irradiation metabolism and the timing of ultraviolet-induced mutations in bacteria, Proc. Intern. Congr. Genet., Montreal, Vol. I, 1958, p. 280.
21. W.D. Rupp and P. Howard-Flanders, Discontinuities in the DNA synthesized in an excision defective strain of Escherichia coli following ultraviolet-irradiation, J. Mol. Biol., 31, 291 (1968).
22. A.M. Rauth, Evidence for dark-reactivation of ultraviolet light damage in mouse L. cells, Radiation Res., 31, 121 (1967).
23. M. Domon and A.M. Rauth, Effects of caffeine on ultraviolet-irradiated mouse L cells, Radiation Res., 39, 207 (1969).
24. M. Domon, B. Barton, A. Porte, and A.M. Rauth, The interaction of caffeine with ultraviolet light-irradiated DNA, Intern. J. Radiat. Biol., 17, 395 (1970).
25. Y. Fujiwara and T. Kondo, Caffeine-sensitive repair of ultraviolet light-damaged DNA on mouse L cells, Biochem. Biophys. Res. Commun., 47, 557 (1972).
26. I.G. Walker and B.D. Reid, Caffeine potentiation of the lethal action of alkylating agents on L cells, Mutation Res., 12, 101 (1971).
27. R. Wilkinson, J. Kiefer, and A.H.W. Nias, Effects of post-treatment with caffeine on the sensitivity to ultraviolet light irradiation of two lines of HeLa cells, Mutation Res., 10, 67 (1970).

28. J.E. Plant and J.J. Roberts, Extension of the pre-DNA synthetic phase of the cell cycle as a consequence of DNA alkylation in Chinese hamster cells; a possible mechanism of DNA repair, Chem.-Biol. Interactions, 3, 343 (1971/72).

29. A. Loveless, Possible relevance of O-6 alkylation of deoxy-guanosine to the mutagenicity and carcinogenicity of nitrosamines and nitrosamides, Nature, 223, 206 (1969).

30. Y. Berwald and L. Sachs, In vitro transformation of normal cells to tumour cells by carcinogenic hydrocarbons, J. Nat. Cancer Inst., 35, 641 (1965).

Chapter 19

CARCINOGENESIS AND DNA REPAIR

J. L. Van Lancker

UCLA Center for the Health Sciences
Los Angeles, California

An hypothesis is never hurtful, so long as one bears in mind the amount of its probability, and the grounds upon which it is formed. It is not only advantageous, but necessary to science, that when a certain cycle of phenomena have been ascertained by observation, some provisional explanation should be devised as closely as possible in accordance with them; even though there be a risk of upsetting this by further investigation; for it is only in this way that one can rationally be led to new discoveries, which may either confirm or refute it.

Schwann

Physical (e.g., UV and X radiation) and chemical carcinogens, except inert polymers, have been shown to cause damage to DNA molecules. UV light, among other lesions, causes the formation of thymine dimers (1). X radiation induces single and possibly double strand breaks and leads to the formation of hydroxy peroxides of thymine (2-11). Some of the known carcinogens are, or are converted to, electrophiles that bind to DNA bases (12,13).

Unless it is repaired, the damage inflicted to DNA by these agents may interfere with its transcription or replication (14,15).

Repair of DNA damaged by UV light, alkylating agents, and carcinogens was demonstrated in bacteria and mammals.

In bacteria a repair mechanism responsive to damage caused by the presence of UV-induced thymine dimers has been discovered and

its enzymic mechanism has been identified at least in part (16).
Classically, the following sequence of steps is believed to be involved: (1) nicking of the radiation-damaged DNA at a point several
bases removed from the dimer by a repair endonuclease similar to one
purified from micrococcus luteus to yield a 3'-PO₄ ending; (b) excision
by a specific repair exonuclease; (c) patching of the gaps by DNA
polymerase; (d) closing of the phosphodiester bonds by polynucleotide
ligase. Kornberg and his associates have, however, proposed an
alternative and simpler mechanism (17). In this model, steps 2 and 3
are both performed by a single enzyme, namely DNA polymerase I,
which exerts its 5' nucleotidase activity and its polymerase activity
sequentially. However, inasmuch as the availability of a free 3'-OH
terminus is a rigid requirement for DNA polymerase and since current
information indicates that all bacterial repair endonucleases yield
3'-PO₄ endings, it is obvious that the DNA polymerase I attack must
be preceded by the catalytic action of a phosphatase. Yet, it can, at
present, not be excluded that several repair endonucleases exist and
that among them some might yield 3'-OH endings.

The interpretation of the role of DNA polymerase I in repair may,
however, need some adjustments because a pol A₁ mutant of E. coli,
deficient in DNA polymerase I, is not as sensitive to radiation as a
mutant (wr A6) of the class wr, mutants which are deficient in their
ability to excise UV-induced pyrimidine dimers from DNA (18,19).
Recent investigations by Cooper and Hanawalt (20), based on the
above observation and utilizing mutants deficient both in the polymerase I and in genetic recombination, have suggested a more complex repair mechanism in which DNA polymerase I is believed to
perform the short patch repair while the rec system will produce the
large patches of repair.

In mammalian systems the development of "non S phase DNA synthesis has been described after exposure to UV irradiation" (21),
administration of carcinogens (22-24), and exposure to alkylating
agents (25). Polynucleotide ligases (26-33) and DNA polymerases
(34-41) have been found and partially purified from various tissues,
but little is known of their role in repair. Although findings made in
patients afflicted with xeroderma pigmentosum have suggested that
the endonucleolitic step is also involved in DNA repair of mammalian
cells, nothing was known of the mammalian repair endonuclease until
Van Lancker and Tomura (42) found such endonuclease activity in rat
liver and reported the purification and some of the catalytic properties
of the enzyme at the 1972 meeting of the American Cancer Society.

Chemical carcinogens are known to react either directly or after
metabolic conversion with many molecular constituents, nucleic
acids, proteins, polysaccharides, molecules containing free SH

groups, etc. (for review, see Refs. 35 and 43). The relationship between chemical binding and the stepwise transformation of a normal cell into a cancerous cell that exhibits survival advantages over all or most other cells in the environment is not known. Surely binding to DNA molecules can be suspected to be critical to the transformation process, but a clear link between DNA damage and oncogenesis has not been conclusively demonstrated. The situation is further complicated by the fact that repair of DNA to which carcinogens are bound has been demonstrated (22-24).

The discovery of a DNA repair defect in patients with xeroderma pigmentosum, who are not only highly sensitive to UV light but who may develop multiple cancers of the skin at an early age, suggests that carcinogenesis and the absence of repair are related.

If alterations of the transcription and translation of the genome into the phenotype are in part or in toto responsible for oncogenesis, then the combination of binding of carcinogens to DNA bases and the partial excision of such bases may be central to oncogenesis in at least two ways. First, because base mispairing could occur during the repair process and, second, because limitations of the repair process would leave some DNA permanently damaged. Unrepaired DNA may either not be transcribable or its transcription may be erroneous. Thus, one could envisage that the phenotypic changes that constitute cancer may develop during the process of oncogenesis, in part or in toto, from a combination of point mutations and deletions which may, under certain circumstances, yield a cancer cell with the survival advantages already mentioned.

Clearly the demonstration of such a pathogenic mechanism is not in our immediate reach, but studies of the properties of the repair endonuclease and of the modulation of its activity in vivo and in vitro may yield evidence excluding or supporting such a mechanism. The factors that modulate DNA repair in vivo or in vitro are not known, but one can postulate at least three conditions that could restrict the activity of the repair endonuclease: (a) the type of injuries inflicted on DNA that are susceptible to the endonucleolitic attack; (b) the effect of the cell cycle and the oncogenic process on the activity of the enzyme; and (c) the possibility that the binding of proteins (histones, acidic proteins, DNA polymerase, repressor) or the state of chromatin may interfere with the endonucleolitic attack.

In this paper we (a) present evidence that the mammalian liver contains an enzyme capable of nicking UV, X irradiated, and carcinogen-bound DNA; (b) report on the effects of potential inhibitors of the enzyme activity; (c) discuss a mechanism of interference with repair that was discovered for X-irradiated DNA, but may well pertain to all forms of DNA damage.

Much of the work presented here has been, or will be published in detail, but this may be an appropriate time to acknowledge Dr. Tomura's collaboration in the purification of the mammalian endonuclease and Dr. Iatropoulos' collaboration in the studies of the role of repression on DNA damage.

Since all cells, including mammalian cells, are constantly subjected to injury inflicted either by physical or chemical agents, it was logical to assume that the repair enzyme found in bacteria might have survived through evolution and would therefore be present in mammalian cells. We made the further assumption that, like other enzymes involved in detoxification, rather than being rigidly specific for the type of injury inflicted on DNA, at least some of the repair enzyme or enzymes would have a broad specificity. Because of possible interference by many other endonucleases or exonucleases, it was felt that the demonstration of crude enzyme activity would not be convincing by itself, and therefore, we proceeded to purify the enzyme. The purification involved preparation of a high-speed supernatant, precipitation with ammonium sulfate, passage through a phosphocellulose column, concentration through diaflo membranes, passage through a G75 Sephadex column, and ultimately through a UV-irradiated DNA cellulose column. In a typical experiment, the enzyme activity, expressed in units per milligram of protein, has been concentrated 10,000 times compared with the activity of the high-speed supernatant. But only approximately one-seventh of activity present in the supernatant is recovered. Approximately 12 different purifications were performed. In all attempts, enzyme activity was recovered at the end, and in all cases except one, the product of the purification yielded a single band on polyacrylamide gel. Elution of the protein associated with the band revealed that it contained endonuclease activity. The level of purification was very similar from one preparation to another, but the yield varied in unpredictable ways.

Three different methods were used to measure the activity of the enzyme. (a) Sedimentation on alkaline sucrose gradients of the substrate before and after treatment with the enzyme. (b) Treatment of [32P]-labeled substrate with endonuclease followed by an alkaline phosphatase attack, a method that measures the number of nicks formed in the DNA. (c) Sequential treatment of the substrate by endonuclease, alkaline phosphatase, and DNA polymerase to measure the ability of the DNA to serve as a substrate for the exonucleolitic attack of the DNA polymerase and the polymerizing activity of DNA polymerase. The substrates were DNA's obtained from mammalian liver after UV or X radiation in vitro, or after the administration of acetylaminofluorene in vivo. In some cases the DNA was labeled with [32P]. To label the DNA, animals were partially hepatectomized and injected repeatedly (18, 20, and 22 hr after hepatectomy) with the [32P] label.

All three procedures used to test the activity of the endonuclease revealed that whereas DNA extracted from the liver of normal rats is not a substrate for the purified endonuclease, the endonuclease causes nicks to appear in DNA irradiated with UV or X rays in vitro and in acetylaminofluorene-bound DNA. DNA containing bound acetylaminofluorene was extracted from liver of rats injected with the carcinogen. In the case of UV-irradiated DNA and acetylaminofluorene-bound DNA, it was possible to demonstrate by using DNA labeled with [^{3}H]thymidine and [^{14}C]acetylaminofluorene that the endonucleolitic attack was followed by the exonucleolitic excision of thymine dimers and guanosine acetoxyfluorene, if the endonuclease-treated DNA was further treated with alkaline phosphatase and DNA polymerase.

Caffeine has been reported to inhibit the activity of dark repair in bacteria (44-46). Similarly, phorbol and anthraline, two co-carcinogens, are believed to inhibit the repair of carcinogen-bound DNA (47, 48). If the active site of the endonuclease specifically binds to thymine dimers, it might be a competitive inhibitor of the enzyme. At present, it has been demonstrated that neither caffeine nor thymidine dimers are inhibitors of the endonuclease. In contrast, phorbol and anthralin were found to inhibit the enzyme, yet the mechanism of such inhibition remains to be uncovered.

It is possible that the repair endonuclease recognizes certain DNA alterations, but not others. For example, if the enzyme is known to cause nicks into AAF-bound DNA, it is not certain whether it would also cause nicks in DNA to which polycyclic hydrocarbons are bound. The fact that in xeroderma pigmentosum some DNA defects caused by carcinogens are repaired while others are not (24) suggests the existence of differences in the ability to repair altered DNA.

Dr. Veronica Maher has kindly provided us with substrate containing various amounts of bound carcinogens. The effects of the endonuclease on these various substrates is now under investigation.

After irradiation of normal rat liver with lethal or sublethal doses, no detectable alterations of the incorporation of precursors in rapidly labeled nuclear RNA or proteins are known to occur (for review, see Refs. 49 and 50). Nor are there detectable morphologic or metabolic changes. If, however, the irradiated animals are partially hepatectomized several days (up to two weeks) after irradiation, there is interference of incorporation of precursors in DNA, rapidly labeled nuclear RNA, and nuclear proteins. In addition, the activities of the enzymes that are normally synthesized after partial hepatectomy are decreased or undetectable after irradiation, a result of interference with their biosynthesis.

Inasmuch as X radiation has been shown to have no effect on translation (51), the findings suggest that X radiation selectively interferes with transcription of the messenger RNA of these proteins indispensable for DNA synthesis that must be synthesized following partial hepatectomy. Such interference occurs even if radiation is administered during interphase. Since the messenger RNA's of those proteins are not likely to be present in nonregenerating liver, it seems logical to conclude that DNA in the regenerating liver is among the primary targets of X radiation.

An explanation for the difference between the effects of X radiation on transcription during interphase and during the cell cycle must be sought in the molecular arrangement of DNA. Although the details of such molecular arrangements are not known, it seems safe to assume that the DNA coding for proteins involved in the last steps of DNA synthesis is repressed in normal liver, but becomes derepressed after partial hepatectomy.

Therefore, it is logical to further assume that damage inflicted to DNA in the repressed state persists while such damage is eliminated from DNA that is in the derepressed state. To explain the restricted expression, after partial hepatectomy, of damage inflicted to DNA irradiated during interphase, the following model was proposed: X irradiation damages all DNA, but derepressed DNA is rapidly repaired, while repressed DNA is not.

The liver is not the only organ that stores damage inflicted during interphase only to express it after the cells have been forced to divide. Studies of the effect of X radiation on organs with normally low or no proliferative activities, but which can be stimulated to proliferate, have yielded similar results. Such systems include kidneys stimulated to grow after unilateral nephrectomy (52), the uterus stimulated to proliferate after the administration of estrogens (53), and lymphocytes stimulated by phytohemoagglutinin (54). In all cases, irradiation during G-0 interferes with DNA synthesis after application of the proliferative stimulus. These findings suggest that in nonproliferative organs of intact mammals, DNA coding for the biosynthesis of proteins involved in DNA synthesis is repressed during interphase. The early observations on the effects of X radiation on antibody formation might well be explained in a similar fashion (55). Formation of antibodies is blocked if irradiation precedes the administration of antigen and continues if irradiation follows the administration of antigen.

Studies by Pollard and Davis (56), in which radiation was applied before and after induction of galactosidase in special strains of bacteria, generally confirm the findings made in the mammalian system, except for the fact that much larger doses of irradiation are needed to affect transcription in bacteria than those in the mammalian system. Thus, radiation applied before induction interferes with galactosidase synthesis while it has little or no effect on the appearance of the enzyme when administered after induction. Similar observations were made by Setlow et al. in bacteria irradiated with UV.

Studies by Stryckmans et al. (57) have shown that the lymphocytes of leukemic patients submitted to extracorporeal radiation were more radioresistant than normal lymphocytes. The radioresistance has been linked to increased turnover of the lymphocytes. These results illustrate the relevance of our hypothesis to radio therapy. It is possible that the survival of lymphocytes depends on constant replacement of one or more species of RNA. Coding for that RNA could take place on a DNA that is alternately repressed and derepressed. If the periods of derepression are short compared with the periods of repression, the lymphocytes would be, of course, highly radiosensitive. If the mechanism controlling repression were lost and as a result either the period of repression is shortened or the repressors are not made, then the lymphocytes would be more radioresistant. Therefore, it is of interest that increased resistance of lymphocytes obtained from chronic lymphocytic leukemia has been observed and that the turnover of the messenger is increased in the leukemic cells. The increased turnover would result from acceleration of transcription that could be caused by modification of the regulation of repression and derepression of the leukemic lymphocyte.

The metamorphosis of what might be an ephemeral working hypothesis into a lasting theory requires the demonstration of (a) the occurrence of damage to DNA, (b) repair of DNA damage, (c) selective repair of derepressed DNA and absence of repair of repressed DNA.

That the administration of X radiation to liver damages the DNA and that the DNA is repaired is no longer in doubt. Within 10 min after irradiation with sublethal or lethal doses, there is a dose-dependent decrease in the ability of the DNA to serve as a substrate for either DNA or RNA polymerase and a dose-dependent decrease in the DNA's ability to hybridize with nuclear RNA. In addition, a dose-dependent amount of double strand breaks develops (15).

Repair of the DNA damage occurs in at least two stages: one that develops within minutes after administration of X radiation, the other that takes weeks to develop. Moreover, part of the DNA damage is not repaired at least up to one week after irradiation. Studies in which liver DNA was first loaded with BUdR by injecting the analog 18, 20, and 22 hr after the partial hepatectomy and was then irradiated in vivo just 30 min before an injection of thymidine, demonstrated that at least part of the thymidine incorporation resulted from non-semi-conservative DNA synthesis. Moreover, up to 4 hr after irradiation,

the incorporation of [³H]thymidine resulting from no "S" phase DNA
synthesis increased with the dose of X radiation administered (58).

When rats are X irradiated with sublethal doses and partially
hepatectomized, even two weeks after the irradiation, regeneration,
as measured by DNA synthesis, is impaired. If, however, the partial
hepatectomy is performed one month after irradiation with 800 R, the
liver regenerates as if it had never been irradiated (59). Therefore,
the damage that interferes with DNA synthesis must have been repaired
sometime between the second and fourth week after irradiation.
Whether this slow repair process results from non S phase or semi-
conservative DNA synthesis, or is the result of another undiscovered
mechanism of repair, is not known.

The demonstration of dose-dependent injuries to DNA after the
administration of X radiation permitted us to follow their eventual
repair at various times after the administration of the dose. The development of double strand breaks and reduction in hybridization and
priming abilities were not repaired as long as one week after irradiation (15). Whether such damage is repaired during the second week
after irradiation remains to be seen.

Although all these findings are compatible with the notion that
X radiation damages DNA and that the DNA damage is repaired in part
very rapidly, they do not prove that repair is restricted to derepressed
DNA and excludes repressed DNA.

Inasmuch as the molecules that cause repression in mammalian
cells are not known, a direct attack on that part of the problem is
impossible. Yet, it was possible to demonstrate that irradiation of
DNA that codes for the proteins that are indispensable for DNA synthesis while such DNA is derepressed does not interfere with DNA
synthesis; this is in contrast to what happens when such DNA is
irradiated while depressed. At 6 hr or 7 days after partial hepatectomy,
the proteins that are indispensable for DNA synthesis are not made;
therefore, the DNA coding for these proteins is likely to be repressed.
Thus, it would seem in keeping with the hypothesis that irradiation
would interfere with DNA synthesis if a second partial hepatectomy
were performed 8 days after the first. If, in contrast, the hypothesis
is correct, irradiation at 18 hr after the first hepatectomy should not
affect DNA synthesis following a second partial hepatectomy performed
8 days after the first. Because, in this case, the DNA coding for the
proteins, indispensable for DNA synthesis, is derepressed and,
therefore, susceptible to rapid repair. The results of such experiments
confirmed our expectations. Irradiation during repression (6 hr or 7
days after the first partial hepatectomy) inhibited DNA synthesis
after the second partial hepatectomy. When, however, the DNA coding

for the proteins indispensable for DNA synthesis was irradiated while derepressed (18 hr after the first partial hepatectomy), no inhibition of DNA synthesis was observed after the second partial hepatectomy. If one cannot consider these findings as conclusively proving our assumption, one must concede that the results do agree with predictions made on the basis of the hypothesis. Moreover, there are biologic observations made under completely different experimental conditions that can be marshalled to buttress the hypothesis. Fahmy and Fahmy (60) found that chromosomal aberration produced by a variety of agents in drosophila larva were most often located in heterochromatic regions, and Evans and Scott (61) showed that when nitrogen mustard and maleic hydrazide were used, 83% of the observed alterations were found in heterochromatin in vicia faba. Hsu and Somers (62) and Natarajan and Schmid (63) have found a similar sensitivity of heterochromatin in mammalian cells. On the basis of these studies, it has been suggested that differences in DNA repair account for the higher sensitivity of heterochromatin.

CONCLUSION

The central question raised by the study of carcinogenesis is that of the conversion of a cell with normal regulation of its rate of proliferation, its mode of differentiation, and its relationship to other cells, to a cell that has lost one or more mechanisms of control in such a fashion that it acquires survival advantages over other cells and thereby succeeds in killing the patient not only by local proliferation, but also by metastasis and invasion.

Inasmuch as the transformation that occurred in the normal cell to make it a cancer cell is transferred from one generation of cells to another, it seems appropriate to assume that the damage must involve the genome. Since UV light, X radiation, and carcinogens modify DNA chemically, it is logical to postulate that DNA is the primary target for an insult that ultimately leads to a stepwise distortion of gene expression that relieves the cell of normal controls of cellular proliferation, maturation, and interreactions. But, because the DNA damage is repaired, at least in part, it also becomes necessary to assess the role that DNA repair plays in carcinogenesis.

We have reported on the properties and the purification of a rat liver enzyme that nicks UV-, X irradiated, and acetylaminofluorene-bound DNA and thereby have helped to clarify, in part, the enzymatic mechanism of DNA repair in mammalian cells. We have also discussed the results of studies of the effects of X radiation on DNA synthesis in regenerating liver tissue and emphasized the complexity of the repair mechanism in vivo. In the intact animals, repair of X irradiated DNA seems to occur in at least two stages; one rapidly following the administration of radiation, another developing weeks after exposure. Moreover, judging from the effect of X radiation on DNA synthesis, it would seem that for reasons that are not yet clear, damage to repressed DNA is not readily repaired.

Even if we have gained some new insights on the enzymic mechanism of DNA repair, many new questions are raised. For example, are all forms of damage to DNA repaired under optimal enzymic conditions? Do some physiologic (such as cell division) or pathologic (e. g., administration of carcinogens) conditions modify the activity of the repair enzyme? Can the repair enzyme be inhibited by either endogenous or exogenous substances? Does the interreaction of DNA with other macromolecules interfere with repair? Finally, if cancer results from point mutation, deletion, or intercalation, are these alterations due to the DNA alteration itself or to the action of the repair enzymes? Because, if it is conceivable that chemical damage to the DNA could result in base mispairing during replication, it is also possible that attempts to repair the damage could cause irreparable strand breaks or base mispairing.

REFERENCES

1. R. Beukers and W. Berends, The effects of UV-irradiation on nucleic acids and their components, Biochim. Biophys. Acta, 49, 181 (1961).
2. P. V. Hariharan and P. A. Cerutti, Repair of gamma-ray-induced thymine damage in Micrococcus radiodurans, Nature New Biol., 229, 247 (1971).
3. W. Szybalski, Molecular events resulting in radiation injury, repair and sensitization of DNA, Radiat. Res. Suppl., 7, 147 (1967).
4. E. C. Pollard, "Physical Considerations Influencing Radiation Response," in The Biological Basis of Radiation Therapy (E. Schwartz, ed.), Lippincott, Philadelphia, 1966, p. 1.
5. F. Hutchinson, "The Inactivation of DNA and Other Biological Molecules by Ionizing Radiations," in Cellular Radiation Biology, Williams & Wilkins, Baltimore, 1965, p. 86.
6. D. Freifelder, Lethal changes in bacteriphage DNA produced by X-rays, Radiat. Res. Suppl., 6, 80 (1966).

7. E. Freese and E. B. Freese, Mutagenic and inactivating DNA alterations, Radiat. Res. Suppl., 6, 97 (1966).

8. K. C. Smith, Physical and chemical changes induced in nucleic acids by ultraviolet light, Radiat. Res. Suppl., 6, 54 (1966).

9. K. V. Shooter, The effects of radiations on DNA biosynthesis and related processes, Progr. Biophys. Mol. Biol., 17, 289 (1967).

10. K. G. Zimmer, Some recent studies in molecular radiobiology, Current Topics Radiat. Res., 5, 1 (1969).

11. A. Wacker, Molecular mechanisms of radiation effects, Progr. Nucleic Acid Res., 1, 369 (1963).

12. E. C. Miller and J. A. Miller, The metabolic activation of carcinogenic aromatic amines and amides, Progr. Exptl. Tumor Res., 11, 273 (1969).

13. E. C. Miller and J. A. Miller, "The Mutagenicity of Chemical Carcinogens: Correlations, Problems, and Interpretations," in Chemical Mutagens. Principles and Methods for Their Detection (A. Hollaender, ed.), Vol. 1, Plenum, New York, 1971, p. 83

14. L. Grossman, J. Ono, and R. Wilson, "The Effects of Ultraviolet Light on Nucleic Acid Coding Systems," in Cellular Radiation Biology, Williams & Wilkins, Baltimore, 1965, p. 107.

15. J. L. Van Lancker, T. Tomura, and K. Ariyama, The effect of X-radiation on DNA sedimentation, hybridization, and template capacity, Cancer Res., submitted, Sept., 1972.

16. J. M. Boyles, "Genetic and Physiological Factors Relating to Excision-Repair in Escherichia coli," in Molecular and Cellular Repair Processes (R. F. Beers, R. M. Herriott, and R. C. Tilghman, eds.), Johns Hopkins Univ. Press, Baltimore, 1972, p. 150.

17. R. B. Kelly, M. R. Atkinson, J. A. Huberman, and A. Kornberg, Excision thymine dimers and other mis-matched sequences by DNA polymerase of Escherichia coli, Nature, 224, 495 (1969).

18. P. De Lucia and J. Cairns, Isolation of an E. coli strain with a mutation affecting DNA polymerase, Nature, 224, 1164 (1969).

19. L. Kanner and P. Hanawalt, Repair deficiency in a bacterial mutant defect in DNA polymerase, Biochem Biophys. Res. Commun., 39, 149 (1970).

20. P. K. Cooper and P. C. Hanawalt, Role of DNA polymerase I and the rec system in excision-repair in Escherichia coli, Proc. Nat. Acad. Sci., 69, 1156 (1972).

21. J. E. Cleaver, "Excision Repair: Our Current Knowledge Based on Human (Xeroderma Pigmentosum) and Cattle Cells," in Molecular and Cellular Repair Processes (R. F. Beers, R. M. Herriott, and R. C. Tilghman, eds.), Johns Hopkins Univ. Press, Baltimore, 1972, p.

22. J. I. Goodman and V. R. Potter, Evidence for DNA repair synthesis and turnover in rat liver following ingestion of 3'-methyl-4-dimethylaminoazobenzene, Cancer Res., 32, 766 (1972).

23. M. W. Lieberman and A. Dipple, Removal of bound carcinogen during DNA repair in nondividing human lymphocytes, Cancer Res., 32, 1855 (1972).

24. R. B. Setlow and J. D. Regan, Defective repair of N-acetoxy-2-acetylaminofluorene-induced lesions in the DNA of xeroderma pigmentosum cells, Biochem. Biophys. Res. Commun., 46, 1019 (1972).

25. J. J. Roberts, "Repair of Alkylated DNA in Mammalian Cells," in Molecular and Cellular Repair Processes (R. F. Beers, R. M. Herriott, and R. C. Tilghman, eds.), Johns Hopkins Univ. Press, Baltimore, 1972, p. 226.

26. T. Lindahl and G. M. Edelman, Polynucleotide ligase from myeloid and lymph tissues, Proc. Nat. Acad. Sci., 61, 680 (1968).

27. J. Sambrook and A. J. Shatkin, Polynucleotide ligase activity in cells infected with simian virus 40, polyoma virus, or vaccinia virus, J. Virol., 4, 719 (1969).

28. S. Spardari, G. Ciarrocchi, and A. Falashi, Purification and properties of polynucleotide ligase from human cell cultures, Europ. J. Biochem., 22, 75 (1971).

29. P. Beard, Polynucleotide ligase in mouse cells infected by polyoma virus, Biochim. Biophys. Acta, 269, 385 (1972).

30. A. M. Pedrini, F. Nuzzo, G. Ciarrochi, L. Dalpra, and A. Falaschi, Induction of polynucleotide ligase in human lymphocytes stimulated by phytohemoagglutin, Biochem. Biophys. Res. Commun., 47, 1221 (1972).

31. T. Lindahl, "Nucleic Acids," in Methods in Enzymology (L. Grossman and K. Moldave, eds.), Vol. 21, Academic Press, New York, 1971, p. 333.

32. B. Kessler, Isolation, characterization and distribution of a DNA ligase from higher plants, Biochim. Biophys. Acta, 240, 496 (1971).

33. U. Bertazzoni, F. Campagnari, and U. De Luca, A convenient solid-state substrate for assays of polynucleotide ligase: The Poly (dA) · [Poly[^{3}H]dT)-Poly(dT)]-cellulose, Biochim. Biophys. Acta, 240, 515 (1971).

34. T.-Y. Wang, Nonhistone chromatin proteins from calf thymus and their role in DNA biosynthesis, Arch. Biochem. Biophys., 122, 629 (1967).

35. G. F. Kalf and J. J. Chih, Purification and properties of deoxyribonucleic acid polymerase from rat liver mitochondria, J. Biol. Chem., 243, 4904 (1968).

36. R. Howk, DNA polymerase from rat liver chromosomal proteins. I. Partial purification and general characteristics, Arch. Biochem. Biophys., 133, 238 (1969).

37. R. Howk and T.-Y. Wang, DNA polymerase from rat liver chromosomal proteins. II. Formation of an enzyme-template complex and association of product with template, Arch. Biochem. Biophys., 136, 422 (1970).

38. J. T. Bellair, The rapid isolation of a regenerating rat liver DNA nucleotidyl-transferase fraction which shows a preference for native DNA as primer, Biochim. Biophys. Acta, 161, 119 (1968).
39. J. F. Chiu and S. C. Sung, DNA nucleotidyltransferase activity of the developing rat brain, Biochim. Biophys. Acta, 209, 34 (1970).
40. J. F. Chiu and S. C. Sung, Solubilization and characterization of particulate form of DNA polymerase from adult rat liver nuclei, Biochem. Biophys. Res. Commun., 46, 1830 (1972).
41. J. F. Chiu and S. C. Sung, Solubilization and characterization of a particulate form of DNA polymerase from adult rat brain nuclei, Biochim. Biophys. Acta, 262, 397 (1972).
42. J. L. Van Lancker and T. Tomura, A mammalian DNA repair endonuclease, Cancer Res., Proc., 13, 112 (1972).
43. J. A. Miller and E. C. Miller, The metabolic activation of carcinogenic aromatic amines and amides, Progr. Exptl. Tumor Res., 11, 273 (1969).
44. M. Vizdalova, E. Janovska, and V. D. Zhestjanifo, Effect of dark-repair inhibitors on the survival of Escherichia coli under different post-irradiation conditions, Intern. J. Radiat. Biol., 20, 49 (1971).
45. E. M. Witkin, "Post-Irradiation Metabolism and the Timing of Ultraviolet-induced Mutations in Bacteria, " in Proceedings, 10th International Congress of Genetics, Montreal, Univ. Toronto Press, Toronto, 1959, p. 280.
46. M. Lieb, Enhancement of ultraviolet-induced mutation in bacteria by caffeine, Z. Vererbungslehre, 92, 416 (1961).
47. D. Gaudin, R. S. Gregg, and K. L. Yielding, DNA repair inhibition: A possible mechanism of action of co-carcinogens, Biochem. Biophys. Res. Commun., 45, 630 (1971).
48. D. Gaudin, R. S. Gregg, and K. L. Yielding, Inhibition of DNA repair by co-carcinogens, Biochem. Biophys. Res. Commun., 48, 945 (1972).
49. J. L. Van Lancker, "Control of Macromolecular Synthesis in Regenerating Liver and Its Alteration by X-radiation, " in Biochemistry of Cell Division (R. Baserga, ed.), Charles C. Thomas, Springfield, Ill., 1969, p.
50. J. L. Van Lancker, Control of DNA synthesis in regenerating liver, Fed. Proc. Fed. Amer. Soc. Exptl. Biol., 29, 1439 (1970).
51. K. Ariyama, N. Fausto, E. Tamvakopoulos, and J. L. Van Lancker, Effects of X-radiation of amino acid incorporation into degenerating proteins, Radiat. Res., 42, 528 (1970).
52. G. Threlfall, A. B. Cairnie, D. M. Taylor, and A. T. Buck, Effect of whole-body X-irradiation on renal compensatory hypertrophy, Radiat. Res., 27, 559 (1966).

53. C. A. Perrotta, Effect of X-irradiation on DNA synthesis in the uterine epithelium, Radiat. Res., 28, 232 (1966).
54. R. Schrek and C. Stefami, Radioresistance of phytohemagglutinin-treated normal and leukemic lymphocytes, J. Nat. Cancer Inst., 32, 507 (1964).
55. E. V. Benjamin and E. Sluka, Antikörperbildung nach experimenteller schädigung des hämatopoetischen systems durch röntgenstrahlen, Wien. Klin. Wochnschr., 11, 311 (1908).
56. E. C. Pollard and S. A. Davis, The action of ionizing radiation on transcription (and translation) in several strains of Escherichia coli, Radiat. Res., 41, 375 (1970).
57. P. A. Stryckmans, A. D. Chanana, E. P. Cronkite, M. L. Greenberg, and L. M. Schiffer, Studies on lymphocytes. X. Influence of extracorporal irradiation of the blood on lymphocytes in chronic lymphocytic leukemia: Apparent correlation with RNA turnover, Radiat. Res., 37, 118 (1969).
58. J. L. Van Lancker, Liver DNA replication, transcription and repair after irradiation and administration of carcinogens, Proceedings Symposium on Liver Regeneration, Paris, 1972, submitted.
59. T. Uchiyama, N. Fausto, and J. L. Van Lancker, Metabolic alterations after total body doses of X-irradiation. The effects of X-irradiation on rapidly labeled RNA, Arch. Biochem. Biophys., 110, 191 (1965).
60. O. Fahmy and M. Fahmy, Gene elimination in carcinogenesis: Reinterpretation of the somatic mutation theory, Cancer Res., 30, 195 (1970).
61. H. Evans and D. Scott, The induction of chromosome aberrations by nitrogen mustard and its dependence on DNA synthesis, Proc. Roy. Soc. (London), B173, 491 (1969).
62. T. Hsu and C. Somers, Effect of 5-bromodeoxyuridine on mammalian chromosomes, Proc. Nat. Acad. Sci., 47, 396 (1961).
63. A. T. Natarajan and W. Schmid, Differential response of constitutive and facilitative heterochromatin in the manifestation of mitomycin induced chromosome aberrations in Chinese hamster cells in vitro, Chromosoma, 33, 48 (1971).